Directory for Older People

REFERENCE ONLY

You'll be surprised what Age Concern can do for you!

You may already know about the work which Age Concern has been doing for over 50 years providing effective care for the older people in this country. But are you aware of the range of other services which Age Concern also offers?

Home & Contents, Motor and Travel Insurance

Age Concern Insurance Services have long specialised in providing affordable insurance for people aged 60 and over. Using the knowledge and experience built up over the years, we have developed a range of policies to meet the various insurance needs of older people.

Pre-paid Funeral Plans

The range of pre-paid funeral plans brought to you by Age Concern can help to avoid rising funeral costs and give you peace of mind that the necessary arrangements have been made in line with your wishes. The plans, recommended as Best Buys in independent surveys, are a proven, careful and considerate way of planning ahead.

Information and advice

Age Concern publishes a wide range of books on housing, health, leisure and much more. Combined with the more detailed information which is available in Factsheet form and a range of other materials, we provide arguably the most comprehensive information service for older people in this country.

Further information on any aspect of our work is available from your local Age Concern organisation, whose name and address will be shown in your local telephone directory. Alternatively, write to Age Concern England, Astral House, 1268 London Road, London SW16 4ER (or telephone 081-679 8000).

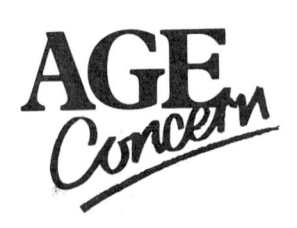

Age Concern

Directory for Older People

A handbook of information and opportunities for the over 55s

Edited by
ANN DARNBROUGH *and* DEREK KINRADE

HEREFORD AND WORCESTER
COUNTY LIBRARIES

R362.60941

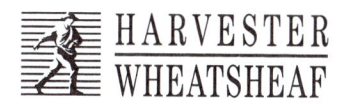

HARVESTER WHEATSHEAF

New York   London   Toronto   Sydney   Tokyo   Singapore

First published 1992 by
Harvester Wheatsheaf
Campus 400, Maylands Avenue
Hemel Hempstead
Hertfordshire, HP2 7EZ
A division of
Simon & Schuster International Group

© 1992 **Harvester Wheatsheaf**

All rights reserved. No part of this publication may be
reproduced, stored in a retrieval system, or transmitted,
in any form, or by any means, electronic, mechanical,
photocopying, recording or otherwise, without prior
permission, in writing, from the publisher.

Designed by Claire Brodmann

Typset in 10/12 pt Garamond
by Mathematical Composition Setters Ltd, Salisbury, Wiltshire

Printed and bound in Great Britain by
Dotesios Ltd, Trowbridge, Wiltshire

British Library Cataloguing in Publication Data

A catologue record for this book is available from the British Library

ISBN 0-7450-1442-9 (pbk)

1 2 3 4 5   96 95 94 93 92

CONTENTS

Foreword vii
Introduction ix
Acknowledgements xi

SECTION ONE *Statutory benefits and concessions* 1

Attendance Allowance (AA); Chronically Sick and Disabled Persons Act 1970; Disability Living Allowance (DLA); Hospital and benefits; Housing Benefit (HB); Income Support (IS); Invalid Care Allowance (ICA); NHS dental treatment concessions; NHS sight test concessions and voucher scheme for glasses; NHS prescription charges concessions; Severe Disablement Allowance (SDA); The Social Fund; State Retirement Pension (SRP); Helpful organisations; Further information.

SECTION TWO *More money matters* 29

Money management; Savings and investment; Raising income or capital from your home; Income from charities; Income tax; Inheritance tax; Wills; Power of attorney; Insurance; Debt; Helpful organisations.

SECTION THREE *House and home* 58

Who's who; What's what; Staying put; Financing improvements and repairs; Help in the home; Buying into sheltered housing; Renting sheltered housing; Housing associations, housing trusts and charitable organisations providing special housing schemes; Home from Home schemes; Residential and nursing homes; Television licence concessions; Household insurance; Helpful organisations; Books and publications.

SECTION FOUR *Equipment for daily living* 107

Categories; Sources of supply; Information services; Equipment centres; Books and publications.

SECTION FIVE *Keeping warm* 121

Financial help; Winter warmth lines; Hypothermia; Warm clothing; Living and sleeping in one room in winter; Eating and drinking for warmth; Keeping active to keep warm; Keeping warm and safe; Heating your home; Insulating your home; Helpful organisations.

SECTION SIX *Keeping safe* 143

Community alarm systems – calling for help; Keeping safe out of doors; Keeping safe indoors; Protecting yourself from fire; Protecting yourself against burglary; Further information.

SECTION SEVEN *Healthy living* 156

Eating for health; Drinking for health; Not smoking for health; Moving and exercising for health; Healthy living holidays; Looking after your body; Alternatives in health care; Continence management; Operations; Helpful organisations; Health care professionals; Private health plans; Publications and resources.

SECTION EIGHT *Planning for death and coping with bereavement* 197

Advance planning for your death; Bereavement; Practical arrangements; Helpful organisations; Further information.

SECTION NINE *Opportunities for volunteering* 214

Voluntary work and social security benefits; Motor mileage allowances and tax; Organisations which welcome volunteers; Publications.

SECTION TEN *Carry on learning* 233

Open learning; Local classes; Universities and colleges; Television; Home study courses; Learning together; Study holidays and courses; Retirement courses; Travelling Fellowships; Helpful organisations; Books and publications.

SECTION ELEVEN *Getting around and about* 245

Travel concessions; Assistance with travel; Low speed scooters and buggies; Driving; The Orange Badge scheme; Community transport schemes; Care with a chair; Books and publications.

Contents vii

SECTION TWELVE Arts, sport and leisure   258

Keeping fit; Activity holidays; Local authority services; Antiques; Archaeology; Archery; Arts; Basket-making; Birdwatching; Bowls; Brass rubbing; Chess; Country dancing; Croquet; Embroidery; Environment; Family history and genealogy; Films and film making; Flower arranging; Gardening; Golf; Heritage and history; Jigsaws; Judo; Meteorology; Music; Netball; Numismatics; Oral history/reminiscing; Orienteering; Painting; Philately; Photography; Radio; Railways; Rambling; Reading; Rowing; Running; Sailing; Skiing; Square dancing; Swimming; Tennis; Short tennis; London theatres and concerts; Windsurfing; Writing; Helpful organisations; Sports Councils; Townswomen's Guilds.

SECTION THIRTEEN *Holidays*   302

Railcards; Insurance; Medical treatment overseas; Your pension and going abroad; Holidays with specialist organisations; Special interest holidays and courses; Publications; Home exchange; Holiday cottages and homes; Helpful organisations; Tourist Boards.

SECTION FOURTEEN *Helpful organisations*   324

SECTION FIFTEEN *Selected further reading*   351

Age Concern England fact sheets; Caring; Common disabilities; Directories; Hospices; Legal aid; Loneliness; Magazines; Retirement guides; Women.

Index   361

FOREWORD

Information is what we all need in our ever more complex and rapidly changing society. For older people the need is often particularly great. They have, of course, already seen more change than any other generation but change is no respecter of advanced years. Indeed, successful adaptation to later life requires coming to terms with some of the greatest shifts of our lives in terms of new opportunities, new problems and new family and social relationships, and physical and emotional changes can all transform our 'map of life' for good and ill.

This *Directory for Older People* provide the signposts to help older people and those who support them to find their way.

The authors have tackled their gargantuan task with thoroughness and optimism and the result is a book which is comprehensive yet accessible. The subjects it covers range from the nitty-gritty details of social security benefits to more life-enhancing subjects such as special interest holidays and theatre booking.

Inevitably such a comprehensive work is also a weighty and not inexpensive production. However, there are many people professionally and personally involved, including advice workers, librarians, personnel managers and family members who can make sure that the invaluable information in this Directory does get through to its ultimate consumers. I urge them to do so. For those who see any part of their role as advising older people, I can think of no better tool.

Sally Greengross
Director
Age Concern England
National Council on Ageing

INTRODUCTION

As older people ourselves, we have very much enjoyed writing this second edition of the *Directory for Older People*. We have found out so much about the opportunities that exist for those of us who are in the third age, and we have taken pleasure in bringing this information together. We hope that our readers will find within the pages of this Directory both help to overcome difficulties and inspiration about activities they may not have considered before.

At last, attitudes to older people seem to be changing, and that word 'ageism' has crept into the language to be used to combat negative discrimination wherever and whenever it arises. No longer are we expected to sit in a corner by the fire and let the world pass us by.

It is very encouraging that 1993 is to be the 'European Year of Older People – and Solidarity Between Generations'. While this is a rather long title, it is nevertheless a splendidly positive one. We hope that this Directory will be a useful contribution to this important year.

In writing this Directory we have tried to cater for the needs and interests of individuals. There are those who are well-off, and those who live in poor circumstances; those who have a disability and those who do not; those who retain their independence and those who do not; those who want to take part in challenging activities and those who prefer to sit at home and take life quietly. We have not, therefore, written this Directory in the belief that 'older people' can be addressed as a single group, or that there are universal ground rules for living as an older person (though there are certainly some things that *everyone* should aim for and some we would all do well to avoid). Rather, this is a storehouse of information from which to make individual choices.

Our emphasis, however, is firmly on the side of living life to the fullest possible extent: taking advantage, wherever possible, of greater freedom and mature experience to expand our lives in new directions. Younger people often find that their lives are largely constrained by the claims of work and family. When these responsibilities are lifted and the pattern of life is changed, many people find themselves in a vacuum. A primary purpose of this Directory is to help people to build new lives: to bring to notice the immense diversity of fresh fields, and the means to take advantage of them. Health and money help, of course, but by no means all life-enhancing strategies require you to be physically active or well-off.

Introduction

Another important purpose of the Directory is to signpost the many sources of help which can alleviate, if not overcome, problems faced by older people: support services, equipment for daily living, and the profusion of organisations and publications which can provide more detailed guidance. We address, to some extent, problems associated with disability because many older people are disabled. More detailed guidance, however, is available in our companion book *Directory for Disabled People*, now in its sixth edition.

Roughly 19 per cent of the population of the United Kingdom is over pensionable age, and that percentage is growing. Life expectancy is also rising: at present it averages over 77 years for men, and roughly four years more for women. People are also retiring earlier, whether by choice or through redundancy. There is, therefore, a large and growing proportion of older people who are not engaged in formal work. A report, *Older Britains*, published by the University of Strathclyde's Centre for the Study of Public Policy concludes that by the year 2021, more than one-third of Britain's population will be over the age of 50. Even more significantly, the number of people over the age of 50 is expected to rise by 5.3 million over the next 30 years, while the number under that age will decline by 2.1 million. While a large proportion of older people can be expected to have made financial provision for their later years, the impact of these figures in terms of total support from taxation is formidable. It seems certain that for very many older people, financial difficulties will continue to occupy centre stage. It is imperative, therefore, that older people in need are made aware of such help as is available, and it is no accident that the Directory opens with a section signposting the main relevant state benefits.

No less important is health, a subject we cover in some detail. Key sections provide guidance on keeping healthy and keeping warm.

Accommodation is also high on the agenda: in a section entitled 'House and Home' we have sketched in the main options. We cover information needed both by people who want to move away in their later years and those who decide to stay put. We have placed some emphasis on suggesting ways in which independence may be preserved, but offer basic guidance on residential and nursing homes.

Later life provides an opportunity to devote more time to leisure pursuits: either activities started earlier or entirely new interests. The sections on arts, sport and leisure and further education provide plenty of ideas and suggestions on how to follow special interests.

Volunteering can lead to exciting new challenges. Very often, expenses are paid and you need not be out of pocket. Our section on volunteering offers guidance to help you to search out exciting possibilities for satisfying commitments.

In whatever you do, we wish you well.

ANN DARNBROUGH

DEREK KINRADE

ACKNOWLEDGEMENTS

The compilation of a book such as this depends upon the cooperation of everybody who has supplied or verified information. Our thanks go to all those people, but in particular to Age Concern England for providing information on almost every subject in the book.

SECTION ONE

Statutory benefits and concessions

We have not attempted to bring out every detail of the benefits and concessions which are available to older people. This would require a book in itself, and there are already a number of excellent guides devoted to this purpose (*see* page 26). Our concern is that many people are wholly unaware of financial help to which they may be entitled. Our objective is to signpost the benefits, outline their purpose and how you may qualify, and point you towards further advice. Because quite a number of elderly people have some kind of disability, we have included the main disability and carers' benefits.

Such are the difficulties of the benefits system that you may need advice on a one-to-one basis from someone who is expert and who can look at your circumstances in the round. This is especially true if you want to do some part-time work while claiming benefit.

Some benefits count as taxable income, while some do not. The relevant details are given at page 46.

Attendance Allowance (AA)

From April 1992, except to the extent described below, AA was replaced by Disability Living Allowance.

AA is a weekly benefit which can be claimed by elderly people who need a lot of help because of illness or physical or mental disability. It is available only to people whose care needs first arise after the age of 65. If you are not yet 66 and your care needs began before your 65th birthday you should claim Disability Living Allowance. AA is not means-tested and does not depend on National Insurance contributions having been paid. You can claim AA if you need a lot of looking after, even if you do not get as much attention or supervision as you need, for example because you live alone.

Residence condition

You must be ordinarily resident and present in Great Britain for a total of at least 26 weeks in the year preceding the claim.

Rates and qualifying conditions

AA is paid at one of two rates:

Higher rate: if you are not expected to live for more than six months, or if you are so severely disabled physically or mentally that you need help from another person both day and night. The help you need must be:

(a) throughout the day: frequent attention in connection with your bodily functions; or continual supervision to avoid substantial danger to yourself or others; and

(b) at night: prolonged or repeated attention in connection with your bodily functions; or another person being awake for a prolonged period or at frequent intervals to watch over you in order to avoid substantial danger to yourself or others.

Lower rate: if you are so severely disabled physically or mentally that you need help from another person during the day as set out at (a) above *or* at night as set out at (b) above.

Normally you must have needed help for at least six months before you can qualify for AA, but this rule is waived if you have a terminal illness.

'Bodily functions', for the purpose of the allowance, include walking and getting about; getting in and out of bed; using a wheelchair; eating or drinking; using the lavatory; washing, bathing or showering; dressing or undressing; shaving; treatment, medication or exercise; using a kidney machine at home or in a hospital self-care unit with assistance from someone who is not employed by the hospital.

The actual rates of payment are reviewed annually and are published in DSS leaflet NI 196.

Notes

1. AA is normally paid in addition to other benefits. It is not reduced because of any savings or earnings you may have and does not count as income in calculating Income Support, unless you are in residential care or in a nursing home.
2. A medical examination is not usually necessary, but may sometimes be required.
3. You cannot be paid AA while you are living in a place which is provided or helped by public money, for example:
   (a) a home run by a local authority;
   (b) a hospital, unless you are a private patient paying all your costs except treatment;
   (c) a private or voluntary home where some or all of your costs are paid by a local authority.
4. There is no provision for AA to be backdated, so you should claim as quickly as possible. You can claim three months in advance of satisfying the six-month rule.
5. AA rules have tended to be strictly applied. It is therefore important that claims are accurate and clear, and give a full and proper picture of the facts. You would be well

advised to study the detail in the *Disability Rights Handbook* (*see* page 26) before applying or to get expert help in completing the form.

Claims

Claim pack DS 2, from DSS, PO Box 51, Heywood, Lancashire OL10 2GG.

Further information (*see also* page 26)

⇒ *The Disability Handbook*
By Mansel Aylward, Peter Dewis and Tim Scott (DSS, 1992), price £11. Available from HMSO bookshops and in libraries.

Chronically Sick and Disabled Persons Act 1970

Section 2 of the 1970 Act is concerned with the meeting of the practical needs of disabled residents by their local authority. This is subject to the authority being 'satisfied' that in order to meet the needs of a disabled resident it must make arrangements for any or all of the following kinds of provision. When it is so satisfied, however, then it is under a duty, under the general guidance of the Secretary of State, to make those arrangements:

(a) the provision of practical assistance in the home;
(b) the provision of, or assistance in obtaining, wireless, television, library or similar recreational facilities;
(c) the provision of lectures, games, outings or other outdoor recreational facilities, or assistance in taking advantage of available educational facilities;
(d) the provision of facilities for, or assistance in, travelling to and from home for the purpose of participating in any services provided under arrangements made with the approval of the authority, or in any similar services which are otherwise provided and which could be provided under such approved arrangements;
(e) the provision of assistance in arranging for works of home adaptations, or the provision of any additional facilities designed to secure the disabled person's greater safety, comfort or convenience;
(f) facilitating the taking of holidays (whether or not provided under arrangements made by the authority);
(g) the provision of meals, whether at home or elsewhere;
(h) the provision of, or assistance in obtaining, a telephone and any special equipment needed to enable the disabled person to use it.

Disability Living Allowance (DLA)

DLA can be claimed by people under the age of 66 who need help with personal care or with getting around or with both, provided that they first needed help before their 65th birthday. Once granted, payment can continue beyond the age of 65.

DLA has replaced both Attendance Allowance for people disabled before the age of 65 (which is, however, still available to people disabled after reaching the age of 65 – *see* page 1) and Mobility Allowance, with automatic transfer of beneficiaries under those schemes to DLA. DLA is, however, somewhat wider in its application than the schemes it has replaced.

To get DLA you must normally have needed help for three months, and must be likely to need help for at least a further six months, but if you are not expected to live longer than six months you do not have to wait for three months.

Residence condition

You must be ordinarily resident and present in Great Britain for a total of at least 26 weeks in the year preceding the claim.

The personal care needs component

The personal care needs component, if allowable, is paid at one of three rates:

Higher rate: if you are not expected to live for more than six months, or if you are so severely disabled physically or mentally that you need help from another person both day and night. The help you need must be:

(a) throughout the day: frequent attention in connection with your bodily functions; or continual supervision to avoid substantial danger to yourself or others; and
(b) at night: prolonged or repeated attention in connection with your bodily functions; or another person being awake for a prolonged period or at frequent intervals to watch over you in order to avoid substantial danger to yourself or others.

Middle rate: if you are so severely disabled physically or mentally that you need help from another person during the day as set out at (a) above *or* at night as set out at (b) above.

Lower rate: if you are so severely disabled physically and mentally that you need help from another person in connection with your bodily functions for a significant portion of the day (about one hour), whether as a single period or the total of a number of periods; *or* if you are over the age of 16 and you cannot prepare a cooked meal for yourself if you have the ingredients.

'Bodily functions', for the purpose of the allowance, include walking and getting about; getting in and out of bed; using a wheelchair; eating or drinking; using the lavatory; washing, bathing or showering; dressing or undressing; shaving; treatment, medication or exercise; using a kidney machine at home or in a hospital self-care unit with assistance from someone who is not employed by the hospital.

Notes on the care component

1. You cannot be paid the care component of DLA while you are living in a place which is provided or helped by public money, for example:
   (a) a home run by a local authority;
   (b) a hospital, unless you are a private patient paying all your costs except treatment;
   (c) a private or voluntary home where some or all of your costs are paid by a local authority.
2. The care component of DLA is normally paid in addition to other benefits. It is not reduced because of any savings or earnings you may have and does not count as income in calculating Income Support, unless you are in residential care or in a nursing home where you are meeting the fees from your own resources.
3. A medical examination is not usually necessary, but may sometimes be required.
4. The care component of DLA replaces Attendance Allowance, the rules concerning which have tended to be strictly applied. It is therefore important that claims are accurate and clear, and give a full and proper picture of the facts. You would be well advised to study the detail in the *Disability Rights Handbook* (*see* page 26) before applying or to get expert help in completing the form.

The mobility needs component

The mobility needs component, if allowable, is paid at one of two rates:

Higher rate: if you meet any one of the following conditions:

– you have a physical disablement such that you are either unable to walk or virtually unable to walk; or
– you have had both legs amputated above the ankle or at the ankle, or you were born without legs or feet; or
– the exertion required to walk would endanger your life or be likely to lead to a serious deterioration in your health; or
– you are both deaf and blind and, because of the effects of those conditions in combination, you are unable, without the assistance of another person, to walk to any intended or required destination out of doors; or
– you are severely mentally impaired and exhibit disruptive behaviour which:
   (a) is extreme; and
   (b) requires another person to intervene and physically restrain you to prevent you causing physical injury to yourself or another person or damage to property; and
   (c) is so unpredictable that you need another person to be present and watching over you whenever you are awake; and

(d) you qualify for the highest rate of the care component.

Lower rate: if you can walk but are so severely disabled physically or mentally that, disregarding any ability you may have to use routes which are familiar to you on your own, you cannot take advantage of being out of doors without guidance or supervision from another person most of the time.

Notes on the mobility needs component

1. The mobility component of DLA stands on its own. It is normally paid in addition to other benefits.
2. You will not be entitled to the mobility component unless you can benefit from 'enhanced facilities for locomotion'.
3. In considering ability to walk, except in the case of double amputees, account will be taken of any artificial aid or prosthesis which you use or which would become suitable in your case.

Rates

Rates are reviewed annually and published in DSS leaflet NI 196.

Further notes on DLA

1. DLA is not reduced because of any savings or earnings you may have.
2. There is no provision for DLA to be backdated, so you should claim as quickly as possible.

Claims

Claim pack DLA1, from DSS, PO Box 50, Heywood, Lancashire OL10 2GF.
The claim form is very long and requires a great deal of personal information. Making a claim can be an embarrassing and essentially negative experience, leaving the person concerned with feelings of inadequacy, particularly if s/he needs help in completing the form.

Further information (see also page 26)

⇒ *The Disability Handbook*
By Mansel Aylward, Peter Dewis and Tim Scott (DSS, 1992), price £11. Available from HMSO bookshops and in libraries.

⇒ *The Way Around Disability Living Allowance and Disability Working Allowance: A critical guide*
(Disability Alliance ERA, Universal House, 88–94 Wentworth Street, London E1 7SA, 1992), price £3.50 including postage and packing.

Clearly charts the allowances introduced in April 1992, with detailed information about the assessment and appeal procedures.

Hospital and benefits

Hospital in-patients

Most Social Security benefits are paid to help with your ordinary needs at home, or the special needs caused by your disability. When you, or your partner or child, are in hospital, some of these needs are met by the National Health Service, so your benefit may go down or stop. But if you are paying the whole cost of accommodation and non-medical services in hospital, your Social Security benefits will not be affected (except for Invalid Care Allowance). DSS leaflet NI 9 gives simple general guidance with tables for each benefit showing what, if anything, happens immediately, after four weeks, after six weeks, after twelve weeks and after a year, if you or a dependant go into hospital. It also points out that if because of a reduction in benefit or loss of earnings you do not have enough money to meet your needs, you can claim Income Support.

Hospital travelling costs

If you have to travel to or from hospital where you receive NHS treatment, either as an out-patient or an in-patient, you may be able to get help with your travel costs. These can be:
(a) normal public transport fares; or
(b) if travel is by private car, the estimated cost of petrol or the equivalent public transport cost, whichever is the less; or
(c) if travel is by a local voluntary car scheme or something similar, the reasonable contributions you make towards transport costs; or
(d) if you have to use a taxi for part or all of the journey (because there is no other way for you to travel), the taxi fare.

In certain circumstances, you will qualify automatically, for example if you are on Income Support or Family Credit, or you are the partner of such a person. You may also be able to get help with travel costs if you and your partner have a low income (*see* DSS leaflet H 11 for details). If you need someone to go with you, you may get help with his or her fares too.

8 Statutory benefits and concessions

If you visit hospital to see a patient who is a close relative, you may be able to get help with travelling costs from the Social Fund if you are getting Income Support.

Further information (*see also* page 26)

DSS leaflet H 11, *NHS Hospital Travel Costs*, which includes information on how to claim.

Housing Benefit (HB)

HB is available to people on low incomes who need help to pay their rent. It is administered by local authorities. It can be claimed if you live in any kind of rented accommodation, public or private. You do not have to be getting other social security benefits or be a British citizen, and you are not necessarily ruled out because you are working.

Most people on Income Support automatically qualify for HB if they pay rent, but they must claim it.

People living in residential care homes or nursing homes cannot get HB in addition to Income Support.

HB is paid only in relation to that part of your rent which you pay just to live in your home. This is called your 'eligible rent', and is not necessarily the same amount as you pay to your landlord. Among other things, local authorities have discretion to make reductions if they consider the accommodation you occupy to be unreasonably large, unreasonably expensive (in the private sector), or in an unreasonably expensive area, provided always that there is suitable and cheaper accommodation available. However, reductions on these grounds should not be made if your personal circumstances are such that it would be unreasonable to expect you to move. *Such circumstances include age, health, disability and special accommodation needs.* If your rent includes charges for extra services such as the provision of fuel or meals, reductions are made in calculating your eligible rent.

If you are getting Income Support and pay rent you will get HB up to a maximum entitlement. This will be all of your eligible rent, unless reductions are made because you have other people living with you who do not depend on you to support them.

If you do not get Income Support, the above entitlement will be reduced by a fixed percentage of any amount by which your net income (apart from some 'disregards') exceeds a prescribed amount (called the 'applicable amount'). The applicable amount consists of a personal allowance, additions for dependent children, and various premiums, *for example for pensioners and disabled people*. In calculating income, savings up to £3,000 are disregarded, but after that, up to £16,000, each £250 or part of £250 is treated as income of £1 a week. If you have a partner to whom you are married or with whom you live as if you were married, your partner's savings are added in. If your savings exceed £16,000 you will not be entitled to HB.

So if your income is low and any savings you have are not over £16,000, it is worth making further enquiries.

Rates

Allowances, premiums and deductions are reviewed annually and are published in DSS leaflet NI 196.

Further information (*see also* page 26)

DSS leaflet RR 1, which includes details of how to claim, or the more detailed RR 2.

- *Guide to Housing Benefit*
By Martin Ward and John Zebedee (SHAC, 189a Old Brompton Road, London SW5 0AR), price £7.95 + 50p postage. Updated annually.

Housing grants for draughtproofing and insulation

See Section 5, 'Keeping Warm'.

Housing grants for improvements, repairs, provision of standard amenities

See Section 3, 'House and Home'.

Income Support (IS)

IS is available to people whose total family income falls below amounts prescribed by law. People who are aged 60 or over will be eligible if they:

(a) are in Great Britain; and
(b) are not working 16 hours or more a week; and
(c) do not have a partner working 16 hours or more a week; and
(d) do not have capital (including a partner's capital) over £8,000.

If both partners in a couple might be entitled to IS either one of them can claim it.

The money you get is the difference between an amount prescribed by law (called the 'applicable amount') and any income (apart from some disregards) you may have from other sources. There are special rules for calculating IS if you live in a residential care home or a nursing home.

The applicable amount consists of prescribed personal allowances, additions for dependent children, premiums (e.g. for pensioners, disabled people and carers), plus any payments for mortgage interest and certain other housing costs not covered by Housing Benefit. In calculating income, savings up to £3,000 are disregarded, but after that, up to £8,000, each £250 or part of £250 is treated as income of £1 a week. If your savings exceed £8,000 you will not be entitled to IS. If you have a partner to whom you are married or with whom you live as if you were married, your partner's savings are added in.

So if your income is low and any savings you have are not over £8,000, it is worth making further enquiries. Fill in the slip in DSS leaflet IS 1, available in post offices, and send it to your local DSS office.

Claimants in residential care homes, nursing homes or Part III accommodation

If you are eligible for IS and go to live in a private or voluntary home where you have to meet the fees from your own resources, you can receive IS to help with the fees. However, a ceiling is put on the amount of fees which will be taken into consideration. In simple terms, you receive a prescribed maximum (or the actual fee if this is lower), plus a personal allowance, minus your 'resources'. In calculating resources, note that there are some major differences from the normal rules, in that Attendance Allowance and Constant Attendance Allowance up to the higher rate of Attendance Allowance, and the personal care component of Disability Living Allowance, count as income.

In the case of residential care homes, the limit is set by reference to the category of care that the home is registered with the local authority to provide. If the home is registered in more than one category, and in the case of nursing homes, the limit is set according to the type of care that is being provided for you.

Maximum support levels are higher in Greater London than elsewhere, but the allowance for personal expenses is the same everywhere.

People living in Part III residential accommodation are entitled to an amount equal to the basic retirement pension rate. Eighty per cent of the allowance goes towards the accommodation and meals costs and 20 per cent is for personal expenses.

Working

The 16-hour-per-week limit was introduced on 7 April 1992. Previously the limit was 24 hours. People working 16 hours or more, but fewer than 24, already claiming IS on the basis of the old limit have transitional protection.

If you are working and you live in a residential care or nursing home or in Part III residential accommodation, because you need care, there is no limit to the number of hours you may work without losing the entitlement to claim IS. Your earnings, however, will be taken into account in the usual way.

Property

If you are going to live in a residential care or nursing home permanently, and you own your own home or part of it, its value or your share of its value will be treated as capital. Assuming this to be more than £8,000, this will debar you from IS unless and so long as the property remains occupied, wholly or partly, by your spouse, cohabitee, or a relative who is over 60 or who is incapacitated. If you decide to sell the property, its value can be disregarded for six months (longer in exceptional circumstances) while the sale is going through. Provided your other capital does not exceed £8,000, you can claim IS in this period.

Spouse's liability

A spouse's income and capital are not taken into account unless your admission to a home is temporary or you are both admitted together. However, if a spouse is capable of contributing towards the fees, this may be taken into account in assessing your IS.

Charges not covered by IS

Where the charges are above the prescribed maximum limit, any payment you receive towards the balance, subsequent to assessment, from charities, relatives or other (e.g. local authority) sources is not taken into account as income.

Rates

Allowances, premiums, deductions, and the ceilings in residential care homes or nursing homes are reviewed annually and are published in DSS leaflet NI 196.

Further information (*see also* page 26)

DSS leaflet IS 20, *A Guide to Income Support*.

Invalid Care Allowance (ICA)

ICA is a weekly cash allowance which can be claimed by people aged 16 to 64 who spend a lot of time caring for a severely disabled person who is getting Attendance Allowance at either rate, Disabled Living Allowance for personal care at the higher or middle rate, or Constant Attendance Allowance at or above the maximum rate with an industrial injuries, war or service pension. It is paid to the person who does the caring, not the person being cared for. You can get ICA irrespective of your sex or whether you are married, whether or not you are related to the disabled person or live at the same address.

ICA is not subject to a means test, is not reduced on account of savings, and does not depend on National Insurance contributions having been paid. You can earn up to a prescribed amount (at April 1992, £40 net of certain allowable expenses) while getting ICA. There are additions for dependants and the benefit includes a Class 1 National Insurance credit which protects the carer's pension rights (if you are a widow and cannot get ICA because you are getting Widow's Benefit, you can nevertheless claim ICA to get the NI credits).

If you are getting Income Support, Housing Benefit or Community Charge Benefit and you or your partner qualify for ICA, you will be entitled to a special carer's premium with those benefits. This applies even if you do not actually get ICA because it overlaps with another benefit.

Benefits being received by the person being cared for will generally not be affected, except that if that person is on Income Support, he or she will not be entitled to the severe disability premium.

ICA can be backdated up to 12 months.

Qualifying conditions

1. You must be aged between 16 and 64 on the date you first qualify.
2. You must be spending at least 35 hours a week (Sunday to Saturday) caring for a disabled person as described above. If, however, you stop looking after the disabled person for a short time, you may still be able to get ICA for weeks when, for example, you need a short holiday, or the disabled person is in hospital (and still getting Attendance Allowance or the Personal Care Needs component of the Disability Living Allowance.), or you are in hospital. (You can take a total of 12 weeks' break in any six-month period, but no more than four can be 'holiday' weeks).
3. You must not be earning (nor expecting to earn) more than £40 a week (April 1992) after certain allowable expenses.
4. You must not be attending, or be on holiday from, a full-time course of education.
5. You must be resident in the United Kingdom, and have been resident there for at least 26 weeks in the 12 months before the date you first satisfy all the other rules for ICA. Special rules apply to people who are in the armed forces and their families, or who are in receipt of tax-free emoluments.
6. You cannot get ICA while you are getting the same amount or more from one of the following benefits:
   (a) Sickness or Invalidity Benefit;
   (b) Unemployment Benefit;
   (c) Unemployability Supplement (paid with an industrial disablement or war pension);
   (d) a training allowance or grant paid out of government funds;
   (e) Industrial Death Benefit;
   (f) Maternity Allowance;

(g) Widow's Benefit (including Industrial or War Widow's Pension);
(h) a State Retirement Pension;
(i) Severe Disablement Allowance.

If the amount received from the above benefits is less than the Invalid Care Allowance, you can claim the difference.

Rates

Rates and maximum permitted earnings are reviewed annually and are published in DSS leaflet NI 196.

Further information (see also page 26)

DSS leaflet DS 700, which includes a claim pack.

Contact the ICA Unit, DSS, Palatine House, Lancaster Road, Preston, Lancashire PR1 1NS.

NHS dental treatment concessions

Everyone is entitled to the following NHS dental treatment free of charge:
- stopping bleeding after extractions;
- repairs to dentures;
- calling a dentist out, either to his/her surgery in an emergency, or for a necessary home visit (but in either of these circumstances you will have to pay for the treatment itself unless you qualify for free treatment as below).

Apart from these services, NHS dental treatment is subject to prescribed charges. Some groups of people, however, are entitled to free treatment. These include people on Income Support or Family Credit or an adult dependant of such a person. You may also be able to get help (full or partial) if you do not get these benefits but are on a low income (see DoH leaflet D 11 for details). If you are a war or service pensioner you may be able to claim a refund of the statutory charges for a dental examination, treatment or dentures needed because of your war or service disablement.

Refunds

If you qualify for free or reduced charge treatment but do not realise this until after you have paid your dentist, you may be able to get a refund.

Further information (*see also* page 26)

DoH leaflet D 11, which includes details of how to claim.

NHS sight test concessions and voucher scheme for glasses

Sight tests

Some groups of people are entitled to free sight tests. These include:
(a) people on Income Support or Family Credit, and their partners;
(b) people who need complex lenses who qualify for an NHS voucher for them (see below);
(c) people who are registered as blind or partially sighted;
(d) people who are diagnosed as having diabetes or glaucoma;
(e) people aged 40 or over who are a parent, brother, sister or child of a person with diagnosed diabetes or glaucoma;
(f) patients of the Hospital Eye Service.

Glasses

Help towards the cost of glasses is given in the form of vouchers. Your optician will complete a voucher form with a code letter covering your prescription. Prescriptions are banded according to their complexity: the more complex the prescription, the higher the value of the voucher. Each code letter carries a maximum voucher value (see DoH leaflet G 11 for details).

If you are in group (a) above, you will automatically qualify for a voucher of the maximum amount. Alternatively, you may qualify for help (all or part of the maximum voucher value) towards the cost of glasses if you are on a low income.

If you are prescribed complex/powerful glasses with at least one lens which has a power in any one meridian of plus or minus 10 or more dioptres, or is made in lenticular form, or is a prism-controlled bifocal lens (your optician will advise), you will be entitled to a voucher (and therefore a free NHS sight test), but its value will be well below the maximum amount.

War pensioners

If you are a war or service pensioner, you may be able to claim back some or all of the cost if your sight test or glasses are needed because of your war or service disability.

Hospital Eye Service

If you are referred to the Hospital Eye Service, and are prescribed glasses as part of your treatment, there are two special vouchers in addition to those available from opticians, and some supplements for special frames or special lenses (*see* DoH leaflet G 11 for details). Some hospitals have their own arrangements for supplying glasses, and there are special arrangements for maximum charges if the glasses prescribed are very expensive.

Sight tests for people who are housebound

People who are eligible for a free NHS sight test and who are also housebound and unable to attend the optician's practice qualify for a free visit and test in their own home under the general ophthalmic services.

Refunds

You can claim a refund on the cost of your sight test where you are claiming on low income grounds and the necessary certificate becomes available only after your sight test. In the case of glasses, however, if you pay for your glasses yourself, you cannot get a refund afterwards even if you were entitled to a voucher unless they were prescribed through the Hospital Eye Service. Make sure you have your voucher before you buy.

Further information (*see also* page 26)

DoH leaflet G 11, which includes details of how to claim.

NHS prescription charges concessions

Some groups of people are entitled to free prescriptions. These include:
(a) men aged 65 or over or women aged 60 or over.
(b) people on Income Support or Family Credit, and their partners.
(c) people receiving a war or service disablement pension who need prescriptions for the disability for which they get a War Pension.
(d) people with one or more of the following conditions:
- a permanent fistula (including caecostomy, colostomy, laryngostomy or ileostomy) which requires continuous surgical dressing or an appliance.
- forms of hypoadrenalism (including Addison's disease) for which specific substitution therapy is essential.

- diabetes insipidus or other forms of hypopituitarism.
- diabetes mellitus, except where treatment is by diet alone.
- hypoparathyroidism.
- myasthenia gravis.
- myxoedema or other conditions where supplemental thyroid hormone is necessary.
- epilepsy requiring continuous anti-convulsive therapy.
- a continuing physical disability which prevents the disabled person leaving home without the help of another person (temporary disabilities, even if they last a few months, do not count).

(e) people on a low income (*see* DoH leaflet P 11 for details).

If you do not qualify for exemption, but need a lot of prescriptions, you can buy a prepaid 'season ticket' covering any number of prescriptions in a given period. This may be for four or twelve months and may cost you less than paying per prescription. Get form FP 95 (EC 95 in Scotland) from a post office or chemist.

Prescription charges do not apply to items which are supplied and personally administered by either prescribing or dispensing doctors.

Refunds

If you qualify for free prescriptions but have already paid a prescription charge, you can reclaim it. But you must have a receipt FP 57 (EC 57 in Scotland) and claim within one month of paying the charge.

Further information (*see also* page 26)

DoH leaflet P 11, which includes details of how to claim.

Severe Disablement Allowance (SDA)

SDA is for people aged 16 or more who are unable to work because of long-term sickness or severe mental or physical disablement. You may be able to get SDA if you cannot get Sickness or Invalidity Benefit because you have not paid enough National Insurance contributions. But you have to have been unable to work for at least 28 weeks before you can qualify. SDA is not means-tested, and does not depend on National Insurance contributions having been paid.

You will not normally get SDA if you are already getting one of the following benefits, unless the SDA would be higher:

(a) Sickness or Invalidity Benefit;
(b) Maternity Allowance;

Severe Disablement Allowance

(c) Retirement Pension;
(d) a widow's benefit of any kind;
(e) Invalid Care Allowance;
(f) Unemployability Supplement paid with Industrial Injuries Disablement Benefit or War Disablement Pension;
(g) Training Allowance from the Employment Department Group or the Ministry of Agriculture, Fisheries and Food.

If you are getting Income Support, it will be reduced by any amount of SDA you get, so there may be no net gain, but it is still worth claiming SDA because there are usually long-term advantages. SDA is reduced if you are in hospital for longer than six weeks.

Residence conditions

You must:

(a) be living in the United Kingdom when you apply for SDA; and
(b) have been in the United Kingdom for at least 24 of the 28 weeks during which you were incapable of work; and
(c) have lived in the United Kingdom for at least 10 of the last 20 years (if you are under 20, for at least 10 years).

Other qualifying conditions

1. You must be unable to work because of sickness or disability (doctor must certify), and have been either:
   (a) incapable of work for 28 weeks in a row; or
   (b) getting SDA at any time in the last 8 weeks; or
   (c) getting SDA previously with no gaps of more than 8 weeks between getting SDA, signing on as unemployed (or getting a training allowance) and making your new claim for SDA;
2. With some prescribed exceptions, you must be at least 80 per cent disabled (in practice 75 per cent or more qualifies). Qualification under this rule can be met in a variety of ways (*see* DSS leaflet NI 252 for details).

Therapeutic earnings

Claimants may, in certain circumstances, derive earnings from work of a therapeutic nature with the approval of their doctor and the DSS without affecting their entitlement to SDA (there are similar provisions for Sickness Benefit and Invalidity Benefit) up to a prescribed weekly maximum (April 1992, £40.50). If, however, Income Support is payable in addition to SDA, any therapeutic earnings over £15 a week would be deducted from your IS.

If you are at retirement age or over (65 for men, 60 for women at the time of writing), you can get SDA only if you were entitled to it on the day before you reached retirement age.

Rates for SDA

SDA consists of a basic allowance with age-related additions. The additions depend on your age when your present period of incapacity for work first began. People under 40 qualify for the higher rate addition, those aged 40-9 for the middle rate addition, and those aged 50-9 for the lower rate addition. But note that people receiving Income Support as well as SDA will have their Income Support reduced by the amount of the increase in SDA. Rates are reviewed annually and are set out in DSS leaflet NI 196.

Further information (*see also* page 26)

DSS leaflet NI 252.

The Social Fund

A much-criticised scheme offering limited help to people with exceptional expenses which it is difficult for them to meet from their regular income.

There are two distinct kinds of benefit: grants available by right in prescribed circumstances with detailed qualification rules, and a cash-limited scheme of discretionary interest-free loans and Community Care grants. Payments from the Social Fund do not depend on National Insurance contributions having been paid, but are means-tested.

Payments by right

These are available, subject to qualification, for maternity expenses, funeral expenses or for heating costs in periods of exceptionally cold weather. The first two grants are limited to people in receipt of specified low income benefits and are reduced by the amount of any capital you have over prescribed levels (currently £500 for people aged under 60, and £1,000 for those aged 60 and over). Cold weather payments of £6 a week are paid automatically to eligible people when the forecast for your local weather station shows that the temperature is likely to average 0 degrees Centigrade (freezing point) or below for a seven day period. However, you qualify for this payment only if you or your partner are on Income Support which includes either a pensioner or disability premium, or an amount for a child under five years of age.

Discretionary payments

Only a limited amount of money has been allocated to this part of the Social Fund, much less than was paid by way of the old Supplementary Benefit single payments and urgent needs payments which the Social Fund replaced. The budget is divided between local DSS offices, each of which is allocated a fixed amount. Within this constraint, Social Fund Officers have to decide which needs can be met and to what extent. If and when the money runs out, it does not matter how desperate your need is. Nor is there any appeal; you are limited to asking the Social Fund Officer to review the decision. There are three types of discretionary payment:

(a) Budgeting Loans;
(b) Crisis Loans;
(c) Community Care Grants.

General exclusions

Certain costs can never be met from the Social Fund. These include the following:

— any need occurring outside the United Kingdom;
— expenses arising from a court appearance;
— removal charges if you are being rehoused under legislation concerned with homelessness or following a compulsory purchase order, a redevelopment or closing order, or a compulsory exchange of tenancies;
— domestic assistance and respite care provided by a local authority;
— repairs to property of public sector housing bodies;
— medical or other health expenses;
— returnable accommodation deposits;
— work related expenses;
— debts to government departments;
— investments;
— expenses for which an award has been made or refused within the last 26 weeks (unless there has been a change in your circumstances).

Budgeting loans

These interest-free loans are intended to help people on Income Support to spread large one-off expenses over a longer period. The minimum loan is £30 and the maximum amount of loans you can have outstanding at any time is £1,000. If you or your partner have capital over £500 (£1,000 if either of you are 60 or over), the loan will be reduced by the excess. You, or your partner, must have been on Income Support for the last 26 weeks, with no more than one break, not exceeding 14 days. The Social Fund Officer must be sure you can afford to repay the loan, usually by weekly deductions (between

5 and 15 per cent) of your Income Support over a period of up to 18 months. If you stop getting benefit, for example because you start work, you still have to repay the loan. You cannot get a Budgeting loan if you or your partner are involved in a trade dispute.

In addition to the general exclusions shown above, you cannot get budgeting loans for:
- mains fuel bills and standing charges;
- housing costs (other than intermittent costs not met by Housing Benefit or Income Support, and rent in advance where the landlord is not a local authority).

Crisis loans

These are for people aged 16 or over who are faced with expenses arising from an emergency or a disaster, and whose resources are insufficient to meet the short-term needs of themselves or their families. They can be claimed whether or not you are in receipt of a Social Security benefit. Crisis loans will, however, be approved only if there is no other way of preventing a serious risk to your or your family's health or safety. The loan is interest-free but must be repaid, either by weekly deductions from benefit or in some other way.

Certain categories of people are not eligible for Crisis loans. These include the following:

(a) residents of Part III accommodation, a nursing home or residential care home;
(b) prisoners or anyone lawfully detained;
(c) members of a religious order who are maintained by it;
(d) hospital in-patients (unless they are to be discharged within the next two weeks);

In addition to the general exclusions shown above, you cannot get a Crisis loan for:
- telephone installation, rental or call charges;
- mobility needs;
- holidays;
- televisions and radios;
- motor vehicle costs (except for emergency travelling expenses);
- housing costs (other than intermittent costs not met by Housing Benefit or Income Support, rent in advance where the landlord is not a local authority, and boarding charges).

Community Care grants

These are for people who are on Income Support, or who expect to get Income Support when they move into the community. They are intended to help people who are facing special difficulty arising from special circumstances and in particular to support the policy of care in the community, primarily to assist individuals and families such as elderly, mentally ill, mentally handicapped, chronically ill and disabled people to re-establish and/or maintain themselves in the community. If, however, you have capital over £500 (or £1,000 if you are aged 60 or more) a Community Care grant will be reduced by the amount of your extra savings.

If you get Income Support you will not have to repay a Community Care grant. If, however, you do not get Income Support when you move into the community, you will have to pay the grant back.

In addition to the general exclusions shown above, you cannot get a Community Care grant for:

- telephone installation, rental or call charges;
- any expenses your local authority has a statutory duty to meet:
- fuel costs and standing charges;
- housing costs.

Further information (*see also* page 26)

DSS leaflet SB 16, *A Guide to the Social Fund*.

DSS leaflet SFL 2, *How the Social Fund Can Help You*.

DSS leaflet D 49, *What To Do After a Death* (funeral payments).

DSS leaflet CWP 1, *Extra Help with Heating Costs When It's Very Cold*.

State Retirement Pension (SRP)

SRP based on National Insurance (NI) contributions can be paid when you reach 'pensionable age' (at present 65 (men) and 60 (women), though a common retirement age may be introduced in the not too distant future), subject to detailed qualification rules. You may be entitled to:

(a) Basic Pension (BP) (dependent on how many qualifying contribution years you have in your working life);
(b) Additional Pension (AP) (see below);
(c) Other additions (see below).

If you are entitled to SRP, you can claim it even if you continue to work, and irrespective of how much you earn. Alternatively, until you reach 70 (men) or 65 (women), you can ask for payment to be deferred or suspended in order to qualify for a larger amount when you do decide to draw it. If you do continue to work beyond pensionable age, you will not have to pay any more NI contributions.

SRP is not paid automatically. It must be claimed. You can do so up to four months before entitlement (you should be sent claim form BR 1 at this time). It is a good idea to do so if you want payment to start on time. If you leave it more than 12 months after becoming entitled, arrears will be limited to 12 months.

Entitlement to SRP is most commonly based on your own NI contribution record, but a widow or widower entitled to Invalidity Benefit who has reached pensionable age can also qualify, as can (for BP only) anyone reaching pensionable age after 5 April 1979 by using the qualifying years of a former spouse. Class 1 (employee), Class 2 (self-employed) and Class 3 (voluntary) contributions can all count in calculating BP. The amount you get depends on how many qualifying years you have in your contribution record in relation to your working life (the period over which you have to meet the contribution conditions for BP: normally 44 years (women) and 49 years (men)). To get the full rate of BP you must have qualifying years for about nine-tenths of the years in your working life. But within prescribed limits you may nevertheless get a reduced BP if you have fewer qualifying years or a shorter working life. The rules about calculations of BP and AP, which are quite complex, are set out in some detail in DSS Notice NP 46.

Additions

Additional Pension (AP)

AP is based on the amount of any earnings as an employee on which you have paid Class 1 contributions, above the level needed for BP, in tax years since April 1978. It is reduced in respect of occupational and/or personal pension received (the contracted-out deduction).

Graduated Pension (GP)

If you paid graduated NI contributions between April 1961 and April 1975 under the then Graduated Pension Scheme, you will be entitled to GP even if you do not qualify for BP or AP.

Invalidity Addition (IA)

You will be entitled to IA if you were receiving Invalidity Allowance with an Invalidity Benefit within eight weeks of reaching pensionable age. This will, however, be reduced by the amount of any AP and/or occupational pension you receive.

Age addition

This will be paid to everyone aged 80 or over (currently 25 pence!).

Additions for dependants

Provided you receive BP you can get additional pension for:

(a) children for whom you are entitled, or treated as entitled, to Child Benefit; and
(b) one of the following (provided their earnings or income from an occupational or personal pension do not exceed a prescribed amount):
 – your wife (unless she already receives BP or some other benefit in an amount equal to the relevant additional pension); or
 – your husband (provided you were entitled to an increase of Sickness Benefit, Unemployment Benefit, or Invalidity Benefit for him immediately before you qualified for your pension); or
 – someone who looks after a child or children for whom you are entitled (or treated as entitled) to Child Benefit.

Married women

At pensionable age, you may, of course, qualify for BP and AP on your own contribution record (this excludes those married women who elected to pay reduced rate contributions up to age 60). Alternatively, you can get BP alone based on your husband's contribution record *if he is getting BP*. This will be roughly 60 per cent of the amount to which he is entitled. If you are entitled to BP in your own right, but the amount is less than you would receive if you relied on your husband's contributions, the two pensions will be combined to give you BP up to the maximum entitlement on your husband's contributions.

As a result of the change to independent taxation in April 1990, a married woman's state retirement pension, even if it is paid jointly and is based on her husband's contributions, is her own income. If she has no other income, her pension will be offset by her personal tax allowance and may thus reduce the couple's overall tax liability.

Widows

If you are widowed after you reach pensionable age, you can claim SRP on your own contributions or on your late husband's contributions or on a combination of the two. If you thus qualify for SRP, you can defer receiving it as described above. Alternatively, you may be entitled to Widow's Benefit. This depends on whether you or your husband (or both of you) were getting SRP when he died, and on whether you have any children.

In claiming SRP, your late husband's contributions can be taken into account even if you remarry. You may also be entitled to:

– any graduated pension earned on your own contributions and/or half of any graduated pension earned on your late husband's contributions;

- additional pension earned on both your own and your late husband's contributions, up to a prescribed maximum;
- increments if you decide to defer your pension (*see* above).

If you are widowed *before* reaching pensionable age, you will similarly be able to claim SRP when you reach that age, but you can rely on your late husband's contributions only if you have not remarried. Alternatively, you can continue to draw any Widow's Benefit to which you are entitled until you reach the age of 65. Having claimed SRP, you can defer drawing it so as to gain increments when it is paid later on. (Whichever choice you make, you can change your mind at any time until you reach the age of 65.)

It will usually be advantageous to claim SRP, in that if you qualify on contributions you may also be entitled to increases by way of graduated pension and additional pension.

If, however, you have not previously qualified for Widow's Benefit or have qualified only at a reduced rate (because you were not old enough when widowed to qualify or to qualify for the full amount), then unless you qualify for SRP on contributions, you will correspondingly not qualify for SRP or will qualify only at the same reduced rate.

Widowers

There is no benefit for widowers comparable to Widow's Benefit, but it may be possible to rely on your late wife's *standard* NI contributions to gain extra pension.

Divorced people

If you are not entitled to full SRP, your former spouse's NI contribution record may be taken into account if it will give you a better pension, provided that you have not remarried before reaching pensionable age. You do not have to wait until your former spouse is receiving his/her pension.

Non-contributory state pensions

You will be entitled to a special pension if you:
(a) are 80 or over; and
(b) satisfy prescribed residence conditions; and
(c) are not entitled to another category of pension (other than one at a lower rate than the special pension).

Payment abroad

Your pension can, on request, be paid to you while you are abroad for as long as you like. But you will not be entitled to annual benefit upratings if you cease to be ordinarily resident in the United Kingdom unless you go to live in one of the European Community countries (including Gibraltar), or one with which the United Kingdom has a reciprocal agreement (Austria, Bermuda, Cyprus, Finland, Iceland, Israel, Jamaica, Jersey/Guernsey, Malta, Mauritius, Sweden, Switzerland, Turkey, former Yugoslavia and the United States).

If you are going abroad for only a short time, you can cash your pension orders when you get back, but remember that you will not be able to cash an order if it is over three months old. If you are going abroad for between three and six months, you can ask to have your pension paid into a bank or building society in the United Kingdom.

See DSS leaflet NI 38 for further details.

Rates

Rates are reviewed annually, and are published in DSS leaflet NI 196. Four months in advance of reaching pensionable age you can ask for a forecast of what pension you can expect to receive.

Further information (see also page 26)

DSS guide FB 6, *Retiring?*, a simplified guide.

DSS guide NP 46, *A Guide to State Retirement Pension*.

DSS guide NI 184, *Over 80s pension*.

DSS guide NI 92, *Earning Extra Retirement Pension by Cancelling Your Retirement*.

▪▶ *You and Your Pension*
(Consumers' Association), price £8.95. Available from Consumers' Association, Castlemead, Gascoyne Way, Hertford X SG14 1LH. For credit card orders, freephone 0800-252100 quoting Dept DFOP.

▪▶ *Your State Pension and Carrying On Working* (Fact Sheet No. 19)
(Age Concern England, Astral House, 1268 London Road,
London SW16 4ER (Tel: 081-679 8000). A free fact sheet which explains the pros and cons of deferring your pension and the increases gained.

Helpful organisations

Advice about benefits is normally best sought locally, where you can meet the adviser and explain and discuss your individual circumstances. In some places there are Welfare Rights Officers, often employed by the local authority, specialising in this field, and in most parts of the country an excellent service on benefits as well as many other matters is provided by Citizens Advice Bureaux.

Many of the organisations featured in Section 14, Helpful Organisations, run information services, and some, such as the RNIB, have specialist advisers on benefits. If you are otherwise in touch with such an organisation, you may find that it can offer particularly personal and sensitive guidance.

The DSS provides the following freephone services:

— Benefit Enquiry Line for People with Disabilities: 0800-882 200.
— Freelines in languages other than English:
   Chinese: 0800-252 451
   Punjabi: 0800-521 360
   Urdu: 0800-289 188
   Welsh: 0800-289 011.

Further information

Books and publications

Department of Social Security leaflets are widely available in post offices, libraries, Citizens Advice Bureaux, social security offices and other advice centres. In case of difficulty, write to the Leaflets Unit, PO Box 21, Stanmore, Middlesex HA7 1AY. A catalogue is available under the code reference CAT 1. Some of the most relevant general guides are mentioned below.

▶ *Disability Rights Handbook*
(Disability Alliance ERA, Universal House, 88–94 Wentworth Street, London E1 7SA, 17th edition, April 1992 to April 1993), price £6.95 including postage, with reduced rates for bulk orders from voluntary organisations and trade unions.

A low priced guide, published annually, which will be invaluable to claimants and advisers alike. Certainly no member of the caring professions or a voluntary organisation should be without a copy. It is expertly written with disabled people in mind and is both clearly set out and wide-ranging, going into the kind of detail and explanation which is not possible in this Directory.

▶ *Disability Rights Bulletins*
Price £3.50 each, issued quarterly to update the *Disability Rights Handbook*. The *Handbook* and the *Bulletins* can be ordered as an inclusive package at a subscription of £12.

Further information

- *A Guide for Blind and Partially Sighted People* (FB 19) (DSS).
  A free guide to benefits available to blind people, partially sighted people and their families. As well as covering the areas where visual handicap is a specific consideration, it also outlines benefits for which all can apply.

- *A Guide to Non-contributory Benefits for Disabled People* (HB 5) (DSS).
  A free guide.

- *A Guide to Reviews and Appeals* (NI 260) (DSS).
  A free guide.

- *National Welfare Benefits Handbook 1992/3*
  (Child Poverty Action Group Ltd, 1-5 Bath Street, London EC1V 9PY, 1992), price £6.50 including postage and packing, £2.50 to individual claimants.

  Written by experienced advisers who have worked at CPAG Citizens' Rights Office. Detailed coverage of means-tested benefits.

- *Rights Guide to Non-Means-Tested Social Security Benefits 1992/3*
  (Child Poverty Action Group Ltd, 1-5 Bath Street, London EC1V 9PY, 1992), price £5.95 including postage and packing, £2.25 to individual claimants.

  Provides expert coverage of benefits for unemployment, sickness, maternity, widowhood, disablement and caring, and pensions. This edition comments on the introduction of Disability Appeal Tribunals from April 1992, and important developments in European law.

  The above CPAG publications are regularly updated by the *Welfare Rights Bulletin*, annual subscription £12, individual copies £1.95.

- *Sick or Disabled?* (FB 28) (DSS).
  A free guide to benefits if you are sick or disabled for a few days or more.

- *Which Benefit?* (FB 22) (DSS).
  A free booklet available in English, Bengali, Chinese, Gujarati, Hindi, Punjabi, Turkish and Urdu. It has brief details on how to make a claim and where to get further advice, and information on National Insurance contributions and how immigration status may affect benefits.

- *Your Benefit*
  (RNIB, 224 Great Portland Street, London W1N 6AA (Tel: 071-388 1266 ext. 2335 or 2336), 1990), price £1 (for individuals).

  This booklet is available in English, Gujarati, Hindi, Urdu and Yoruba. The English version is published in large print, tape, Braille and Moon versions.

Statutory benefits and concessions

▶ *Your Rights 1992/3*
(Age Concern, Astral House, 1268 London Road, London SW16 4ER, 1992), price £2.50 including postage and packing.

SECTION TWO

More money matters

Money management

Planning for your later years should, of course, start well before retirement. With the numbers of elderly people steadily rising, both in real terms and as a proportion of Britain's total population, it is probably unrealistic to expect that state benefits will ever provide more than a basic (and meagre) living. As far as you are able (and we do realise that many people can do little to help themselves), you need to plan for the future to provide out of present income a reasonable standard of living in retirement in a way which takes into account the steady decline in the value of money. Given the pattern of inflation, it is not enough to put some money by in an old sock.

When you do reach retirement, it is even more important to organise your financial affairs so as to provide the best possible provision for the years ahead (recognising that they may well be many) within a secure framework: to consider what your resources are, whether they can be enhanced, and to budget those resources. A good starting point is simply to list your annual income and expenditure. If you have previously had a job and are comparing your pre- and post-retirement situation for the first time, you may actually find this somewhat reassuring: things may not be as bad as you feared. Although there will be a sharp drop in income, there will also be reductions in expenditure: for example, less tax, no National Insurance or pension contributions or work related expenses, and, when you do travel, some special concessions. Hopefully, any mortgage commitments will also have been paid off or considerably reduced. Conversely, of course, you are likely to be at home more and your heating and lighting costs will rise. But whatever result the figures provide, the fact that you have weighed up your financial position and set it out clearly will give you an informed basis for further action: perhaps to reduce spending (in which case you will have a better idea of where savings can usefully be made), or to decide that you need to seek additional income, perhaps from a part-time job, from savings or investments, or, if you own your own house, from realising part of its value. There is, of course, no one answer: how you spend (or save) your money is ultimately a matter of personal choice, constrained by personal circumstances, but there are some ground rules you might usefully follow.

Savings and investment

If you have not thought about it before, on retirement you may have to consider what to do with your money, whether from savings, from an insurance policy which has matured, or from a lump sum gratuity from your employer. There may also be a change of direction. If you have enjoyed a regular income from work, and have hitherto looked to building up your savings, you may find that this process has to go into reverse: that you now need to derive income from capital. You are faced by choices and it is important to recognise that there may be no one answer: you may need to diversify your savings and investments to meet different needs and contingencies. There are many factors to consider. In the paragraphs which follow, we mention only a few, and the less sophisticated, of the many possibilities, and offer only general advice. More detailed guidance is available in many specialist books, some of which are mentioned at page 37.

You may need professional advice. There are dangers here. An investigation by the Consumers' Association reported in *Which?* in February 1992 clearly indicated that the quality of financial advice is variable. In particular, financial advisers work on commission, and the less scrupulous may be tempted to steer your investments towards what is more lucrative for them in terms of commission rather than what is best for you. Some investments are also very risky. We think you should try to gain a clear idea of what is on offer and whether it meets your needs, and consider it carefully before you commit yourself. We also think that you are entitled to know whether you will be charged a fee or how much of your investment will disappear as your broker's commission.

It is also important to be aware that under the Financial Services Act 1986, measures have been introduced to regulate UK-based companies, with a compensation scheme against default (offshore funds are not covered by these compensation arrangements, which are described on page 36). You can at least check whether a financial adviser is fully authorised under the Act. One of the most significant rules is that a sharp distinction is drawn between representatives who are 'tied' to one particular company and those who operate independently. Tied agents recommend the products of their own principal, if they are suitable, whereas independent intermediaries should have a wide knowledge of financial institutions from which to make their choice. Both should carefully consider the individual circumstances and needs of their clients and offer 'suitable advice'.

Ethical investment

In many investment funds, we have no control over the use to which our money is put, whereas, we suggest, this should be a prime consideration. It is now possible to invest through financial managers who aim to avoid investments in activities which they consider to be socially or environmentally damaging. There are a growing number of businesses offering 'ethical investment'.

The difficulty is knowing which to choose. We rarely make commercial recommendations, preferring to suggest the principles which should govern your choice. The criterion here is essentially that your concern is to direct your money to worthy objectives rather than to obtain the maximum possible return on your investment. In that connection you should want to know just where your money will go, rather than the kinds of company that will be avoided. We must, nevertheless, mention that guidance is commercially available from EIRIS (Ethical Investment Research Service), 504 Bondway Business Centre, 71 Bondway, London SW8 1SQ (Tel: 071-735 1351). Since 1983, EIRIS has been building up its information on all major UK companies. Individuals seeking ethical investment advice are invited to complete a questionnaire as to what they regard as unethical and submit it with a list of their present shareholdings. You then receive a 'portfolio screen' showing how your present shareholdings match up to your ethical crieria. Additionally you can request details of company groups which meet your ethical criteria. Charges for this service are as follows:

– Portfolio screen on up to 20 present shareholdings: £36.00
– As above, plus list of 50 acceptable company groups: £63.25
– Portfolio screen on up to 30 present shareholdings plus full acceptable list updated quarterly: £178.25

EIRIS also publishes a range of books on ethical investment and a quarterly newsletter, *The Ethical Investor*, subscription £10 a year for individuals. Details will be sent on request.

We will also mention The Ecology Building Society, 18 Station Road, Crosshills, Keighley, West Yorkshire BD20 7EH (Tel: 0535-35933), which is opposed to the wasteful use of land and resources sometimes encouraged by orthodox lending policies. It aims to contribute to the regeneration of rural areas and inner cities and to promote a more ecological way of life. It thus lends on such properties as organic smallholdings and farms, houses which incorporate special energy saving or energy efficient features, and derelict but sound houses which would otherwise have been abandoned.

Further information on ethical investment

Socially Responsible Investment
By Sue Ward (Directory of Social Change, Radius Works, Back Lane, London, NW3 1HL, 1986), price £7.95 + £1.50 postage.

Could I be liable for capital gains tax?

In certain circumstances, this is a possibility. Capital gains tax (CGT) is charged on the gain made when you give away, exchange or sell something you own which has increased in value since you acquired it. Thus if you sell shares at a profit you may become liable to CGT. Since 6 April 1988 tax on capital gains has been the same as that paid on income, and net gains are treated as the 'top slice' of income and charged accordingly at income tax rates. If your other income is very low and you have some unused income tax reliefs and allowances, these cannot be set against net gains.

There are, however, some special concessions. Only gains since March 1982 are taxed, and any increase in value which is attributable to inflation since then is discounted in calculating your net gain. There is also an exemption limit for each tax year (1992/3: £5,800 for individuals). The effect of these concessions is that taxpayers can benefit if they are able to invest for growth rather than income. Some income can be taken simply by cashing in investments from time to time.

You may get relief from CGT if you sell your business or shares in a family-owned company because you are retiring at age 55 or over, or because you are ill. Inland Revenue leaflet CGT 6 *Retirement: Disposal of a business* will tell you more. Two capital gains tax leaflets are available from tax offices: CGT 14, *An Introduction to Capital Gains Tax*, and CGT 15, *A Guide for Married Couples*.

Further information on capital gains tax

▶ *Inheritance Tax and Capital Gains Tax*
By Paul Lewis (Saga Publishing Ltd, The Saga Building, Middelburg Square, Folkestone, Kent CT20 1AZ), free to Saga Club members – *see* page 345).

▶ *Which? Way to Save Tax*
(Consumers' Association, Castlemead, Gascoyne Way, Hertford X, SG14 1LH, published annually in August), price (1991/2) £11.95.

Does investment income count as part of my taxable income?

Generally, yes (National Savings certificates, TESSA and Premium Bond winnings are exceptions). If your total income is high enough to be liable to tax, this may mean not only that your investment income is reduced by the tax charge but that the higher tax allowances available to people aged 65 and over are affected. In these circumstances, you may wish to consider investing, at least to some extent, for growth rather than income, taking advantage of the capital gains tax concession, and periodically cashing in part of your investment if you need income.

Further information on income tax and its effect on investment income is given on page 44.

How safe will my money be?

Generally speaking, the higher the potential return the greater the degree of risk. If you cannot afford to lose money or are simply someone who does not like to take risks, you can opt for an absolutely dependable borrower (that is what they are!), such as a bank, building society, local authority, rock-solid insurance company, National Savings or the government. The problem with these 'safe' options, however, is that if you need to draw out the interest to help with your living expenses, there is no capital growth: the amount of your savings remains the same, while because of inflation the value of your savings in terms of what the money will buy is steadily eroded.

Many savings plans are available, including a number which provide for a regular monthly income to be drawn. The normal principle is that the interest rate is higher when the savings are substantial and/or are put in for a guaranteed period and/or where notice is required before withdrawals. Interest rates, of course, are generally variable, but some schemes offer a fixed rate and there is an obvious advantage if you can lock into one of these when the rate is high.

Building societies

Building societies offer a variety of schemes. If you want a reasonable return and need easy access, you should find a plan suited to your needs. They provide a convenient home for money which you may need quickly, but you can do better if you have a substantial amount by investing long-term. Smaller societies usually pay higher interest, but you may have to balance this against the inconvenience of not having a branch office near enough to visit.

Banks

Banks offer deposit accounts of various kinds, the advantages and disadvantages of which are similar to building societies. The interest rates are generally lower, but you may find it more convenient to hold money short-term at the bank which keeps your current account.

National Savings

National Savings are another safe option, with a diversity of schemes:

Investment accounts yield, at the time of writing, 9.5 per cent interest per annum. The minimum deposit is £5, and the maximum holding £25,000. Although interest counts as part of your income for tax purposes, no tax is deducted at source. A month's written notice is required to make withdrawals.

Income Bonds offer a slightly better rate (10.25 per cent per annum at the time of writing), which is paid as a monthly income. Again, tax is not deducted at source. Holdings are in multiples of £1,000; the minimum holding is £2,000 and the maximum £25,000. Three months' written notice is required for repayment and interest is limited to half-rate if repayment is made within the first year.

Savings Certificates offer interest which is entirely free of tax at a compound rate which is guaranteed for five years. Interest is earned for each completed period of three months. At the time of writing, the 37th issue certificate is available. It offers 8 per cent per annum compound interest where the certificates are held for the full five years (£46.94 added to every £100 invested). The mimimum purchase is £25 and the maximum holding is £7,500, except that you can reinvest mature Savings Certificates up to a further £10,000. Repayment is quite prompt in response to a written form request. The certificates can be cashed in before their full term, but the interest earned is then lower, and no interest is given if repayment is made within the first year (except for reinvested certificates).

Capital Bonds offer interest which is added annually to the value of the bond. At the time of writing, Series C bonds are available. These offer a gross return which averages out at 11.5 per cent per annum if you hold your bond for a full five years (£72.34 on every £100 invested). Although the interest counts each year as taxable income, tax is not deducted at source. Capital Bonds, with a high rate of interest, paid gross, will therefore show a very good long-term yield for non-taxpayers who do not need income. Holdings are in multiples of £100; the minimum purchase is £100 and the maximum total holding of Capital Bonds from Series B onwards is £100,000. Three months' written notice is required for repayment. If cashed in before their full five year term, the interest earned is lower, and no interest is given on bonds cashed before the first anniversary of payment.

First Option Bonds Introduced in 1992, these lump sum bonds offer a guaranteed fixed rate of interest, net of tax, for one year at a time. They are intended for investors who are liable to tax at the basic rate (higher rate taxpayers would have to pay additional tax on the interest earned). The 'option' is simply that at the end of each year, you can leave your money invested or cash it in. The minimum investment is £1,000 and a small bonus is paid where the value of the bond does not fall below £20,000. The maximum investment is £250,000.

Leaflets explaining the various schemes in greater detail are available in post offices, where interest rate charts are displayed and where you can also obtain the appropriate application and repayment forms. If you would like further information about National Savings products you can telephone during normal office hours as follows:

South: 071-605 9461
North West: 0253-715666
North East: 091-374 5023
Scotland: 041-636 2950
Northern Ireland and Wales: 0800 868 700

How can I make my money grow?

Even interest-only savings will, of course, grow if you do not draw out the interest. But this may not be possible, and even if it is the rate of growth may not keep pace with inflation, particularly if the interest is taxed.

An alternative is to consider buying 'securities' (the Stock Exchange term for stocks and shares). At the bottom of the risk ladder are government securities ('gilts'). These are held for a fixed period, pay a fixed rate of interest and provide a guaranteed return, that is, the face value of the stock. The interest is taxable but any capital gain is tax-free. Whether you gain or lose in capital terms will depend on the price you pay at purchase. Gilts which offer a high rate of interest when prevailing rates are low will command a high price and *vice versa*. You may therefore choose to maximise interest or capital, depending on your need for income and your tax liability. The previous day's market price for a gilt can be found in those newspapers which publish financial information. You can sell gilts before the redemption date, but the price you get will depend on the market: if interest rates have gone up since you purchased them, you will receive less than you paid. Personal investors may find it convenient to buy and sell gilts through the National Savings Bonds and Stock Office, Blackpool FY3 9YP (Tel: 0253-697333). Details are given in leaflet DNS 708, *Government Stock*, available in post offices.

If you are prepared to take risks, you can buy shares ('equities') in commercial companies. The ordinary shareholders jointly own the company and have a vote in determining how it is run. If the company succeeds, they share that success. The shares will rise in value and the shareholders will normally receive a 'dividend' (how much depends on the size of the profit and the amount which the directors decide to keep back to build up reserves). But the potential for growth must be balanced against the possibility of contraction. There are losers as well as winners. If you are inexperienced, you would be wise to seek advice from a reputable broker or consultant. The degree of risk varies and can be reduced by spreading your investments, either by choosing a number of shareholdings or by investing in a managed fund. Fund managers will spread your money widely, using their specialist expertise. The best-known such investments (but by no means the only type) are unit trusts. Over the years, unit trusts have generally shown a much better return than investments on interest, though it can take some years for them to show a good return and management charges are quite high. There are well over a thousand unit trusts from which to choose and most allow for income to be drawn by way of six-monthly distributions. Tax is already deducted, but can be reclaimed by non-taxpayers.

Can I maximise my income at the expense of capital?

Yes, by purchasing an annuity. This involves the payment of a lump sum to an insurance company which then pays you an income for life. The amount of income depends on the capital sum provided, but also on your age (i.e. your life expectancy) and the interest rates prevailing when you purchase the annuity. The older you are and the higher the prevailing rates, the higher your income will be. Various schemes are available and you would be well advised to 'shop around'. Whether, in cash terms, you do well depends, of course, on how long you live and go on drawing income, which none of us can predict with any certainty. It's a gamble, though since you'll be dead if you lose you may not be too worried about that! Another consideration is that income is normally fixed, though some annuities provide for extra income year by year and some can be passed on to a surviving spouse. Although tax is deducted at source, it can be reclaimed if you are not, in fact, liable to tax.

'Capital Protected' annuities return some of the capital in the event of death within five years, but the income they provide is slightly less.

Investment protection

A degree of risk in investment is inevitable, and the only protection against it is caution or total abstinence. At what has been described as the 'slow and steady' end of the market, where the aim is for a modest return, the risk may be small, but at the other extreme, for example in the commodities sector, where there is a play for large and quick profits, the risk is obviously significantly greater. But investors cannot calculate nor be expected to take responsibility for a degree of risk represented by a dishonest or an insolvent firm.

The Financial Services Act 1986 is designed expressly to regulate the provision of financial services and to protect investors, as far as possible, against the perils of malpractice and default. Firms which are carrying on investment business under the Act are now required to be authorised and to operate in accordance with strict rules. The general activities of banks and building societies (such as administering deposit accounts) are not covered by the Act. However, if your bank or building society gives investment advice on life insurance or unit trusts, then it should be a member of a regulatory body as this is an activity which requires authorisation. Life insurance is covered by the Act but general insurance (such as motor insurance) is not. Businesses will be authorised only if they are found to be 'honest, solvent and competent to advise or act for you'. Your first line of defence, therefore, is to ensure that you deal only with authorised traders. If you are in any doubt, the Securities and Investment Board (SIB) keeps a register of those businesses which it has authorised. You can check through Prestel, by writing to the SIB at Gavrelle House, 2-14 Bunhill Row, London EC1Y 8RA, or by telephoning the Board's special number for Register enquiries, 071-929 3652.

A particularly important aspect of the protection arrangements is 'the final safety net', the Investors' Compensation Scheme. This cannot, of course, compensate you against an ordinary investment risk, but in respect of investments made after 27 August 1988 it does offer protection if you lose money because a fully authorised firm has gone into liquidation. If you suffer a loss following advice given by a financial adviser and it is established that you were given negligent advice, you should be able to claim that money back from the firm. If the firm is unable to repay the money it owes you, it is likely that the firm would then go into liquidation as it would be unable to pay its debts. Once it had been established that the firm had gone into default you would then be able to make a claim under the Compensation Scheme. If an authorised financial adviser which has collapsed was holding money on your behalf, it should be safe: the rules require that funds from private investors be held in a separate account and as such they should not be affected by a liquidation. But if, in fact, an authorised firm cannot meet its obligations to you, you can claim compensation for the whole of amounts up to £30,000 and 90 per cent of up to a further £20,000.

The SIB publishes a series of free booklets for investors which are well worth reading:

- *Financial Services: A guide to the new regulatory system*
- *The Central Register*
- *The Investors' Compensation Scheme*
- *How To Spot the Investment Cowboys*

Further information on savings and investment

There is, of course, a vast range of literature and data outputs devoted to investment. For the older person wanting to gain a basic understanding of the subject and to provide for the future in the best way, we would suggest three books in Woodhead-Faulkner's Moneyguides series:

- *Family Finance: How to make your money go further*
  By Sue Thomas, 1987, price £4.95.
- *The Share Owner's Guide: How to invest profitably and safely in shares*
  By J.T.Stafford, 1987, price £4.95.
- *Unit Trusts: A guide for investors*
  By Sara Williams, 1988, price £5.95.

The series is available from Woodhead-Faulkner Ltd, Campus 400, Maylands Avenue, Hemel Hempstead, Herts. HP2 7EZ.

Also useful in setting out the ground rules are:

- *Which? Way to Save and Invest*
  (Consumers' Association, Castlemead, Gascoyne Way, Hertford X, SG14 1LH), price £10.95.
- *Your Taxes and Savings 1992–3*
  (Age Concern England, Astral House, 1268 London Road, London SW16 4ER), price £4.50.

Raising income or capital from your home

If you are one of those retired people whose only significant capital asset is the home in which you live, you may wish to consider ways in which you can raise money from it. There are various ways of doing this, though most have significant disadvantages and some are extremely risky.

Selling up

If you don't mind the upheaval and the change of location, and particularly if your present home is bigger than you need, you may wish to consider moving either to a smaller, lower priced property or into rented accommodation. This has two distinct advantages: it can raise a significant amount of money, while at the same time reducing your future living expenses. You will, on the other hand, need to take account of the costs of moving: estate agent's fee, survey, legal expenses, removal, etc. The Office of Fair Trading, 15–25 Bream's Buildings, London EC4A 1PR has produced a simple (though inconveniently shaped) free guide, *Buying and Selling a Home*, to help you through the problems you may experience when working with an estate agent. It reflects recent changes in the law designed to give consumers greater protection, and explains the various kinds of agency agreements.

Raising money from your home while staying put

There are also a number of financial schemes on offer which allow you to take capital or income against the equity in your home. It is important to be aware that, with the exception of home reversion plans, all of these are credit transactions in one way or another: you borrow money against the value of your home. As with any credit transaction the terms need to be carefully considered and, above all, understood before you commit yourself: some schemes have proved to be positively dangerous. The schemes on offer vary considerably and we strongly recommend that you seek independent financial and legal advice before locking yourself into a deal of this kind.

One welcome recent development is the Safe Home Income Plan (SHIP) Campaign in which a number of companies offering home income plans for older people have come together to produce a code of practice. Key features of the code will be a requirement to provide clear and adequate information about the pros and cons of the schemes and clearance by the client's solicitor before the transaction is finalised. Details about the SHIP Campaign are available from Cecil Hinton, SHIP Campaign, Hinton and Wild (Home Plans) Ltd, 374 Ewell Road, Surbiton, Surrey KT6 7BB (Tel: 081-390 8166).

Home income plans

Normally, an interest-only loan is advanced against a proportion of the value of your home. You remain fully the owner of the property. The loan is used to provide an annuity (*see* page 35) which provides an income for life. Part of this income is used to pay the loan interest (which is reduced by MIRAS tax relief at the base rate); the remainder comes to you. The loan itself is repaid from the proceeds of the sale of your home when you die or give up ownership of your home (or, in the case of joint participants, when the second partner dies).

Points to watch

You will wish to consider the pros and cons of a home income scheme very carefully. We suggest that, if you decide to go ahead, you should look at all the available schemes and take independent financial and legal advice before you commit yourself to any one of them. The following are some of the main features to be taken into account.

- The interest rate may be fixed or variable. If variable, the balance of income due to you will fall if interest rates rise. Interest rate changes in recent years have been such as to make this a significant factor. You need to be clear about the rate of interest on the loan, *expressed as an annual percentage rate* (APR), and what the income derived will be. The basic question is whether you are prepared to pay interest at this rate to generate the level of income you will receive.
- The repayment of the loan will, of course, reduce the amount your beneficiaries will receive. And your home will normally have to be sold to pay off the loan when you (or your surviving partner) die.
- If you are receiving a state means-tested benefit such as income support or housing benefit, the extra income will result in you losing part or all of your entitlement and related concessions.
- The plan may restrict your freedom to move house. A move is likely to cause problems and affect the interest you receive.
- Annuities have some drawbacks (*see* page 35). In particular, the return can be poor if the holder(s) die(s) early.
- There are likely to be arrangement, survey and legal fees.
- There is a minimum age for individuals and for couples; in many plans this is around 70 and 150 respectively.
- The realisable proportion of the value of your home varies from plan to plan.
- There is normally a minimum and a maximum loan, which varies from plan to plan.

There are several financial institutions offering home income plans. Details are given in Age Concern England's fact sheet No. 12, which is regularly updated. Inclusion in that fact sheet, however, does not constitute a recommendation, and any claim suggesting Age Concern endorsement of a particular company or scheme should be ignored.

Home reversion schemes

In these schemes you sell your home to the reversion company but you (and any surviving partner) retain the legal right to live there as a tenant for life, usually rent-free. You receive a proportion of the value of your home (depending on your life expectancy) outright and not as a loan, but this is usually not more than 50 per cent and may be a good deal less. The amount concerned may come to you as a lump sum or be used to purchase an annuity (*see* page 35). In some schemes it is possible to sell off only part of the property.

Points to watch

You will wish to consider the pros and cons of a home reversion scheme very carefully. We suggest that if you decide to go ahead, you should look at all the available schemes and take *independent* financial and legal advice before you commit yourself to any one of them. Those companies providing annuity income are registered with LAUTRO; those providing a lump sum do not have to be registered, and greater care is necessary to check out the merits of the plan. The following are some of the main features to be taken into account.

- Annuities have some drawbacks (*see* page 35). In particular, the return can be poor if the holder(s) die(s) early.
- Your beneficiaries will not inherit your home.
- There is likely to be a significant arrangement fee (usually about 1.5 per cent of the value of the property).
- It may not be possible to sell your property to a reversion company if you have only a leasehold interest.
- If you are receiving a state means-tested benefit such as income support or housing benefit, the lump sum or extra income could result in you losing part or all of your entitlement and related concessions.
- You are likely to remain responsible for repairs and maintenance.
- The plan may restrict your freedom to move house; this needs to be checked beforehand.
- Some schemes allow for compensation if you find you cannot continue to live at home and have to surrender possession.
- Some schemes periodically supplement the lump sum or annuity income as property prices rise.
- There are minimum age requirements for individuals and for couples; these vary from scheme to scheme.
- The realisable proportion of the value of your home and the extent to which it is discounted varies from plan to plan.

There are several reversion companies offering schemes of this type. Details are given in Age Concern England's fact sheet No. 12, which is regularly updated. Inclusion in that fact sheet, however, does not constitute a recommendation, and any claim suggesting Age Concern endorsement of a particular company or scheme should be ignored.

Investment bond income schemes

These schemes can be risky in that money from a building society interest-only loan (at variable interest and without MIRAS tax relief) is advanced with your home as security i.e. its sale can be forced to meet the debt if you are unable to repay the loan. The loan is invested in an insurance company bond with the hope that the annual growth in the value of the bond will be sufficient both to cover the interest on the loan and to provide you with some income. The sad fact is that interest rates may rise so high and the growth in the bond be so low (there may even be a loss) that no income is generated and the interest charge cannot be met, or fully met, in this way. In such circumstances, the building society may have to take money from the bond itself or defer part of the interest and add it on to the loan. The results can be dire.

Unfortunately, in the past, some of the marketing literature for these schemes gave little or no indication of the risks. Schemes were sold on the basis of historically high investment returns, with no warning of the volatility of the stock market or the unpredictability of interest rates and property values. In practice, all of these factors have in recent years moved quite dramatically against those who succumbed to such marketing, and significant numbers of elderly people have been seriously disadvantaged. Regulatory bodies have sought within their rules to ensure redress in such cases and have given clear advice to their members about the marketing of such products, making it clear that, in the context of the requirement to offer 'best advice', bond-based home income plans are likely to be suitable for only a very small minority of investors, even within the narrow market (the over-70s) at which such plans are aimed.

Roll-up loans

These are interest-only loans (at variable interest and without MIRAS tax relief) advanced with your home as security (i.e. its sale can be forced to meet the debt if you are unable to repay the loan). Instead of you paying the interest, it is 'rolled-up' (i.e. added on to the loan). You do not have to repay the loan or the interest on it unless or until the property is sold. If you remain there for the rest of your life, neither the loan itself nor the interest need be repaid in your lifetime, except in the circumstances explained below.

Points to watch

The expectation behind such schemes is that, generally, the value of your property will appreciate over the period of the loan so as to offset, at least in part, the impact of the growing debt. This is, however, a dangerous assumption. You will wish to consider the pros and cons of a roll-up loan very carefully. We suggest that if you decide to go ahead, you should look at all the available schemes and take *independent* financial and legal advice before you commit yourself to any one of them. The following are some of the main features to be taken into account.

– The interest rates are usually set somewhat above building society base rates.
– There are significant potential dangers. When interest rates are high, the deferred interest mounts up very quickly. Age Concern England calculates that at the interest

rates prevailing in July 1991, the total amount a borrower would owe under one of the schemes would double about every five years. At the same time, property prices may not grow as they did before 1989; indeed, they may fall. It is possible, therefore, that after some years the value of your property may not be sufficient to repay the loan and the accrued interest. In some schemes, if a point is reached when your debt (original loan plus accrued interest) reaches a certain proportion of the value of the property (typically 60 to 75 per cent), you will be required to start paying the interest. Age Concern England cautions that it would seem highly risky for a person aged 65 or over to borrow as much as 25 or 30 per cent of the property value in one lump sum.

– If you are receiving a state means-tested benefit such as income support or housing benefit, the loan could result in your losing part or all of your entitlement and related concessions.
– The repayment of the loan and accrued interest will, of course, be a charge on your estate, and will reduce the amount your beneficiaries would otherwise receive.
– Particularly beware of a roll-up loan which is conditional upon part or all of the loan being invested in a specified way.

There are several building societies offering roll-up loans. Details are given in Age Concern England's fact sheet No. 12, which is regularly updated. Inclusion in that fact sheet, however, does not constitute a recommendation, and any claim suggesting Age Concern endorsement of a particular company or scheme should be ignored.

Further information

▶ *Using Your Home as Capital*
By Cecil Hinton (Age Concern England, 1268 London Road, London SW16 4ER (Tel: 081-679 8000), 1991), price £3.50 including postage and packing. [New edition Summer 1992, price £4.50.]

This book, which is updated annually, gives detailed information on the possibilities for capitalising on the value of your home to obtain a regular additional income. It includes an explanation of interest rates, how state benefits are affected, how the schemes are taxed and what happens if you move home. The advantages and disadvantages of the various schemes are considered.

Income from charities

There are a great many charities that can be approached for help if you are in need. Most of them will expect that you have tried all possible statutory sources and family connections first. It may help if a social worker or your doctor can support your application; indeed many societies will accept an application only if it comes from a professional. You will need to search out those charities which are most relevant to your individual needs. Some charities will consider only one-off grants, while others cater only for continuing support, for example to help meet the costs of residential care. You might also look for a charity with which you can claim some connection. This might be a local trust particularly concerned with the needs of elderly or disabled people in its area, or the local branch of a national organisation such as Round Table, Rotary, Foresters, Buffaloes, or Lions. Or, if you have a particular disability, there may be a national organisation specifically concerned to help those who are so disabled; some, such as the Multiple Sclerosis Society, have local branches with funds of their own.

Another possible source of help are those charities and benevolent funds set up to look after the members of a particular group and their families. These include trade and professional organisations (e.g. the Civil Service Benevolent Society, the Royal Agricultural Benevolent Institution), trade unions, welfare societies associated with a particular religion (e.g. Jewish Care), and those for 'gentlefolk' or professional people generally (e.g. Distressed Gentlefolk's Aid Association, Friends of the Elderly and Gentlefolk's Help, Guild of Aid for Gentlepeople, and the Royal United Kingdom Beneficent Association). If you have or have had any such connection, either directly or through a member of your family, such charities are a potential source of assistance.

In much the same way, many elderly people have a personal or familial connection with an ex-service organisation, either in this country or overseas (e.g. the Not Forgotten Association, the Officers' Association, the Royal Air Forces Association, the Royal British Legion, and SSAFA).

Finally, there are those national charities whose objectives are specifically identified with the needs of elderly or disabled people, such as Counsel and Care for the Elderly, and RUKBA. Please note, however, that Help the Aged, which funds many community-based groups and projects, is prevented by its terms of reference from making grants to individuals.

Further information

▶ *The Association of Charity Officers*
c/o RICS Benevolent Fund Limited, 1st floor, Tavistock House North, Tavistock Square, London WC1H 9RJ (Tel: 071-383 5557).

The Association encourages liaison and co-operation between its member charities, of which there are now about 250. It maintains a directory of all its members, many of whom are professional and trade benevolent funds, and will try to help enquirers locate possible sources of charitable help.

▶ *Charity Made Clear*
By Auriel James (Petal Publishing, 25 Portview Road, Avonmouth, Bristol BS11 9LD, 1992), price £4.95.

This book, written by the founder of Charity Search (see below), is primarily intended to show ordinary people and those concerned with the welfare of others how to find charitable help for individuals. It explains the underlying structure of the charity field and demonstrates the importance of the background of individuals who find themselves in financial difficulty if their predicament is to be resolved. The author argues that once the basic principles of linking those in need with relevant established charities is understood, the problems of finding them relief are considerably simplified.

Charity Search
25 Portview Road, Avonmouth, Bristol BS11 9LD (Tel: 0272-824060).

Charity Search is a free advice service for elderly people in genuine financial difficulties that links them with established charities that might help them. An experienced team responds promptly and sympathetically to enquiries, either by telephone or letter, on a national basis.

A Guide to Grants for Individuals in Need
(The Directory of Social Change, Radius Works, Back Lane, London NW3 1HL, 1992), price £14.95.

This well-known guide should be available in your local reference library or CAB. There are currently about 1,700 trusts in the Guide with a combined grant total of about £86 million. Sources of help are listed under five main headings: occupation, services and ex-services, disability, geographical area, and other national charities. The information provided covers the beneficial area, who is eligible, the usual size of grants, the types and number of grants made, the annual grand total, the person to contact and any other relevant facts. The book also contains much useful advice and a model application form. At the very least, in any application, you should include your name, address, telephone number, income, spending, savings, property, any special difficulties, how much you need and what for, why you are approaching this particular charity, and what other sources of help have been tried, including information on which statutory sources have been approached.

Inevitably, the Guide points out, even if you are successful, it can take some time between application and grant. You should apply as early as possible, and never after the need has been met. It is most unlikely that any charity will make a retrospective grant, for instance, recompense you for something you have already bought.

Income tax

Older people are, of course, liable to pay income tax if their gross taxable income exceeds their tax allowances.

Investment income

Most investment income counts as taxable income, though there are some limited exceptions to this: TESSA, Premium Bond winnings, National Savings certificates. Taxable investment income may be paid gross, whence it forms part of your income to be assessed for tax, or with tax deducted at source. If you are a non-taxpayer (i.e. your total gross income – including investment income – is offset by allowances) you may prefer a form of investment which pays a gross return, but even if tax has been deducted at source there is a mechanism to reclaim it (see below).

Interest on bank and building society accounts is normally taxed at source. But if your gross income (including *gross* interest) does not exceed your tax allowances, so that you are not liable to pay income tax, you can ask your bank or building society to pay the interest without first deducting tax. There is a special form, R85, for this purpose, which can be obtained from banks, building societies, post offices and tax offices.

If tax has been deducted at source when you are not liable to pay tax or are liable to pay on only part of the investment income or interest, you can ask the Inland Revenue for a refund. This will be made at the end of the tax year, or interim repayments can be made earlier provided the amount of tax repayable is £50 or more. Further information is given in Inland Revenue leaflets IR 111 and IR 112.

In the case of a married couple, the impact of tax on investment income can be reduced where partner A is liable to tax but partner B has an income below his/her allowances. Tax liability can then be reduced by transferring, as an outright gift, assets from partner A to partner B. There can be a similar saving where one partner is liable to tax at the higher rate and the other is below the higher rate threshold.

Pensions

Retirement pensions and occupational pensions normally count as taxable income, but the amount by which a pension awarded on retirement through disability caused by injury on duty or by a work related illness (e.g. pneumoconiosis, asbestosis, etc.) or by war wounds, exceeds the pension which would have been awarded if retirement had been on ordinary ill-health grounds is not treated as income for income tax purposes. Similarly, a pension awarded solely on account of such retirement is not treated as income.

As a result of the change to independent taxation in April 1990, a married woman's state retirement pension, even if it is paid jointly and is based on her husband's contributions, is her own income. If she has no other income, her pension will be offset by her personal tax allowance and may thus reduce the couple's overall tax liability.

Further information is given in Inland Revenue Leaflet IR4, *Income Tax and Pensioners*. This answers many of the questions pensioners ask about their income tax. It gives some general explanation on matters which often cause misunderstandings, as well as describing some of the tax allowances which may be claimed and the way in which National Insurance pensions and other pensions are taxed.

Letting rooms

The second 1992 Finance Bill introduced an exception from income tax on payments of up to £3,250 per annum for the letting of rooms in one's own house.

Lump sums on leaving employment

Liability to tax depends on why the payment was made. Special rules apply if your contract of employment gives you the right to receive the lump sum. The following payments are not usually taxed if they are under £30,000:

- redundancy payments
- payments for loss of office
- payments in lieu of notice
- ex-gratia payments.

If your employer pays you a lump sum because your illness means that you cannot continue in your job, it may be completely free of tax even if it is more than £30,000, but your employer should seek prior authorisation from the tax office.

Lump sums paid under the rules of most pension schemes are free of tax whatever the amount.

State benefits

Liability is as follows:

Taxable

- retirement pension, including any invalidity addition
- widow's pension, widow's allowance and widowed mother's allowance
- unemployment benefit
- income support paid to those who are unemployed, on strike or involved in a trade dispute
- invalid care allowance
- industrial death benefit (if paid as a pension).

Not taxable

- sickness benefit (but statutory sick pay is taxable)
- invalidity benefit, including invalidity allowance
- severe disablement allowance
- industrial disablement benefit
- disability living allowance

- disability working allowance
- housing benefit
- maternity allowance (but statutory maternity pay is taxable)
- child benefit and one-parent benefit
- income support paid to those who are not unemployed, on strike or involved in a trade dispute
- Family Credit
- Christmas payment to pensioners
- guardian's allowance
- child's special allowance
- war widow's pension
- Social Fund payments.

Personal allowances

Personal allowances are higher for people aged 65 to 74 (1992/3: £4,200) and even higher for those aged 75 or more (1992/3: £4,370). However, these higher allowances are reduced if your total *gross* income exceeds a specified amount (1992/3: £14,200). For every £2 over the limit you will lose £1 of the allowance down to the level of the basic personal allowance (1992/3: £3,445). Personal allowances cannot be transferred between husband and wife, but the transfer of assets from one partner to another, as an outright gift, as described above, may reduce the loss of age-related allowances by cutting back the income of the donor partner.

Further information is given in Inland Revenue Leaflet IR4A, *Income Tax Age Allowance*. A guide to all the income tax personal allowances (leaflet IR22) can be obtained free from any office of HM Inspector of Taxes or from PAYE Enquiry Offices, where information and help on specific problems can be obtained.

Married couple's allowance

A married man who lives with his wife can claim this allowance (1992/3: £1,720). However, if he has insufficient income to take advantage of all or part of the allowance, any unused allowance can be transferred to his wife.

The allowance is higher if either partner is aged 65 to 74 (1992/3: £2,465) and even higher if either partner is aged 75 or more (1992/3: £2,505). However, if the man's total gross income exceeds a specified amount (1992/3: £14,200) and, the man having first reduced his personal allowance as explained above, there is still an excess of income, the higher married couple's allowance will then be reduced, again by £1 for every £2 of income, down to the level of the married couple's allowance appropriate to someone aged under 65 (1992/3: £1,720).

The transfer of assets from husband to wife, as an outright gift, as described above, may reduce the loss of age-related allowances by cutting back the husband's income.

Example (using 1992/3 rates)

Man aged 75 (his wife aged 73); his income £16,700.
   Personal allowance   £4,370
   Married couple's allowance £2,505
Amount by which income exceeds specified amount £2,500
Amount by which allowances will be reduced £1,250
Personal allowance reduced by £925 to £3,445
Married couple's allowance reduced by £325 to £2,180.

Widow's bereavement allowance

This special allowance to widows (1992/3: £1,720) can be offset against taxable income in the tax year of their husband's death and the following year. No special allowance is available to widowers, but they can claim the full married couple's allowance in the tax year of their wife's death.

Further information is given in Inland Revenue leaflet IR23, *Income Tax and Widows*.

Further information

▪ *Age Concern England fact sheet no. 15*
Available from 1268 London Road, London SW16 4ER, free.

▪ *Tax and Pensioners*
By Paul Lewis (Saga Publishing Ltd, The Saga Building, Middelburg Square, Folkestone, Kent CT20 1AZ), free to Saga Club members – *see* page 345.

▪ *Which? Way to Save Tax*
(Consumers' Association, Castlemead, Gascoyne Way, Hertford X, SG14 1LH, published annually in August), price (1991/2) £11.95.

▪ *Widows' Benefits and Tax*
By Paul Lewis (Saga Publishing Ltd, The Saga Building, Middelburg Square, Folkestone, Kent CT20 1AZ), free to Saga Club members – *see* page 345).

▪ *Your Taxes and Savings 1992–3*
(Age Concern England, 1,268 London Road, London SW16 4ER), price £4.50.

Inheritance tax

This tax applies to estates valued above a prescribed limit at the time of the owner's death. It may also apply to transfers of possessions which would reduce the value of your estate when you die, for example if you gave your house to a daughter or son as a present. The rules are complex, so if you are thinking of transferring your home or business to your children or otherwise giving away capital, you would be well advised to seek professional advice. It is desirable to consider any strategy as to the disposal of your estate in the context of your will and to seek the guidance of a solicitor. The following notes are intended only as general pointers to the main features and implications of the tax.

The rates for 1992/93 are: up to £150,000: nil; thereafter: 40%.

No tax is charged on an estate passing to a UK-domiciled spouse or on bequests to UK charities.

Although a substantial band of estate is liable at a nil rate, inheritance tax can nowadays easily affect people who, though not rich, own their own homes. As can be seen, the tax rates bite quite heavily once the nil rate band is exceeded.

For married couples, the bright spot is that each has a separate nil rate entitlement. If part of either's estate is to pass to someone other than a surviving spouse, or against the possibility that both die together, it normally makes sense to divide the whole estate – including the marital home – between the partners. This both reduces the estate liable on the death of one of the partners and confers a nil-rate exemption on each of the individual parts of the estate. This does not, however, entirely overcome the problem. Usually, to meet the needs of the surviving spouse, most of the estate will pass to that spouse. Although no tax arises on estate passing to a spouse, the surviving partner will end up with the bulk of the total estate and only one nil-rate band allowance. Beneficiaries of the surviving spouse may then face a significant inheritance tax bill. One interesting solution would be for the surviving spouse always to remarry and redivide the estate, but for the purposes of this guidance we will assume that this does not happen and that the situation of the surviving spouse becomes that of any other individual person.

The main route to reducing tax liability is to bring forward the making of bequests, so that they are made in the bequeather's lifetime rather than at death. There is an obvious merit in this quite apart from the avoidance of tax, in that the beneficiary has the use of the money earlier: this can be particularly helpful to children who are just starting to make their way in life. However, this must, of course, be balanced against your own future needs. It is important to be aware that gifts can only reduce liability to inheritance tax if they are made outright and unreservedly.

There are four kinds of gift:
1. *Gifts exempt from tax*
   (a) gifts up to a prescribed amount (1991/92: £3,000) made by any one individual in each tax year (if not fully utilised in any one tax year, these can be used over and above the allowance for the next tax year – but no further);
   (b) gifts of a prescribed amount made to a bride or groom on marriage (at the time of the wedding or just before), for example, for 1991/2:
      (i) each parent   £5,000
      (ii) each grandparent £2,500

(iii) any other person   £1,000;
(c) gifts to UK charities;
(d) small gifts up to a prescribed amount (1991/2: £250 each) to individual donees in any one tax year (these cannot be on top of other gifts to a donee);
(e) gifts to the donor's spouse;
(f) gifts which form part of the donor's normal expenditure payable out of income (these can include the premiums on an insurance policy on your life – or joint lives – in favour of your beneficiaries to help them to pay any future inheritance tax liability).

2. *Gifts made more than seven years before death (Potentially Exempt Transfers – 'PETs')*
Such outright gifts are excluded from your estate if seven years elapse after they are made. Should death occur earlier, the gift is counted in with the estate but the rate of tax charged on the gift is reduced progressively if made more than three but less than seven years before death. It is possible, however, that the gift, because it is treated as the bottom 'slice' of the estate, will come within the nil-rate band. The reduction of tax on gifts made more than three years before death cannot, of course, apply to a gift within the nil-rate band.

3. *Chargeable transfers*
These are outright gifts of a kind which do not qualify as PETs, for example gifts to companies or to discretionary trusts. They can be set against your nil-rate tax band, and the amount by which the nil-rate band has been reduced is reinstated if you are still alive seven years after the gift was made.

4. *Gifts with reservation*
These are gifts made with some reservation of benefit (e.g. if you transfer ownership of your home to one of your children, but continue to live in it). If made after 17 March 1986, they do not qualify as gifts for inheritance tax purposes unless and until the reservation is withdrawn.

Further information about inheritance tax

- Booklet IHT1, *Inheritance Tax*, from the Capital Taxes Offices at Minford House, Rockley Road, London W14 0DF, or 16 Picardy Place, Edinburgh EH1 3NB, or Law Courts Building, Chichester Street, Belfast BT1 3NU.

- *Inheritance Tax and Capital Gains Tax*
By Paul Lewis (Saga Publishing Ltd, The Saga Building, Middelburg Square, Folkestone, Kent CT20 1AZ), free to Saga Club members – *see* page 345.

- *Which? Way to Save Tax*
(Consumers' Association, Castlemead, Gascoyne Way, Hertford X, SG14 1LH, published annually in August), price (1991/2) £11.95.

Wills

A will is simply the formal expression of how you want your property to be divided up when you die. If you do not make your intentions clear in this way, you will be said to die 'intestate', and your estate will be divided up by strict rules of law. These vary between England and Wales (on which the following text is based), Northern Ireland and Scotland, but the essential message remains the same: that if you do not make a will your property may be divided up in a way which is not what you would wish.

By way of example of what can go wrong, if you are married and have children, and your estate is worth more than £75,000, under the intestacy rules your surviving spouse will be entitled only to £75,000, plus your household and personal effects. The remainder is divided equally: half to your children, and the rest in a trust for them in which your spouse will have only a life interest and from which he or she can have only the income which it yields. Such a disposal may be quite contrary to your wishes, and, if your estate includes a house worth more than £75,000, it could result in your home having to be sold.

Intestacy can bring many other problems, some of which you may be quite unable to anticipate. It makes sense to make your wishes crystal clear in a will.

It follows that your will should be drawn up in a way in which your intentions are explicitly stated and cannot be misinterpreted. A will is a legal document with numerous technical requirements, and there are many pitfalls for the layperson. You can make your own will, but our view is that the DIY will is appropriate only in simple circumstances and for those able to grasp exactly what is required. Although a solicitor will naturally charge a fee, this seems to us money well spent for ensuring that the disposal of a much greater amount is properly expressed. Apart from this, a solicitor may be able to draw your attention to possibilities and provisions which have never crossed your mind. His/her help may be essential if inheritance tax planning is an integral consideration. If necessary, your local Citizens Advice Bureau can give you information about solicitors in your area.

Making a will also enables you to specify your executors: those who will manage your estate. We use the plural deliberately, because appointing two executors allows flexibility so that each can take on different parts of the administration of your estate; if there are going to be complex matters to handle or inheritance tax problems, you may wish one of them to be a professional person such as your bank, an accountant or a solicitor. You will, in any event, want them to be competent people and, if your will sets up a trust, you will want to appoint a person or persons on whom you feel you can totally depend. You should, of course, have the permission of prospective executors before you name them in your will: no one is bound to act as an executor, and even a named executor can renounce the appointment. An additional advantage of naming two people is that it guards to some extent against the eventuality of one of them dying, but you can also provide for substitute executors if the first team is unable or unwilling to act. An executor can be named as a beneficiary, and can also claim the expenses of administering the estate against the estate. But a trustee appointed to hold and manage property for a beneficiary may not benefit in any way from that property.

You can revoke a will by making a new will which specifies that it revokes all previous wills and codicils, or by deliberately destroying your will (but this must be done by you or on your direction in your presence). If you marry or remarry, any previous will becomes invalid unless it has been made in anticipation of the marriage and written accordingly. The position on divorce is more complicated: it does not automatically invalidate a will but does negate any bequest to, and appointment as executor of, the former spouse. We think that you will want in these circumstances to make a new will. It is desirable, in any event, to keep your will under review from time to time to take account of changed circumstances. *But never make alterations on the original document either by way of insertion or deletion.* Some changes can be made by adding a supplementary codicil (which must be witnessed in the same way – though not necessarily with the same witnesses – as the will itself). Alternatively, or if the changes are substantial or complex, you can make a new will, remembering to include the clause which revokes previous wills and codicils.

Keep your will in a safe place: somewhere where it certainly will be found. If it has been drawn up by a solicitor, it is usual for the solicitor to keep the original and provide you with a copy. Age Concern England, Astral House, 1268 London Road, London SW16 4ER (Tel: 081-679 8000) publish a leaflet, *Instructions for My Next of Kin and Executors Upon My Death*, price 25p, which can be left in a convenient place to advise your family where to find your will and other important documents, and to pass on other information and requests.

Further information about wills

- *Making your will*

    A very useful article in *Which?*, the magazine of the Consumers' Association, June 1991. Libraries keep back issues.

- *Making Your Will*
    (Age Concern England, Astral House, 1268 London Road, London SW16 4ER.)

    Fact sheet No. 7, free in response to a 9" x 6" s.a.e.

- *Making and Changing Your Will: A practical guide*
    (Age Concern England, Astral House, 1268 London Road, London SW16 4ER.)

    A simple guide in non-technical language.

- *Wills and Probate*
    (Consumers' Association, Castlemead, Gascoyne Way, Hertford X, SG14 1LH), price £9.95.

    In our view an indispensable guide to the subject. Regularly updated, it is written for the layperson and includes advice on making your own will, inheritance tax and the administration of an estate.

=▶ *Don't Leave Your Money to Chance*
(Money Management Council, 18 Doughty Street, London WC1N 2PL, 1989.)

A free fact sheet. Please send a s.a.e.

Power of attorney

Circumstances may arise in which you may wish to appoint an 'attorney': someone to act on your behalf in financial matters, if, for example, you are going into hospital or abroad for an extended period. A 'power of attorney' is conferred by completing a legal document, normally with the help and advice of a solicitor. It is important to be aware that an ordinary power of attorney loses its validity if the person who created it no longer has the mental capacity to manage his/her own affairs. If you wish to appoint an attorney against this possibility, you will need to complete a special form called 'Enduring Power of Attorney'. This enables you, while you are mentally capable, to decide for yourself who you would like to act for you should you become mentally incapable of handling your own affairs. Subsequently, if your attorney thinks that you have become or are becoming mentally incapable, he/she should apply to *register* the enduring power of attorney with the Court of Protection (*see* below) to have the right to act (or continue to act) under it.

While it is not essential, you would be well advised to seek legal advice on how to go about completing an enduring power of attorney, particularly if you have substantial assets. The power given can be *general*, authorising the attorney to carry out any transactions on your behalf which you are legally able to delegate, or *specific*, authorising the attorney to deal only with specified aspects of your affairs. Either a general or a specific power can be made subject to restrictions and conditions (e.g. excluding the power to sell the house in which you reside, or to direct that the attorney is not to act unless and until the power is registered). You can also make a number of enduring powers, appointing different attorneys to do different things.

The form of enduring power of attorney can be obtained from stationers who supply legal forms (*not* from the Court of Protection nor the Public Trust Office) and must conform in all respects to the Enduring Power of Attorney (Prescribed Form) Regulations 1990. Further guidance is available from the Public Trust Office (Enquiries and Acceptance Branch), Stewart House, 24 Kingsway, London WC2B 6JX, which publishes a free booklet, *Enduring Powers of Attorney*.

Where no enduring power of attorney has been made, anyone who considers that the affairs and property of someone else may require protection because of his or her mental incapacity can ask the Court of Protection for help. The Court is located at Stewart House, 24 Kingsway, London WC2B 6JX and is an office of the Supreme Court. Its function is to protect and manage the financial affairs and property of people who, because of a mental disorder, are unable to manage for themselves. The Court's control is regulated by the Mental Health Act 1983 and the Court of Protection Rules Act 1984. The Protection Division of the Public Trust Office, on behalf of the Court, deals with the management of the affairs of the person under protection in conjunction with a *Receiver* appointed by the Court. In practice, referrals are made by, among others, relatives, friends, medical authorities, solicitors and accountants. Provided that the Court has received medical evidence confirming incapacity and is satisfied that there is a need for a Receiver to be appointed it will so order. A pamphlet, *Court of Protection*, and a booklet, *Handbook for Receivers*, are available from the Protection Division, Public Trust Office, Stewart House, 24 Kingsway, London WC2B 6JX.

The Court of Protection charges annual fees for its services. These are fixed by Parliament and are based on the clear annual income of the person under protection.

Different (though similar) arrangements apply to Scotland and Northern Ireland.

Note

This is an area which continues to give rise to concern, in that the definition of mental incapacity is very vague and open to wide interpretation. Moreover, Receivers are often relatives, who, though they will mostly be people of integrity and goodwill, may in some cases be tempted to manage the affairs of the person under protection to their own advantage. Pressure of work on the Court's limited staff and practical difficulties in supervising the activities of Receivers can mean that the best interests of the person under protection are, in practice, not always adequately safeguarded.

Insurance

We will not deal generally with insurance matters in this directory, except to say that retirement is one of those points in life when you should perhaps step back and consider whether you are as adequately insured as you would wish: is your life insurance now enough should you or a partner die after pension age? Any policies which you took out when you were younger no doubt seemed quite large at the time, but how do they look against today's money value? There is a different question to be asked about any home and contents policies you may have, but the effect is likely to be the the same. If they have not been reviewed regularly they will scarcely reflect current values, nor the probability that you now have more cherished possessions than in earlier years. To help you to consider, or reconsider, your insurance cover, the Association of British Insurers, 51 Gresham Street, London EC2V 7HO, has produced a range of leaflets on various aspects of insurance any of which will be sent in response to a stamped addressed envelope. There is also an insurance information service offering information and advice during business hours on 071-600 3333. Advice is also available from the Association's ten regional offices situated in Belfast, Birmingham, Bristol, Glasgow, Leeds, Liverpool, Manchester, Newcastle upon Tyne, Norwich and Southampton.

Insurance for pets

▶ *Pet Protect Ltd*
55 High Street, Epsom, Surrey KT19 8DH (Tel: 0372-739490)

This company offers insurance with a difference. The Pet Protect 7 Star Plan, which is underwritten by Aegon Insurance Company (UK) Ltd, covers healthcare for cats and dogs. For an annual premium of £59.95 (per pet, of course) the following cover is provided:

1. Up to £2,000 for veterinary fees;
2. Up to £750 death benefit if your pet dies as a result of illness or accident;
3. Up to £750 of the cost of advertising and reward to try to trace and recover your pet if it is lost;
4. Up to £750 boarding kennel fees for your pet if you have to go into hospital for more than two days;
5. Up to £750 for loss of your pet by theft or straying;
6. Up to £2,000 holiday cancellation should your pet need emergency surgery up to seven days before your holiday;
7. Up to £2,000,000 third party legal liability should your pet cause an accident or injury.

This cover is for pets aged 2 months to 10 years.

There is no limit to the number of claims in a year within the above amounts, but benefits on veterinary fees and kennel boarding fees are subject to the policyholder paying the first £20 of the total claim or course of treatment. Preventative treatment such as vaccinations is not covered.

Pets should be in good health, have no vicious tendency, and not be used in any business, trade or profession.

A specimen copy of the policy is available on request.

Debt

An unpleasant subject, but one that has to be faced realistically. We have, unfortunately, gone through a period of easy credit: when borrowing has been positively encouraged and lenders of all conditions have been only too ready to offer loans. Credit, of course, has its place. Vast numbers of people are thankful that they have been able to finance major purchases in this way: not least those who own their own homes thanks to a mortgage taken out when they were young. But there is a downside. Perils such as overcommitment and unexpected disability or unemployment have blighted the lives of many ordinary people and made it impossible for them to meet their repayments.

At the other end of the scale are those who simply do not have enough money to live on: including many thousands of elderly people on small fixed incomes faced with steeply rising costs, particularly for the necessities of life.

56   *More money matters*

The problem in all these situations is that things are liable to go from bad to worse: those who have loans that they cannot repay discover that arrears and interest charges not only pile up but escalate; those who need to borrow money simply to get by find that they are regarded as a bad risk and can get credit only at high, sometimes extortionate, rates of interest. The Social Fund has been inadequate to meet the full range of need, and loan sharks prey on the poorest of the poor.

We will not say that there are easy solutions to these problems, but they can certainly be eased and at least contained. We recommend a free booklet published by the Office of Fair Trading, Field House, 15–25 Bream's Buildings, London EC4A 1PR under the title, *Debt: A survival guide*. This begins with the advice that you need to tell the people to whom you owe money (your creditors) as soon as you have problems. Ignoring their letters and demands can only make things worse. It then sets out a six-step action plan for dealing with your personal finances, cautions against borrowing again to get out of debt, and explains your legal rights (particularly if the credit charges appear to be extortionate). The booklet goes on to outline court procedures if proceedings are taken against you, and provides a detailed chart on which to set out your financial position.

You can also seek advice from a Citizens' Advice Bureau or a money advice centre, if there is one in your locality, or you might, if necessary, be able to get free advice from a legal aid solicitor.

An organisation committed to helping people in debt is:

▶ *National Debtline*
The Birmingham Settlement, 318 Summer Lane, Birmingham B19 3RL
(Tel: 021-359 8501).

This is a national advice service to which anyone in England and Wales with debt problems can turn for advice. Every caller is given expert advice on the telephone, and this is backed up by a self-help information pack, *Dealing with Debts*, sent free of charge, and packed with information: how to work out your personal budget, how to decide priority debts and how to deal with them, including working out offers of payment to creditors, and how to cope with court orders. The writing is clear and concise and the advice is very practical and comforting in its concern for the reader's problems.

Helpful organisations

▶ *The Money Management Council*
18 Doughty Street, London WC1N 2PL.

This independent educational charity publishes a range of information to promote awareness and education in personal and family finance. Its materials are addressed to people who are financially inexperienced and unused to using professional financial advice. Of special interest are the leaflets *All Change for Pensions*, *Who Will Give Me*

Best Advice?, *Don't Leave Your Money to Chance* and *Savings and Lump-sum Investment*. There is a recommended reading list, *Savings and Investment*.

▶ *Occupational Pensions Advisory Service (OPAS)*
11 Belgrave Road, London SW1V 1RB (Tel: 071-233 8080).

An independent voluntary organisation giving free help to members of the public concerned about their pension rights on all matters about pension schemes (other than state schemes) including personal pensions.

SECTION THREE

House and home

Most of us, as we grow older, are likely to spend more time in our homes. We therefore want our homes to be warm, comfortable, easy to manage, appropriate to our needs, and secure. It is probably quite important that we are near shops and other community facilities, or at least near public transport services that will take us there.

This Section describes some of the housing options open to older people. On retirement, many of us decide to move to what we consider to be more attractive areas, seeking to get away from an environment chosen principally to be near to work. There are suddenly wider horizons and the opportunity, perhaps, to move to the home of one's dreams. For other older people, whose lives have been altogether harder, there are fewer options as the problems of coping with existing living accommodation become even more difficult. We will look, therefore, at a wide range of alternatives, including a number of sheltered housing schemes.

If you own your own home, you may decide to 'trade down' and move to a smaller, and hopefully cheaper, property, purpose-built with older people in mind, where some services are provided and where you will be relieved of some routine physical work. This kind of move, though it may be difficult to achieve with the housing market as it is at present, could bolster your capital reserves as well as fulfilling other objectives. Alternatively, with the prospect of an even greater release of capital, you may choose to move to rented accommodation in one of the sheltered schemes provided by a housing association or voluntary organisation. A number of such developments offer privacy in your own home, while making available various communal facilities which allow you to mix as you like with other residents. Having some facilities in common may mean that your private accommodation is relatively small, and this is something to consider carefully if you have a lot of treasured furniture and possessions.

However, you may decide that you would rather not move away from the locality where you have friends and good neighbours and have put down roots. The snag then may be that your accommodation is difficult and inconvenient to manage as you get older: perhaps it is large and expensive to heat, or involves climbing a lot of stairs. Fortunately, there are some helpful schemes provided by several housing associations and other agencies. These help you to stay put by providing practical advice on how your housing can be made more convenient for you and how you can pay for any necessary alterations.

The important message in approaching any of these options is to consider them very carefully. Do not be rushed into making a change which perhaps need not be taken for some years. Be sure that you know exactly what is involved and that it is what you want.

Who's who

Housing for elderly people is provided by local authorities, housing associations, charitable organisations and private developers.

Local authorities

Among the priority needs for accommodation specified by the Housing Act 1985 are those of 'a person who is vulnerable as a result of old age, mental illness or handicap or physical disability or other special reason, or with whom such a person resides or might reasonably be expected to reside' (section 59(1)(c)). Some local authorities, in seeking to meet the needs of older people, provide special housing and have designated staff within their Housing Departments to deal with sheltered housing applicants. As well as having their own properties, local authorities usually have powers to nominate applicants for sheltered housing in their area to housing associations. Your local authority will know which housing associations work in your area and how to contact them.

Housing associations

These are non-profit-making organisations, run by voluntary committees, which provide housing, either by the improvement of existing properties or by constructing new buildings. They operate throughout Britain, in inner cities, towns and remote rural areas. The accommodation they provide is primarily for rent, but they also make available homes for sale through special schemes to help people on lower incomes who wish to become home owners. Housing associations now own, manage and maintain a variety of properties which together provide homes for well over a million people. They may be registered with the Registrar of Friendly Societies or with the Charity Commissioners, or they may be companies which are also registered as charities. To be entitled to receive public funds, housing associations must be registered with the Housing Corporation, which supervises the initial spending and the subsequent management of any public investment.

Often, housing associations work in co-operation with specific voluntary organisations. They also work closely with local authorities, taking referrals from them.

The great advantage that housing associations have over local authorities is flexibility. They do not have to be tied to strict allocation procedures and restrictive residential requirements. Local authorities, of course, have a responsibility to provide accommodation for a wide cross-section of the community. Housing associations, on the other hand, can choose either to concentrate on certain specialist fields or to provide more general family accommodation, or, indeed, to combine the two. They are thus in a position to complement provision made by local authorities, and also to provide housing for those whose needs cannot be met by local authorities to any extent. Among the special need groups who can benefit from the housing association movement are one-parent families, and elderly and disabled people.

The Housing Act 1988 deregulated rents for new tenants. While existing tenants continue to enjoy secure tenancies, with rents determined by the Rent Officer, almost all tenancies which started after 15 January 1989 have a lesser standard of legal protection, and are not subject to statutory rent control. Housing associations must, however, have a policy to ensure that the rents of accommodation provided with the help of public funds can be afforded by people on low incomes, and do not exceed market rents.

Private developers

These often specialise in building property specially designed for older people, including many sheltered housing schemes. They usually entrust the management of such schemes to a management company or to a housing association. We do not list such developers, or recommend any company in particular. Details are readily available from The New Homes Marketing Board, 82 New Cavendish Street, London W1M 8AD (Tel: 071-580 5588), while particulars of schemes under construction are provided in the magazine *Retirement Homes and Finance* (*see* page 105).

What's what

Sheltered housing

This is purpose-built for older people and forms part of a scheme of grouped, self-contained accommodation provided with various estate management services.

The sale of sheltered housing by builders and developers registered with the National House-Building Council is subject to a detailed code of practice (*see* page 73).

Sheltered housing is provided by local authorities, housing associations and private developers, and is available to rent or to buy. Estates usually include a common room available for residents, a guest room and laundry. Some housing may be built to 'wheelchair' or 'mobility' standards (see below), and can also be 'warden assisted', the warden being either on-site or available from a central point via an intercom or alarm system. A warden's duties typically include: summoning help in an emergency; keeping a neighbourly eye on residents; reporting repairs or maintenance problems; and helping to organise social activities. Wardens do not, however, provide help with shopping, cleaning or cooking, nor provide personal care such as help with dressing or bathing.

Sheltered housing provides opportunities to share communal facilities while also having varying degrees of privacy. Tenants retain their independence while having the security of available support. Actual services vary: for example, in some schemes all meals may be taken in a communal dining room, whereas in others only a main midday meal is provided, while in some tenants are responsible for preparing all their own meals.

Sheltered housing is usually located within easy reach of shops and other local community facilities.

Rents will include contributions to communal facilities, regardless of how often you use them, as well as to other services such as a resident warden, alarm call system and so on. Most sheltered accommodation is provided by housing associations or benevolent and/or charitable institutions of one sort or another. Some provide extra care when this is needed. It is clearly very important to make sure, if possible, that you will not lose your accommodation in the event of illness or if you come to need extra care.

Mobility housing

This is built to conventional space standards, but includes such features as a ramped entrance and wide doors; it will be best suited to those who can walk a little, and do not need to use a wheelchair all the time or at all.

The important feature of mobility housing is that it obviates the need to cope with steps or stairs. This can be achieved in: bungalows; ground-floor flats in low-rise blocks; flats with lifts to upper levels; two-storey houses with bathroom and bedroom at ground level; and two-storey houses with a staircase on which a stairlift can be installed.

Wheelchair housing

This is specially designed for people who use wheelchairs. Important design considerations are: a level or slightly ramped approach to the entrance with no threshold obstruction; internal planning for wheelchair manoeuvre, with passageways 1,200 mm wide and suitable doors – either 900 mm doorsets or sliding doors with a 775 mm opening; a kitchen planned for wheelchair manoeuvre, with space to turn the wheelchair and access to equipment and storage; a bathroom planned for use from a wheelchair, with a shower or bath allowing a person to transfer from a wheelchair; a lavatory planned for transfer from a wheelchair; switches, window controls, door furniture and other fittings placed so as to be comfortably reached from a wheelchair; windows placed to give views out from a wheelchair; and a garage or carport (if provided) with undercover access to the dwelling.

Staying put

Not all of us want to up and off when we retire. We have put down roots in our communities and we feel at home. We doubt whether we would find it easy to make new friends in unfamiliar places, even if the surroundings were more beautiful. This is not unreasonable. There is a lot to be said for staying with old friends and neighbours, and remaining part of the community we have shared during our more active lives.

We may, however, need to have help in our home. Or we may need adaptations to make our accommodation easier to live in. Making such changes can be expensive, particularly for people on low fixed incomes, and can be complicated to arrange. Fortunately, there are a number of organisations and groups in many areas who offer advice and practical help.

Care and Repair and Staying Put schemes

These are particularly important. Many such schemes help elderly home owners to stay in their homes in comfort and security. The agencies concerned give sensitive advice to each individual to suit their particular needs. Information is given about repair problems and costs, reliable builders, help available from the DSS to pay for building work, and other grants and loans. As well as giving advice, agencies will handle applications and paperwork on behalf of elderly clients, and will check that building work is up to standard. Help is available for any job, from replacing a few slates to full renovation and improvement works.

Building repairs and adaptations are carried out where they are needed. Care and Repair schemes normally employ three workers to advise elderly people and to arrange financial and building help. These staff liaise with service providers such as local authorities, building societies and trusts, and also develop a list of well-tried builders. Sometimes community programmes or voluntary labour are also used for small repairs. Ideally, the building work should be carefully monitored. This combination of organising finances and building work for small and large jobs is the outstanding feature of these projects.

Anchor
Anchor House, 269a Banbury Road, Oxford OX2 7HU (Tel: 0865-311511).

Anchor's Staying Put service is designed to help older home owners to improve and repair their houses so that they can continue to live in them in greater comfort and security.

The Staying Put team is able to advise on the feasibility of carrying out the work you wish to have done and may also suggest other work which you should also consider. Once you have decided what to have done, the team will advise you on the selection of suitable contractors and help you to secure estimates. If the extent or complexity of the work requires the services of a surveyor or architect the team will help you to select one. He or she will be responsible for advising on the technical aspects. For smaller jobs the team itself will monitor the contractors and help you cope with the disruption of having work done. The Staying Put team is skilled in devising financial packages which are affordable and will advise you of the most suitable ways of paying for the work, including helping you to apply for grants where these are available. The team may be able to advise you on how to use the value of your house to pay for the work.

The Beth Johnson Housing Association Ltd
Three Counties House, Festival Way, Stoke-on-Trent ST1 5PX (Tel: 0782-219220).

This Association's Staying Put project can help you with your repairs and adaptations to your home to enable you to 'stay put' in your own home. They will help you obtain grants and low cost loans as well as any other benefits to which you may be entitled. They are able to specify the work you need and to recommend a reliable builder. They will also visit you in your own home, help with paperwork, and draft letters if you wish.

The project's main efforts are currently concentrated in Newcastle under Lyme.

Care and Repair Ltd
22A The Ropewalk, Nottingham NG1 5DT (Tel: 0602-799091) (London Office: 175 Gray's Inn Road, London WC1X 8UX).

Care and Repair Ltd is a friendly society set up by Shelter and the Housing Associations Charitable Trust in order to develop and support Care and Repair projects, as well as forming and pressing for policies which will improve provision for elderly owner occupiers and private tenants. In 1991, Care and Repair Ltd was chosen by government to be the national co-ordinating body for Home Improvement Agencies.

Although not all Care and Repair projects are directly associated with Care and Repair Ltd, there are a considerable number of established schemes throughout England, Wales and Scotland and advice can be given about the availability of schemes in your locality.

Care and Repair schemes in Scotland are working in over twelve areas. For further details contact Care and Repair Scotland, 53 St Vincent Crescent, Glasgow G3 8NQ (Tel: 041-204 2154). Age Concern Scotland has five projects and has published a leaflet describing them.

Care and Repair in Wales has eighteen agencies helping elderly people in similar ways. For further details contact Care and Repair Cymru Ltd, 109 St Mary's Street, Cardiff CF1 1DX (Tel: 0222-387232).

North British Housing Association Group
11th Floor, Unicentre, Lords Walk, Preston PR1 1DP (Tel: 0772-24441).

This Association has worked with Anchor (see above) on a Staying Put scheme in Bolton, and with the experience gained has now set up its own scheme in the Blackburn area. *Home Ground*, as it is known, will offer help and advice on identifying what work needs to be done, locating a suitable contractor, and sorting out the financial aspects. The

Association has used money from its General Reserve to finance a team of three trained members of staff to carry out the work.

▶ *Northern Ireland Housing Executive*
The Housing Centre, 2 Adelaide Street, Belfast BT2 8PB (Tel: 0232-240588).

Among its services, the Housing Executive can help people to move to more suitable accommodation or to repair, improve or adapt their homes.

▶ *Orbit Housing Association*
Regional offices: Midlands Region – 5/7 Dormer Place, Leamington Spa, Warwickshire CV32 5AA (Tel: 0926-32255); London and Home Counties Region – 23 Ewell Road, Cheam, Surrey SM3 8DD (Tel: 081-661 9921); Eastern Region – 14 St Matthew's Road, Norwich NR1 1SP (Tel: 0603-614348); West Region – 5 Beaufort Park, Woodlands, Almondsbury, Bristol BS12 4NE.

The Orbit Care and Repair Service offers practical advice and guidance to elderly home owners who need help to repair or improve their homes. The advice is free and without obligation. Orbit will only make a charge for more complex repairs or alterations to your home, but they will, in any case, discuss any charges with you, before you decide to go ahead with the repairs to your home.

Orbit's Care and Repair staff will: survey your home and advise on repairs needed; arrange grants and loans; put you in touch with a reliable builder; oversee the work as it is carried out; help you through every stage, until the work is finished.

To find out if there is an Orbit Care and Repair Service in your area contact the appropriate Regional Office as above.

Choosing your own contractors

If there is no Care and Repair or Staying Put scheme available in your area, or you prefer to make your own arrangements, it is important to be very careful who you choose to carry out building, maintenance and repair work. Some traders try to take advantage of older people, overcharging and carrying out shoddy work. Given the opportunity, slick salespeople may use high pressure selling techniques to persuade you to enter into contracts for goods and services which you do not need and cannot afford. Some firms may take a deposit and 'forget' to do the work, or go out of business, or simply disappear. Others, notoriously, will take on more work than they can handle, flitting from one job to another, leaving work unfinished and subjecting customers to long delays. Be particularly on your guard against people who come to your home uninvited and who seek to persuade you there and then that certain work needs doing. Above all, do not part with money by way of a deposit to people you know nothing about, or rely on the word of a doorstep salesperson that it is safe to sign documents, when you have not read them or do not fully understand their terms.

Most reputable, professional tradespeople belong to a trade association and work to a code of conduct. If anything does go wrong, you can complain to the relevant association, which should be prepared to intervene between you and the firm concerned and will hopefully put the matter right.

The golden rule is to make sure that you are in control, that you decide what work you want to have done, and that your requirements and a firm commitment to a work programme are put into writing. If the work is extensive, you may need to take the advice of an architect or a surveyor, in which case you may find it helpful to consult the Centre for Accessible Environments (*see* page 102). When choosing a firm to carry out the work, try to take advice from people you trust and 'shop around', getting several estimates.

The Office of Fair Trading, Field House, 15–25 Bream's Buildings, London EC4A 1PR (Tel: 071-242 2858) has a very useful, easy to read, free leaflet, *Home Improvements*, which describes in greater detail the pitfalls often associated with arranging home improvements. In addition to general advice, it explains the importance of contracts (and of reading them before you sign!), cancellation rights (which apply only in limited circumstances), guarantees (which may be worthless) and your legal rights. There is also a useful list of relevant trade and professional bodies, some of whom have sound guarantee schemes or codes of practice.

Home adaptations and equipment

There is a wide range of useful equipment to enable you to adapt your home to your particular needs and requirements and to make it easier to manage. Grabrails, lifts and stairlifts are obvious examples. You can also buy prefabricated, purpose-built add-on rooms, such as lavatories and bathrooms, which are relatively easy to install.

If you have a disability, you may find it useful to seek the help of an occupational therapist. He or she will be able to help you cope with any practical problems arising from your disability, and to advise you about adaptations which could help you with everyday living tasks.

For further information, see Section 4.

Planning permission

Normally, unless your home is listed, you can carry out works of maintenance or improvement which do not increase the size of the house (even though they may alter its external appearance) without any need to apply for permission. For example, you may knock down an interior wall to make one large room, or convert a scullery into a kitchen or a bedroom into a bathroom without having to apply for planning permission. You do not always require planning permission even to build on an extension, so long as it will not increase the volume of the house by more than a permitted amount.

The Planning Department of your local authority will be glad to give you general information and advice on any development you have in mind. A useful booklet *Planning: A Householder's Guide; What you need to known about the planning system*, is available free from the Department of the Environment, PO Box 135, Bradford, West Yorkshire, BD9 4HU, or by telephone from the Public Enquiry Unit, 071 276 0900. Also invaluable for any significant alteration to a property is *A Simple Guide to Planning Applications*, by Robert Cooke, available from Ian Henry Publications Ltd, 20 Park Drive, Romford, Essex RM1 4LH (Tel: 0708-749119), price £4.95.

Financing improvements and repairs

Paying for renovations and alterations to our homes to make them more manageable can be a problem. If you own your own home, there are a number of schemes (explained on page 37) to release part of the capital value of your house. Another possibility is a 'maturity loan' from a building society. Such loans may be advanced to older home owners on an 'interest only' basis (the loan itself being repaid when the house is sold or you leave it permanently). We suggest, however, that you would be well advised to explore all other options before saddling yourself with expensive borrowing.

If your improvements/repairs are being undertaken under a Care and Repair or Staying Put scheme, the staff of the scheme will advise you about possible sources of funding. These may include grants from charities or trade and professional benevolent societies (*see* page 42) and, in some circumstances, local authority grants (*see* below).

The Royal British Legion runs a Property Repair Loan Scheme, which makes loans to ex-servicemen and -women at an interest rate of only 5 per cent per annum. Widows and widowers of ex-service personnel can also apply. The loans, which are charged on the property by way of a mortgage, must be for repairs/adaptations to freehold property, and the maximum loan is £5,000. Applications should be made via local British Legion branches.

If you are disabled, then if your local authority is satisfied that to meet your needs it must provide assistance in arranging for works of home adaptations or additional facilities to secure your greater safety, comfort or convenience, then the authority is under a statutory duty to do so (Chronically Sick and Disabled Persons Act 1970, section 2).

Local authority grants in England and Wales

Since 1 July 1990, a new system of grants has operated in England and Wales. The grants are all means-tested, so that in many cases the applicant will have to make a contribution towards the cost of the work, something which undoubtedly deters many applicants in genuine need. The means-test and required contribution vary according to the type of grant and the circumstances of the applicant. Subject always to the means-test, the grants are either discretionary (it is for the local authority to decide whether

Financing improvements and repairs

to provide grant aid or not) or mandatory (the local authority must provide grant aid). However, even mandatory grant aid may be held up if the local authority has used up its budget allocation. The combination of the stringent means-test and limited local authority funding has, in practice, led to many people being denied help.

If you intend to seek a grant, you must obtain the agreement of your local authority before the work is begun. Council staff will be able to tell you whether or not you are likely to get a grant, what sort of help can be sought and how to apply. When any delay occurs it is important for the applicant to reapply, usually every six months.

The main types of grant are described below.

House renovation grants

Mandatory

Subject to means testing, to qualify for mandatory house renovation grant aid the dwelling concerned must currently be unfit for habitation, and the work proposed must improve the standard and be the most satisfactory way of doing so. It is appropriate for properties which are structurally unstable, in a state of serious disrepair, or so damp as to endanger health. Mandatory grants can also be sought where adequate lighting, heating and ventilation cannot be provided, or if the property lacks certain basic amenities: a wholesome piped water supply; proper cooking facilities; a suitably located toilet; a suitably located bath or shower and wash-hand basin with hot and cold water; and an effective system for draining foul, waste and surface water.

Discretionary

Subject to means testing, discretionary grants can be sought for necessary repair and improvement work which, although quite extensive, falls outside the criteria for mandatory grant aid. The kind of work covered includes: putting the dwelling into reasonable repair; providing separate living accommodation by conversion; providing adequate thermal insulation; providing adequate space heating; providing satisfactory internal arrangements; ensuring that the dwelling conforms with government specifications or other statutory requirements.

Whether mandatory or discretionary, a test of financial resources will be applied to decide how much you are considered to be able to afford to pay from your own resources and how much of the cost of the works can be covered by a grant.

Minor works assistance

This assistance can be given to owner occupiers and private sector tenants (including housing association tenants) who are in receipt of family credit, community charge benefit, housing benefit or income support.

Assistance will usually be in the form of a grant, which could cover the cost of the works (including labour) if you employ a contractor, or the cost of the materials used for doing the work. Instead of a grant, however, your local authority may sometimes provide you with the materials to carry out the works. Minor works assistance is always discretionary and it is therefore up to the council whether to give you any help in this way. Much will depend on the local authority's own resources. The maximum grant payable on any one application is £1,000 (and no more than £3,000 over a three year period).

Minor works assistance is available for the following purposes: to provide or improve thermal insulation; to repair, improve or adapt a property occupied by someone over 60 (including safety and security safeguards); to adapt a property to enable someone over 60 to move into another person's home; to carry out 'patch and mend' repairs to a property in, or soon to be in, a clearance area, usually where the property is eventually to be demolished.

Disabled facilities grants

Disabled facilities grants are designed to help make the homes of disabled people more suitable for them to live in, and to help them to manage more independently in the home.

Applicants must either be registered (or registrable) as a disabled person or have such a disabled person living in their home. Owner-occupiers, tenants (both council and housing association) or landlords on behalf of tenants can apply. In London and metropolitan areas you should contact your local authority; elsewhere in England and Wales, your County Council.

Subject to means testing, there are mandatory and discretionary disabled facilities grants:

Mandatory
The proposed work must be necessary and appropriate to make the dwelling suitable for the disabled person. This will usually be a matter for assessment by an occupational therapist from the local authority social services department. In addition, the proposed work must be reasonable and, depending on the age and condition of the dwelling, practical.

Subject to these criteria, grants are available for the following types of work: improving access into and out of the dwelling; improving access to the living room, bedroom, kitchen and bathroom; providing suitable kitchen and bathroom facilities; adapting the heating and lighting controls; improving and adapting the dwelling so that the disabled person can care for a dependant.

Discretionary
The proposed work must be necessary to make the dwelling suitable for the accommodation, welfare or employment of the disabled person. It is up to the individual local authority to decide if it considers the work relevant. Discretionary grants are limited and will not provide the same level of financial assistance as mandatory grants.

Help in the home

As well as having our home adapted and renovated to our needs, as we grow older we may also need some help in the home if we are to 'stay put'. There are a number of services on which you can call.

Social workers

A social worker will visit you in your home if you request a call. He or she will be able to advise about available services, and to arrange for any service you need. A social worker would be able to put you in touch with or advise you about any of the services mentioned below. The telephone number of your Social Services Department will be in your telephone book under the name of your local council. Social Services will then arrange for a social worker to call.

Home care

Domestic assistance, where this is needed to relieve the domestic situation in the home when someone in the household is elderly, sick or handicapped, may be provided by a local authority. Most local authorities make a charge for this service, and this is often based on the means of the household and the number of hours the home carer is in attendance.

The home care service is intended to provide back-up help and cannot usually be stretched enough to enable a handicapped elderly person to live at home if continuous personal help is needed.

Laundry service

Where there is a laundry service in a particular area for people with incontinence problems or for those too handicapped to manage laundry, it will usually be run by the local Social Services Department. However, in some areas the service may be run by the District Health Authority. Where a laundry service does not exist as such, extra practical help may be given through the Home Help Service.

Disposing of waste

Soiled incontinence pads, dressings and other nursing waste which cannot be disposed of normally and which arises from the care of a sick and handicapped person at home should be collected by the local authority refuse disposal service.

This service is sometimes provided by the District Health Authority, but more commonly by the Environmental Health Department, which is listed in the telephone book under the name of your local council.

Meals-on-wheels

These are administered by local councils, and one hot meal a day may be delivered by volunteers. The service is usually limited to a number of days per week. There may be a charge.

District nurses

District nurses are employed by District Health Authorities and provide nursing care and medical treatment at home. They may help with incontinence problems and with bathing among their general duties. Anyone needing their services should contact their doctor.

Day centres

Day centres provide a hot meal, warm surroundings and social contact for part of the day.

Practical help

Some areas have schemes to help elderly and disabled people with minor repairs, redecoration or gardening. Some of these use volunteers and therefore cut down a lot of the cost. Generally you will only have to pay for the cost of materials and not for the labour. For details of any local schemes contact your Citizens Advice Bureau, local council or Age Concern group.

Community Service Volunteers – Independent Living Projects

The Independent Living Projects are a flexible and relatively low cost form of non-professional care, which match full-time Community Service Volunteers (CSVs) with individuals and families who need a particularly high and concentrated level of support to enable them to remain within their own community and to be able to continue to live as independent a life as possible. Some assignments are arranged for a specified period of time. Others are long-term, and as one volunteer completes her/his period of service (at least four months), arrangements are made for another to take her/his place.

Families and individuals in all sorts of difficult situations can find the scheme useful. Some of these may be elderly people who need fairly regular care, particularly elderly people with disabilities.

CSVs are young, untrained people, committed to helping where they can. Their role is to enable, not to impose care. They can undertake physical care and offer genuine support, but they need expert direction from the individual or family with whom they are working.

Projects are expected to be organised through and supported by the local social services, health authority or other statutory or voluntary agency. Potential users are asked to consider how much care is required, then to judge the number of volunteers needed. An external supervisor, with an overall view of the project, is nominated to offer regular support for the CSV before any placement can begin. The CSV's pocket money (at £21 a week), board (or food allowance of up to £25 a week), lodging and travelling expenses and a retainer fee must be met by the appropriate agency (this may be the local authority) and/or the CSV user.

If you are interested in the idea of using the help of CSVs, please contact: CSV, 237 Pentonville Road, London N1 9NJ (Tel: 071-278 6601) or CSV Scotland, 236 Clyde Street, Glasgow G1 4JH (Tel: 041-204 1681).

Older people can themselves become volunteers – for details of the Retired and Senior Volunteer Programme (RSVP) see Section 226.

Buying into sheltered housing

A wide range of properties and developments is now available to retired people who can afford to buy their own homes. Some of the accommodation is built by private developers and some by housing associations. Often the commercial developers arrange for the developments to be managed by housing associations or other agents. If and when the properties are resold it is the managing agency which is likely to be involved.

Most housing of this kind is sold on a long lease (normally 99 years), to ensure that a development planned for retired people will continue in that way. The resale of properties can be controlled so that each new buyer is another retired person (usually over 55 years of age).

It is essential that before you sign a leasehold agreement you understand what your rights are as a leaseholder and in the event of resale. You should seek professional advice before you sign anything.

A variety of services is made available at each development, typically alarm systems, communal rooms, laundry facilities, and the upkeep of the outside of the properties and of the gardens. Most developments are situated near local communities and shops.

Apart from full-price purchase, there are a number of options which involve a smaller capital outlay:
- buying a life interest (some developers): cost varies with age at entry.
- part-exchange of your present home (some of the larger developers).
- buying at a percentage of the full price (some developers): only a percentage is recoverable on resale.
- shared ownership (some housing associations and local authorities): usually you pay rent on the part you do not own.
- a special leasehold scheme designed for elderly people (a few housing associations): usually you pay 70 per cent of the full price, the balance being subsidised by the Housing Corporation; conversely only 70 per cent is recoverable on resale.

The terms of any such schemes vary and must, of course, be carefully considered. Legal advice is, in our view, essential if you are contemplating a special scheme in the private sector. Age Concern England's fact sheet No.24 (free in response to a large s.a.e. from the address shown at page 103) gives initial information on most of these options.

In considering any purchase you need to have careful regard to the *full* cost, including any loan or mortgage interest, service/management charges, repair/maintenance expenses and insurance premiums, bearing in mind that all or any of these costs may rise over the years.

In the case of sheltered housing, the NHBC Code (*see* below) requires the provision of a Purchaser's Information Pack, giving information about the builder and management organisation, the purchaser's legal rights, services, charges, and conditions applicable to resale.

Finding special housing to buy

Information on properties available from local authorities, voluntary organisations and housing associations can be sought from housing departments and advice centres, and local Age Concern groups. Details of local housing associations and special schemes can also be sought from:

- The Housing Corporation, 149 Tottenham Court Road, London W1P 0BN (Tel: 071-387 9406) and its regional offices.

- The National Federation of Housing Associations, 175 Gray's Inn Road, London WC1X 8UP (Tel: 071-278 6571).

- The Scottish Federation of Housing Associations, 40 Castle Street North, Edinburgh EH2 3BN (Tel: 031-226 6777) and its regional offices.

- The Welsh Federation of Housing Associations, Norbury House, Norbury Road, Fairwater, Cardiff CF5 3AS (Tel: 0222-555022).

⇒ The Northern Ireland Federation of Housing Associations, 88 Clifton Street, Belfast BT13 1AB (Tel: 0232-230446).

⇒ Age Concern's fact sheet No.24, referred to above, has details of some of the firms and organisations offering special purchase schemes.

⇒ The Elderly Accommodation Counsel's database (*see* page 102) has detailed information on non-public sheltered housing. A search fee of £5 is normally charged.

⇒ Sheltered Housing Services Ltd, 8–9 Abbey Parade, North Circular Road, London W5 1EE (Tel: 081-997 9313), an independent national marketing company, provides a specialist service to anyone actively searching for a retirement home to purchase. The company claims to offer the greatest choice available from one source, with over 300 new developments and 400 resales. A one-off charge of £4.50 is payable, but this is refundable if you purchase through the company's efforts.

⇒ The magazine *Retirement Homes and Finance*, published every two months (£1.30), always contains a section devoted to individual schemes.

Further information

Age Concern England fact sheet No.2 gives an outline of the main points to consider if you are thinking of buying special housing.

⇒ *A Buyer's Guide to Sheltered Housing*
(Age Concern England, 1989, available from Central Books, 99 Wallis Road, London E9 5LN (Tel: 081-986 4854)), price £2.50 including postage and packing.

This guide covers in detail the factors to watch out for when considering a purchase. The guide looks first at the financial aspects of buying and running sheltered housing, then at its location, design and facilities, and the role of the warden. The main section covers the legal points concerned with buying, occupying and reselling, including information on management organisations, the service charge, repairs and maintenance, and what happens if you become frail.

⇒ *Housing Options for Older People* (*see* page 105)

⇒ *National House-Building Council Sheltered Housing Code of Practice*
(NHBC, 58 Portland Place, London W1N 4BU), price £6, including postage and packing.

Renting sheltered housing

Most sheltered housing for rent is provided by housing associations, voluntary organisations and local authorities.

It is likely to be very difficult to secure a tenancy in local authority accommodation other than by transfer from an existing tenancy.

Housing associations and voluntary organisations extensively provide special housing for older people. Many of these, unfortunately, have long waiting lists. Moreover, waiting lists are not necessarily operated on a first-come, first-served basis: when vacancies arise, places may be allocated to those in greatest need. Some areas, obviously, are better supplied and/or are less in demand than others. You can apply direct.

There are more than 2,300 groups of almshouses in the United Kingdom, providing 26,000 separate homes for elderly people, and such accommodation continues to be built. Almshouses are normally reserved for local people, but it is also worth making enquiries if you have a special reason for wishing to take up residence in another area.

Private sheltered accommodation is made available, to a limited extent, by a number of specialist developers. Rents on the open market, however, are no longer controlled and you would need to be sure that you could afford the full cost, including any service/management charges, bearing in mind that these are likely to increase over the years. You would also be well advised to seek advice from a solicitor, Citizens Advice Bureau or housing aid centre to ensure that your legal rights under the tenancy agreement are adequate.

Selling up your home to go into rented accommodation

Again, it is important to seek specialist help to discuss the pros and cons of selling up, and to look at possible rental and other costs. If you are considering the possibility of claiming Housing Benefit (for details *see* page 8) you need to be aware that the capital you gain from the sale of your home will affect your entitlement.

Finding special housing to rent

Information on voluntary organisations and housing associations can be sought from housing departments and advice centres, and local Age Concern groups.

Details of local housing associations can also be sought from:

▶ *The Housing Corporation*
149 Tottenham Court Road, London W1P 0BN (Tel: 071-387 9406) and its regional offices.

▶ *The National Federation of Housing Associations*
175 Gray's Inn Road, London WC1X 8UP (Tel: 071-278 6571).

- *The Scottish Federation of Housing Associations*
  40 Castle Street North, Edinburgh EH2 3BN (Tel: 031-226 6777) and its regional offices.

- *The Welsh Federation of Housing Associations*
  Norbury House, Norbury Road, Fairwater, Cardiff CF5 3AS (Tel: 0222-555022).

- *The Northern Ireland Federation of Housing Associations*
  88 Clifton Street, Belfast BT13 1AB (Tel: 0232-230446).

- Age Concern (*see* page 103) will send you details of housing associations etc. with special accommodation for older people in any given county in response to a 9" x 6" s.a.e.

- The Almshouse Association, Billingbear Lodge, Wokingham, Berkshire RG11 5RU (Tel: 0344-52922) can give you the address of local almshouse charities throughout the United Kingdom.

- The Elderly Accommodation Counsel's database (*see* page 97) has detailed information on non-public sheltered housing. A search fee of £5 is normally charged.

- The magazine *Retirement Homes and Finance* contains a regular index of properties for older people. It is published six times a year and is available at bookstalls such as W H Smith, price £1.30 per issue.

Scheme to help tenants move home

- *Housing Organisations Mobility and Exchange Services (HOMES)*
  26 Chapter Street, London SW1P 4ND (Tel: 071-233 7077).

  HOMES is funded by the government to provide a national framework through which people can move home in the local authority and housing association sectors. Its main purpose is to make it easier for people to move home or find housing which is more appropriate to their needs. Council and housing association tenants can either be helped ('nominated') to move by their landlords or arrange a move themselves via mutual self-help exchange schemes ('swaps').

  The schemes which HOMES runs may be able to help you if you need to move in order to provide or receive support from relatives or friends, or to take up an offer of employment. Other good reasons for moving will also be considered. In the case of exchanges, there are no eligibility criteria, although permission from both landlords needs to be obtained before an exchange can take place.

The schemes are free of charge to tenants. There is no guarantee that a move will happen, and the amount of time applicants have to wait depends on the type of property they are looking for and the part of the country to which they wish to move.

Details of how the different schemes work are available from the above address.

Further information

▶ Age Concern (*see* page 103) fact sheet No.8, *Rented Accommodation for Older People*, free in response to a 9" x 6" s.a.e.

▶ *Housing Options for Older People*: see page 104.

Housing associations, housing trusts and charitable organisations providing special housing schemes

We describe below some of the main special housing organisations. The list is not comprehensive and you would be well advised to make local enquiries as described on page 59.

▶ *The Abbeyfield Society*
186–92 Darkes Lane, Potters Bar, Hertfordshire EN6 1AB (Tel: 0707-44845).

Homes to rent
Abbeyfield is a federation of voluntary local societies, each with charitable status, which set up and manage family-sized houses, where seven to nine elderly people have their own bed-sitting rooms. Each house aims to be financially self-supporting, with residents paying their own way. Operating costs are reduced by the extensive work of local volunteers, and also by minimising the use of interest-bearing loans for the improvement and purchase of properties. The greatest possible use is made of public funds for capital purposes, and when these grants are not available as much charitable money as possible is found.

Abbeyfield describes its purpose thus: '...to provide the elderly with their own homes within the security and companionship of small households, which can become focal points for goodwill and friendly contact within the community'.

Houses are situated in the communities from which the residents are usually drawn. Many of the houses are specially designed and built; some are converted from Edwardian villas, Georgian terrace houses or suburban semis (perhaps two knocked together); occasionally village schools and ex-public houses are adapted.

In selecting residents, loneliness is the primary consideration. No one is below pensionable age, and the majority are over 75. Residents have rooms of their own which they can furnish as they wish and which they look after. A housekeeper, residing in each house, cares for the residents, runs the house and provides and prepares the main meals. The housekeeper is supported by a house committee, a group of volunteers responsible for the day-to-day running of the house and the well-being of the residents and staff.

The Society encourages local people to volunteer to become involved with a particular house and with the individual residents who may welcome companions from the local community who can also provide practical help with shopping, car rides, leisure pursuits and so on.

Abbeyfield has developed and is expanding its provision of 'Extra Care' houses for those who can no longer look after themselves in their own room in a supportive house. Needs vary but Abbeyfield say that 'devoted care rather than professional nursing solves most of the problems with, of course, full 24-hour cover'. In an 'Extra-Care' house, a rather larger number of residents – say 20 to 25 – can be housed and cared for in an environment where help is available round the clock over such personal matters as dressing and undressing, bathing and toilet requirements, and just getting around.

There are now 1,000 Abbeyfield houses spread throughout the United Kingdom – from Black Isle in the North to Mullion in the South, from Lowestoft in the East to Strabane in the West.

The Abbeyfielder is the magazine of the Society which gives news of houses and the residents, and discusses national and regional policy.

Anchor

Anchor House, 269a Banbury Road, Oxford OX2 7HU (Tel: 0865-311511).

Homes to rent or to buy

Anchor is a housing trust with charitable status which provides housing and care for older people in need by means of sheltered housing for rent and sale, a 'Staying Put' scheme and other forms of help and community care. Over the last 20 years Anchor has built over 22,000 sheltered flats in towns and cities all over England. The flats are let to older people who for pressing social, health and financial reasons need security and support. All flats are centrally heated, have their own bathroom and are located in buildings with resident wardens. Some accommodation has been especially designed for residents who use wheelchairs. The warden checks daily with each resident either by a personal visit or by the use of an alarm/intercom system.

Anchor's sheltered housing has a range of communal facilities, including a laundry, hairdressing, guest room, library/quiet room and a lounge. Anyone may apply directly to Anchor via its regional offices, providing they are over retirement age and not in full-time employment. Anchor does, however, consider special cases where disability is involved.

Astra Housing Association

Refuge House, 64–6 Stuart Street, Luton, Bedfordshire LU1 2SW (Tel:0582-429398).

Homes to rent
The Association houses mainly elderly people and has schemes throughout England and Scotland. The accommodation includes independent, self-contained flats, sheltered housing schemes (with some communal facilities) and residential homes where residents have their own room with washbasin and lavatory, sharing a bathroom and a kitchen to make snacks. Meals are provided.

The Beth Johnson Housing Association Ltd
Three Counties House, Festival Way, Stoke-on-Trent ST1 5PX (Tel: 0782-219200). Area offices in Telford and Stafford.

Homes to rent
BJHA provides flats to rent for elderly people in North Staffordshire, Shropshire and South Cheshire. This accommodation falls into two main categories:

Category I – for those who are generally fit, active and independent and who may experience only occasional emergencies when they need to be able to call for help from others. These are self-contained, centrally heated flats mainly in groups of 10–20.

Category II – Often known as warden-supported or sheltered accommodation, for those who, while still independent, are now less fit and active and need convenient general lounges in which to 'mix and meet' with others, without having to go outside to do so, and the reassurance of a warden who will check daily that they are all right. These are self-contained, centrally heated flats in groups of 24–60 with communal lounge, laundry, guest room and resident warden.

All flats are fully self-contained and comprise living room, kitchen, bedroom (single or double) and bathroom. A very small number of flats have two bedrooms. Kitchens are fully fitted, with electric cooker and refrigerator provided.

A central alarm network provides emergency cover to all the Association's sheltered housing schemes. The system provides 24-hour cover whenever wardens are off-duty or on holiday. When the alarm is raised, tenants can speak to operators at Air Call who have detailed records on each tenant, and the necessary action can then be taken.

Castle Rock Housing Association Ltd
2 Wishaw Terrace, Meadowbank, Edinburgh EH7 6AF (Tel: 031-652 0152).

Homes to rent or to buy
This is a non-profit-making organisation, providing purpose-built sheltered and amenity housing for rent, and purpose-built and modernised general and sheltered housing for sale.

Homes to rent are situated in Edinburgh, Midlothian and East Lothian. These self-contained flats are designed for retired people. Most developments have one and two person accommodation. Castle Rock describes its accommodation as either 'sheltered' or 'amenity' housing.

Sheltered developments have a communal lounge, laundry, garden/sitting out area, and a guest bedroom. Wardens are resident at each complex and each flat has an alarm call intercom to the warden's house.

Amenity housing is designed to the same standard, but communal facilities may not be provided. A regular weekly visit from a non-residential warden is arranged where possible and there is a telephone contact number. Off-site warden call-out may be arranged in some developments.

A further scheme in Midlothian provides 'care' housing for elderly people – bedsits plus communal facilities. Meals are provided, but not nursing care.

In many schemes there are one or two specially adapted flats for wheelchair users.

Retirement homes for sale are located at Edinburgh, Haddington and North Berwick (East Lothian). Each development has a manager, some of whom are resident.

Church of Ireland Housing Association (NI) Ltd
74 Dublin Road, Belfast BT2 7HP (Tel: 0232-242130).

Homes to rent
The Church of Ireland Housing Association has charitable status and its aims are the provision of housing for elderly people throughout Northern Ireland. It undertakes schemes for people who are more active and also for those who need sheltered housing. Allocations are made on the basis of the Association's own points system.

Locations include: Eglinton and Portstewart in Co. Londonderry; Bushmills, Co. Antrim; Helen's Bay, Co. Down; Cairnshill Court, Belfast; Dundonald (this includes a sheltered housing scheme with a resident supervisor, and retirement bungalows); and Manor Drive, Lisburn (which has sheltered accommodation and retirement flats). The Association has also recently completed schemes in Newtownbreda, Belfast and in Magheralin.

Country Houses Association Ltd
41 Kingsway, London WC2B 6UB (Tel: 071-836 1624).

Homes to rent
This Association, registered as a charity, was founded in 1955 with two aims:

1. To save, for the benefit of the nation, houses of historic importance, architectural interest, or of beauty which may otherwise decay through the inability of individual owners to keep them maintained.
2. To create within the houses apartments for letting as residential accommodation.

Properties include: Albury Park, Guildford; Aynhoe Park, Banbury; Danny, Hurstpierpoint; Flete, Ermington, Plymouth; Gosfield Hall, Halstead; Greathed Manor, Lingfield; Great Maytham Hall, Cranbrook; Pythouse, Tisbury; and Swallowfield Park, Reading.

Apartments range from bed-sitting rooms to three-roomed suites all with *en suite* bathrooms. Charges from £150 per week cover all meals, hot water, cleaning, heating, lift service, and an internal telephone service. Residents also loan the Association a fixed sum, which may range from £20,000 to £60,000, according to the type of apartment chosen. The loan is returnable, less 3 per cent p.a., when the apartment is vacated and relet.

Residents furnish their own apartments. There are a few apartments where pets may be kept.

Derwent Housing Association Ltd
Phoenix Street, Derby DE1 2ER (Tel: 0332-46477; answerphone 0332-32982).

Homes to rents or to buy
The Association is a non-profit-making organisation registered with the Housing Corporation and the Registrar of Friendly Societies. Its main objective is to provide accommodation for those in need whether through rent or sale.

Among the groups of people in need that the Association seeks to help are elderly people from both public and private sectors who require smaller accommodation, and elderly people wishing to move into an area to be near relatives. The Association has a number of Category I developments for active elderly people and Category II warden-aided developments where priority is given to those less active elderly persons who can, in the main, lead an independent life, but who will benefit from the security of a warden-aided scheme. The Association is currently developing a 'Frail Elderly' scheme in Nottingham and the accommodation should be ready for occupation during the latter part of 1992.

All the Association's properties are newly built, and include, in addition to accommodation for rent, elderly persons' flats and bungalows for sale on long leases and shared ownership.

The Association's properties are located in Derbyshire, Nottinghamshire and North West Leicestershire.

Disabled Housing Trust
Norfolk Lodge, Oakenfield, Burgess Hill, West Sussex RH15 8SJ
(Tel: 0444-239123).

Homes to rent or to buy
The Trust is a registered national charity providing specialist housing for physically handicapped people. Residents make their own decisions and run their own lives, but at the same time they receive individual care and attention and there are staff available to help if needed. Accommodation offered is of two kinds:

- Sheltered housing – self-contained bunglaows or flats intended for those disabled people and their families who are capable of independent living but who feel a need for additional security. A few are for sale, but most are rented.
- Residential accommodation – individual bed-sitting rooms, giving privacy and independence, for those requiring additional care for whatever reason. All have *en*

suite bathrooms. Full board is provided but residents also have either their own cooking facilities or the use of a shared kitchen.

Communal facilities include a lounge and dining room with a licensed bar.

All the Trust's developments are built to wheelchair standards and connected to a sophisticated alarm and communication system. Special equipment is provided for bathing; grab rails and hoists are installed where needed. There are electronic aids such as self-opening and -closing doors, hoists and automatic lavatories.

An individual care programme is agreed by the Trust with each resident. Many of the staff have nursing qualifications and all are trained in looking after disabled people. A counsellor is available to give advice and help on personal matters. The services of a physiotherapist and chiropodist are provided free, and other specialist services can be arranged where needed.

Developments are at Burgess Hill and Eastbourne. Burgess Hill houses 50 residents with sheltered housing consisting of 17 bungalows, and residential accommodation providing 19 bed-sitting rooms. Eastbourne houses up to 50 disabled people, and comprises 15 sheltered housing flats, and residential accommodation in 22 bed-sitting rooms (including three doubles).

The Trust also offers residential rehabilitation for those who have suffered a brain injury, in two purpose-built units, one in Milton Keynes and the other in Leeds.

English Churches Housing Group
Sutherland House, 70–8 West Hendon Broadway, London NW9 7BT
(Tel: 081-203 9233).

Homes to rent
English Churches Housing Group is a non-profit-making association with charitable status. Its aim is to provide homes for those in housing need; to provide an efficient and effective service to people who become their tenants; and to provide support and help for those tenants in need. The Association has a strong equal opportunities policy, and the tenant allocation policy is based on that.

The Association has over 3,500 units of accommodation for elderly people spread throughout England. Roughly half of the developments for elderly people have resident wardens, and a few have facilities for wheelchair users.

The English Courtyard Association
8 Holland Street, Kensington, London W8 4LT (Tel: 071-937 4511).

Homes to buy
The Association is a non-profit-making company aiming to provide specialised luxury accommodation for elderly retired people. The cottages and flats are normally for sale on long leases of 150 years. The occupier, though not necessarily the owner, has to be a person of retirement age.

Developments are based on the traditional courtyard plan of almshouses and consist of terraces and courts of two storey cottages and flats. These have a VHF 'bleeper' alarm system. The grounds are landscaped to create the atmosphere of a country house garden. There are properties in Wiltshire, Worcestershire, Somerset, Sussex, Dorset, Suffolk, Kent, Devon, Northamptonshire and Berkshire. Prices start at about £100,000.

▶ *The Five Counties Housing Association Ltd*
Three Counties House, Festival Way, Stoke-on-Trent ST1 5PX (Tel: 0782-219200).

Homes to buy
This Association, a sister association to The Beth Johnson Housing Association, has developed purpose-built bungalows and apartments at 70 per cent of cost for elderly home buyers. There are two leasehold schemes at Riversmead (warden service) and Spinneymead (where each bungalow has an emergency alarm system) in Newcastle under Lyme.

The Association also has long-term agreements with several housing associations/organisations for the management/maintenance of existing accommodation, including schemes for elderly people in Staffordshire and Shropshire.

▶ *Fold Housing Association*
3 Redburn Square, Holywood, Co. Down BT18 9HZ (Tel: 0232-428314).

Homes to rent or to buy
This Association builds sheltered housing for elderly people throughout Northern Ireland, having about 1,800 units under management in 61 schemes.

The Association also builds leasehold housing for sale to elderly people in which the purchaser pays 70 per cent of the cost of a flat, the balance being met by a government grant.

▶ *Friends of the Elderly and Gentlefolk's Help*
42 Ebury Street, London SW1W 0LZ (Tel: 071-730 8263).

Homes to rent
Friends of the Elderly have 12 homes situated in Wimbledon; Moulsford near Wallingford, Oxfordshire; Alton, Hampshire; Coulsdon, Woking and Haslemere, Surrey; Malvern, Worcestershire; and Nynehead, near Taunton, Somerset. Some of these homes have nursing wings where short- or long-stay patients may reside, and one is for the care of frail elderly people.

In the homes residents are asked to furnish their own rooms, including carpets, curtains and bedding – these are single bed-sitting rooms or, in the case of a married couple, two rooms. Sometimes little flatlets are available for couples in some of the homes. Residents are described as having freedom to come and go as they please. We are informed that lunch and supper in the dining room are the only fixed points of the day. Laundry facilities are provided. Residents make their own breakfast and tea in the pantries and all food is provided. Television and telephones can be installed in the rooms. In addition, there is a large colour set in each home, situated in either the drawing room or the TV room.

In order to pass for selection the Homes Committee has to ensure that the candidate is not only medically fit and capable of leading an independent life, but will also contribute to the general life in the home. There is no fixed rule about applicants' ages, but 75 would be a recommended minimum age. In cases of illness, residents are cared for in the nursing wings of their own home, at no extra charge, or in one of the Society's nursing homes.

Regarding fees, applicants are asked to give details of their income and capital and they pay only what they can afford. Sufficient money is always left for personal needs. The wardens and staff of the homes are not informed of the amount paid by a resident.

Guardian Housing Association Ltd
Anchor House, 269A Banbury Road, Oxford OX2 7HU (Tel: 0865-311711).

Homes to buy
The Guardian Housing Association is a registered housing association and is a charity in association with Anchor Housing Association and Anchor Housing Trust. Guardian provides and manages sheltered accommodation throughout England for older people able to buy their own property. It offers a range of properties from shared-ownership to outright sale. It is presently responsible for over 5,000 properties throughout England.

The Guinness Trust
17 Mendy Street, High Wycombe, Buckinghamshire HP11 2NZ (Tel: 0494-535823).

Homes to rent
The Trust, a registered housing association with charitable status, provides warden-supervised flats for elderly people as part of larger, general purpose housing estates in many parts of the country. Each estate is the responsibility of a resident estate manager who advises tenants, collects rents, arranges repairs and ensures that the estate is clean, tidy and well maintained. Most estates have additional resident staff who carry out minor repairs, maintain the grounds and provide an emergency service night and day for seven days a week.

The Trust will only consider applicants who are on a low income, who are in real need of housing, and who can manage their own home. No waiting list is maintained except for those who can reasonably be housed within twelve months.

Enquiries for accommodation should be made to the Trust's area offices located at Stratford (East London), Horley, Welwyn, Exeter, Washington (Tyne and Wear), Manchester and Nottingham.

The Trust also runs two residential homes in London (at Stratford and Camden), and another at Torpoint (Cornwall).

Hanover Housing Association and Hanover Housing Ltd
Hanover House, 18 The Avenue, Egham, Surrey TW20 9AB (Tel: 0784-38361).

Homes to rent or to buy
Hanover Housing Association is non-profit-making, with charitable status, providing and managing accommodation for rent to older people throughout England and Wales. An integral part of the Association's service to tenants is the resident warden, and all dwellings are connected to the warden's residence by a communication system.

The estates generally consist of self-contained one-bedroomed dwellings, but there are also some bed-sitters and two-bedroomed units.

Hanover Housing Limited, which does not trade for profit, provides leasehold housing for sale to retired people. A warden lives on the estate, and emergency alarms are installed in each property. Some developments have a common room, a small kitchenette, a laundry and a guest room.

Hanover (Scotland) Housing Association Ltd
36 Albany Street, Edinburgh EH1 3QH (Tel: 031-557 0598).

Housing to rent and to buy
Hanover (Scotland)'s aim as a non-profit-making organisation is to provide housing for elderly people who are physically able to lead independent lives, or who need no more support than that which a resident warden can provide. Tenants are normally aged 60 or over.

Most property consists of unfurnished rented flats (on a monthly tenancy), each of which is completely self-contained with its own bedroom, living room, kitchen and bathroom. On some schemes two-bedroomed accommodation is available. There are a few schemes with bed-sitters. A warden is resident on every scheme and there is an emergency alarm system. In addition, there is a central alarm service which can be linked in to the warden call service or to individual telephone systems in private dwellings. Tenants are normally allowed to keep one pet.

Hanover (Scotland) also manages a number of developments providing sheltered housing for sale. Prospective buyers must normally be aged 60 or over and wholly able to lead an independent life. A resident warden service is provided.

An alternative to outright purchase is provided in the form of shared equity accommodation. Under this arrangement, flats are available for part purchase. Proprietors enjoy all the normal rights of occupation, but at a reduced capital cost which may be affordable by households who cannot raise the full purchase price.

Help the Aged – Housing and Care Division
St James's Walk, London EC1R 0BE (Tel: 071-253 0253).

Homes to rent
As well as providing general help and advice to older people concerned about housing

matters, Help the Aged also has its own Housing and Care Division. The accommodation includes extra-sheltered and semi-sheltered housing.

Extra-sheltered accommodation provides 24-hour staff cover and the option of a lunch. Semi-sheltered accommodation generally has an alarm system and is regularly visited by regional staff and care advisers.

Accommodation may consist of studio flats, apartments, cottages, or bungalows. Communal facilities include a lounge/dining room and a laundry room.

Developments are located at Chester; Colchester; Corbridge (Northumberland); Huddersfield; Lindfield and Rustington, Sussex; Lowestoft; Luton; and Woking, Surrey.

The Gifted Housing Plan, which is unique to Help the Aged, is a scheme whereby people can donate their property to the charity and continue to live there. Later, if the former owner wishes, he or she is given priority to move to alternative accommodation within Help the Aged. In return for the donation of the property, Help the Aged takes over the responsibility for the cost of repairs, maintenance, external decoration, gardening, rates, and buildings insurance. Before entering such a scheme it would be important to take legal advice to ensure the arrangements were completely satisfactory in respect of your particular needs.

Heritage Housing Ltd
36 Albany Street, Edinburgh EH1 3QH (Tel: 031-557 0598).

Homes to buy
This is a non-profit-making housing association formed by the Hanover (Scotland) Housing Association as a completely independent association to develop and build sheltered housing for sale to elderly people. Hanover (Scotland) takes over management of schemes on completion. Developments are located at Abedeen, Ayr, Broughty Ferry, Cupar, Dunblane, Edinburgh, Glasgow, Gullane, Inverness, Milngavie, Peebles, Stonehaven and Troon.

James Butcher Housing Association
James Butcher House, 39 High Street, Theale, Reading RG7 5AH (Tel: 0734-323434).

Homes to rent and to buy
This Association (non-profit-making and a charity) provides rented subsidised accommodation mainly for older people in the counties of Berkshire, Buckinghamshire, Gloucestershire, Hampshire, Oxfordshire, Surrey, Sussex and Wiltshire. As well as the residents' private homes there are also communal facilities within the developments. These include a lounge and gardens. Hairdressing and chiropody facilities are also available.

The majority of dwellings consist of either one-person bed-sitting rooms or two-person, one-bedroomed, self-contained flats. However, single person flats with a separate bedroom are being included in all new developments.

In sheltered schemes wardens are available for help. Sheltered flats are not usually allocated to persons who have gone beyond their late 80s other than as Additional Care accommodation. This type of accommodation is available to elderly people who can no longer cope easily with day-to-day chores, but who are nevertheless ambulant, continent and able to deal with personal care. All meals are provided and there is a flat cleaning and laundry service.

The Association also provides retirement leasehold (99 years) housing in sheltered environments for older people. The day-to-day management of each scheme includes the employment of a warden, external maintenance of buildings and grounds, insurance, and any other services considered necessary. Housing schemes are available in the counties of Berkshire, Gloucestershire, Hampshire, Oxfordshire, Surrey and Sussex.

All accommodation consists of one- and two-bedroomed self-contained apartments and bungalows. Each development has communal gardens maintained by the Association. The majority of schemes have a guest bedroom and laundry facilities and may include a residents' lounge. Pets may be kept, but special permission must first be sought.

▪▶ *Jephson Homes Housing Association Ltd*
Jephson House, Blackdown, Leamington Spa, Warwickshire CV32 6RE (Tel: 0926-339311).

Homes to rent or to buy
Jephson is one of the United Kingdom's leading housing association groups, originally formed to provide homes for elderly people. They now build and manage new homes for letting, leasing, sale and shared ownership for a wide variety of clients – elderly people, families, couples, single people and those with special needs.

Each Jephson sheltered development has a resident or visiting warden and 24-hour emergency alarm facilities. Properties consist, in the main, of two-bedroomed bungalows and one- or two-bedroomed flats for sale or rent.

New retirement developments for sale are being marketed at Leamington Spa, Warwick, Caversham, Arlesford and Egham.

▪▶ *Kirk Care Housing Association Ltd*
Registered Office: 3 Forres Street, Edinburgh EH3 6BJ (Tel: 031-225 7246).
Area Offices: 533 Baltic Chambers, 50 Wellington Street, Glasgow G2 6HJ (Tel: 041-221 3445); 58–60 Church Street, Inverness (Tel: 0463-240344).

Homes to rent
Kirk Care (a non-profit-making company) was formed in 1973 to provide sheltered housing for elderly people in Scotland. The Association's principal aim is the provision of specially designed rented accommodation for older people in the form of sheltered and amenity housing developments throughout most areas of Scotland. Every sheltered development has a resident warden, and in amenity housing a locally based

representative is appointed as a link between tenants and the Association's offices. The call systems in all cases incorporate a link to a remote alarm centre which will summon assistance in emergency sitations during the warden's absence (in the case of amenity housing, at any time).

Kirk Care is currently exploring with local authority social work departments plans to provide continuing care to tenants who become extremely frail, so that many will not require to move into residential accommodation.

Future developments are designed and planned with continuing care in mind and again in liaison with social work departments. A sheltered development currently under construction at Girvan incorporates eight care units for physically frail persons, who will be cared for by a resident housekeeper. Meals will be provided. Kirk Care has pioneered a project at Alloa to provide domestic style accommodation for elderly people suffering from moderate to severe dementia. This is a co-operative venture with Central Regional Council, the social work department, and Forth Valley Health Board, and will offer continuing care in their own area to persons whose only alternative would be a long-term hospital ward some distance from their homes.

Joint projects have also been undertaken – in Inverness with the Church of Scotland, for persons recovering from alcohol and other addictions, and with the Leonard Cheshire Foundation, for severely physically disabled people. At Lochinver, the Association's small sheltered development was constructed along with the Assynt Centre – a local base for social and medical services serving that part of Sutherland.

Merseyside Improved Homes
46 Wavertree Road, Liverpool L7 1PH (Tel: 051-709 9375).

Homes to rent or to buy
This housing association provides nearly 17,000 homes in the Merseyside area. The bulk of applicants are people on low incomes. Elderly people, mostly on their own, now form a significant proportion of people entering MIH accommodation. As well as the provision of rented accommodation, which is the main activity, MIH is currently involved in leasehold schemes for the elderly (LSE) and shared ownership for the elderly (SOFTE). An associated company, MIH Harbour Housing Association Ltd, has recently introduced a resales service which will help existing elderly tenants to sell their homes.

Methodist Homes for the Aged
Epworth House, Stuart Street, Derby DE1 2EQ (Tel: 0332-296200).

Homes to rent
MHA Housing Association runs 22 sheltered housing schemes in the United Kingdom for elderly people (not necessarily Methodists). There is a 24-hour warden service and MHA seeks to ensure continuing care for tenants as they become more frail. MHA also maintains 37 residential homes and two homes for physically and mentally frail people. In all, MHA cares for nearly 1,900 elderly people.

Nationwide Housing Trust Ltd (Development Arm of Nationwide Building Society)
Correspondence address: Moulton Park, Northampton NN3 1NL (Tel: 0604-794189).

Homes to buy
The Trust has a wide variety of property available, including sheltered retirement homes (flats, bungalows, cottages and houses). Facilities vary from development to development, but usually incorporate a 24-hour emergency call system, resident manager and communal facilities.

The Trust offers an equity share scheme on some retirement developments, which can reduce the cost of purchase by up to 50 per cent.

Developments are located throughout the country. The Trust occasionally also has details of resale properties.

North British Housing Association Group
4 The Pavilions, Portway, Preston PR2 2YB (Tel: 0772-824441).

Homes to buy or to rent
NBHAG is a non-profit-making organisation and is now one of the leading associations in the country, with over 30,000 homes in management, including those managed for other bodies. Its primary objective is to provide good quality, properly managed accommodation and appropriate support services for rent or sale which is affordable to those in housing need. Over the years, it has gradually become involved in the provision of care and support services, particularly for older people. It now provides and manages over 1,000 places for people with special needs, many in partnership with statutory and voluntary organisations. The Association also has over 6,000 sheltered housing units and a national community alarm service.

NBHAG has regional offices in Manchester, Nottingham, Newcastle upon Tyne, Preston, London (Hendon) and Bradford.

North Housing
Ridley House, Regent Centre, Newcastle upon Tyne NE3 3JE (Tel: 091-285 0311).

Homes to rent or to buy
North Housing provides sheltered housing (houses, flats and bungalows) for older people to rent in North East, North West, and South East England and the East Midlands. Any specific adaptation needed by the intending resident will be carried out, including the installation of stair lifts, bath chairs, showers and reduced height kitchen units. Communal facilities are incorporated. Some flats are adapted for the use of people in wheelchairs. Properties either have resident wardens living on site or 'travelling wardens', and there is an alarm system.

North Housing also provides sheltered housing for sale to older people, with similar facilities.

Northern Counties Homes
Princes Buildings, Oxford Court, Oxford Street, Manchester M2 3WQ (Tel: 061-228 3388 or 061-228 3333 (24 hours)).

Homes to buy
Northern Counties Homes is part of Northern Counties Housing Association Ltd (see below). Apartments are sold on a long leasehold for residents of retirement age or on some developments from the age of 55 years.

Dogs and cats are not usually allowed in any apartments.

All apartments and bungalows are constructed to a high specification, and have an emergency 24-hour call system as a standard feature.

New developments are located in many areas of the North West, with resales available on many existing schemes. New apartments are currently in Cheadle, Heaton Mersey, Chorlton-cum-Hardy, Woodley, Sale and Bolton.

Northern Counties Housing Association Ltd
Princes Buildings, 15 Oxford Court, Oxford Street, Manchester M2 3WQ (Tel: 061-228 3388).

Homes to rent or to buy
This Association has sheltered housing schemes for older people to rent, with resident wardens and communal facilities, throughout the North of England. Special facilities are available in some schemes for frail elderly people where special support is provided by extra staff from social service departments. Care in the Community schemes have also been developed for disabled people, giving round-the-clock care and nursing support.

Resident wardens are available in sheltered developments which would also have communal residents' sitting rooms and other facilities. Some developments are classified as category one and are intended for those people who are more active. On these there would be no resident wardens or communal rooms. Some developments are a mixture of 'sheltered' and 'category one' and on these the category one residents would be able to share the communal facilities with those living in sheltered accommodation.

The Association also provides leasehold dwellings for sale for older home buyers. Properties are situated in the North of England between Carlisle and Nottingham.

Northern Ireland Co-ownership Housing Association Ltd
Murray House, Murray Street, Belfast BT1 6DN (Tel: 0232-327276).

Homes to buy
The aims of the Association are to help people to own their own homes by initially part-buying (at least 50 per cent of the value of the property) and part-renting the property of their choice. NICHA purchases the property on behalf of the person joining the scheme and then shares ownership with her or him. The Association purchases approximately 1,000 properties each year on behalf of its applicants.

Any kind of property can be considered for co-ownership, provided that the purchase price is not more than £36,000. Property less than ten years old must have NHBC cover.

The price ceilings are reviewed regularly, and these figures will be effective until 31 March 1993.

Although the scheme is primarily intended for first time buyers looking for family-type accommodation, the scheme is appropriate for people at any stage of their lives, and the Association is happy to accept elderly persons on an equity-sharing basis. Each application received is assessed on its own merits, taking into account the property applied for and the capacity of the applicant to maintain the financial commitment. However, as the promotion of home ownership is the scheme's main aim, the Association must also consider any potential the applicant has to increase that financial commitment at a later date, thereby increasing her or his equity share and eventually achieving full ownership of the property.

Orbit Housing Association
44–5 Queens Road, Coventry, West Midlands CV1 3EH (Tel: 0203-632231).

Homes to rent or to buy
Orbit aims to provide flats or houses to rent for those in the greatest need in the community, including early retired people and elderly people. On larger estates there is usually a resident caretaker, who is responsible for the upkeep of the estate and its grounds. In sheltered housing for elderly people a resident warden provides a good neighbour service to the tenants. Many schemes have guest rooms, and other communal facilities may include a common room and a laundry.

Orbit also provides accommodation for people in special need. This includes hostels, cluster flats, and group homes for people with some special disability or requirement, either in self-contained accommodation or in shared housing.

Orbit accommodation is located in the Midlands, London, the South East, the South West and East Anglia.

Orbit is also developing housing schemes to enable elderly owner occupiers, whose homes are too large or difficult for them to maintain, to move into smaller accommodation better suited to their needs. Some projects include bungalows, others include flats, and there are a variety of facilities which may be available in some of the schemes.

The specially-designed accommodation is intended to enable you to retain your independence in your own home for as long as possible.

Orbit also runs leasehold schemes for elderly people. In the first case you purchase a 60-year lease but pay only 70 per cent of the market value, receiving 70 per cent of the market value when you leave. In the other, you purchase a lease, probably for 99 years, but in this instance you pay a higher proportion of the market value – 99 per cent instead of 70 per cent – and therefore receive a similarly higher percentage at the end of your occupation.

A Resident Manager will be on hand to help as required, though not to provide personal help with dressing, washing, etc.

Orbit Spa Housing Association Ltd
44–5 Queens Road, Coventry, West Midlands CV1 3EH (Tel: 0203-632231).

Homes to rent
Orbit Spa is the charitable member of the Orbit Housing Group. It provides homes to rent throughout the same areas as Orbit Housing Association (above).

A short waiting list of applicants for tenancies is kept. Applicants are only accepted on to the waiting list if there is a real possibility of an offer of rehousing being made within a reasonable period of time.

Presbyterian Housing Association (NI) Ltd
Lowry House, 27 Hampton Park, Belfast (Tel: 0232-491851).

Homes to rent
The main aim of the Association, which has charitable status, is to provide sheltered housing for elderly people throughout Northern Ireland. Accommodation is available to all who are genuinely in need of sheltered housing regardless of their religious beliefs. Sixteen different schemes have been completed, which provide accommodation for around 500 tenants, with more accommodation being provided all the time.

Accommodation usually consists of one- and two-person apartments. Communal facilities may include a sitting room, a launderette and a kitchen. Apartments each have a lounge, bedroom, kitchen, bathroom, store and entrance hall. Equipment provided to each apartment includes a refrigerator, a door entry system and an emergency alarm.

Existing developments are located in Belfast, Craigavon, Bangor, Millisle, Carnmoney, Maghera, Ballycastle, Comber, Portstewart and Cruglin. The Association also administers a hostel for frail elderly people.

Quaker Social Responsibility and Education
Friends House, Euston Road, London NW1 2BJ (Tel: 071-387 3601).

Homes to rent
A list *Accommodation for Elderly People under Quaker Auspices* is available from the address above. Each housing scheme is run completely independently and should be contacted directly for information about fees and waiting lists; most are available to non-Quaker residents although priority is often given to Friends, and to those who live in or near the locality or have relatives or friends there. There is no maximum age common to all homes. In general, state of health and degree of need for the sort of care provided are more important than age.

Different facilities are available in each scheme, which may consist of single or double rooms, self-contained flats, bungalows and cottages. Accommodation may be furnished or unfurnished. Some or all meals may be provided. Some nursing care is provided. In many schemes there are communal facilities, including lounge, laundry and guest room. Two schemes are for women tenants only – in Bury St Edmunds and Plymouth (for women who have lived in Devon or Cornwall).

Schemes are in: Avon, Buckinghamshire, Cambridgeshire, Cheshire, Cumbria, Devon, Dorset, Hertfordshire, Hampshire, Kent, Lancashire, Leicestershire, Nottinghamshire, Oxfordshire, Somerset, Suffolk, Surrey, Sussex, West Midlands and Yorkshire, as well as Northern Ireland (Belfast) and Ireland (Dublin).

Retirement Lease Housing Association
19 Eggar's Court, St George's Road East, Aldershot, Hampshire GU12 4LN (Tel: 0252-318181).

Homes to buy
This Association provides and manages housing schemes (flats and bungalows) specially designed for retired but active elderly owner occupiers. Property is sold on a leasehold basis – 60 or 99 years. RLHA schemes will have a resident warden and a 24-hour alarm call system. On some schemes there may be a launderette, a guest room and a common room.

The Royal Air Forces Association
Portland Road, Malvern, Worcestershire WR14 2TA (Tel: 0684-892505).

Homes to rent
The Association, which is a registered charity, works closely with the Royal Air Force Benevolent Fund. It is a membership organisation, having some 110,000 members and 635 branches worldwide. The assistance given by the Association is wide ranging and includes offering professional advice on pensions, legal matters and housing, as well as handling day-to-day welfare problems. The Association has some 635 voluntary welfare workers and its welfare support is not confined to its membership but extends to serving and ex-Air Force non-members and their dependants.

The Association has sheltered housing schemes in Storrington, Sussex, Bolton, Lancashire and Moffat, Scotland. Three further sheltered housing schemes (Eagle Lodges) have been developed and provide accommodation with the extra care of a 'live-in' housekeeper. Eagle Lodges are now operational in Melton Mowbray, Southport and Bexhill-on-Sea, and there are plans for another in Wales.

The Association also has a residential home for disabled people, Sussexdown, which is situated nine miles from Worthing. Full 24-hour nursing service is provided, as well as physiotherapy and occupational therapy.

The Royal British Legion Housing Association Ltd
PO Box 32, St John's Road, Penn, High Wycombe, Buckinghamshire HP10 8JF (Tel: 049-481 3771).

Homes to rent
This non-profit-making Association with charitable status, while having a direct responsibility to ex-service people, will nevertheless consider applications for rented accommodation from others needing sheltered housing.

Schemes of grouped flats are situated throughout England, Wales and Scotland. Each scheme has its own resident warden and communal rooms are available for the use of residents.

Housing is now managed locally so as to be more responsive to people's needs.

The Shires Housing Association Ltd

Three Counties House, Festival Way, Stoke-on-Trent ST1 5PX (Tel: 0782-219200; Fax: 0782-213234).

Homes for sale

This Association, a sister organisation of The Five Counties Housing Association, has developed purpose built bungalows and flats for older people in Newcastle under Lyme, Nantwich and Market Drayton. Each scheme has an emergency call system which will provide 24-hour support cover, and is surrounded by communal gardens.

The Sutton Housing Trust

Sutton Court, Tring, Hertfordshire HP23 5BB (Tel: 0442-891100).

Homes to rent

The Trust is a registered charitable housing association which provides good quality rented accommodation on estates with resident management and maintenance staff for people on low incomes in housing need. The Trust owns over 14,000 properties in 32 towns throughout England. Most of the estates incorporate small flats or bungalows which are particularly suitable for occupation by elderly people. At Crownhill, Plymouth the Trust manages an elderly person's village.

In November 1991, the Trust managed a total of 1,053 properties within 24 sheltered housing schemes and four warden-assisted schemes for retired people. The sheltered housing schemes comprise self-contained flats which are linked by a two-way speech alarm system to the resident warden's office and in some cases to a community alarm system when the warden is off-duty. Each sheltered scheme has communal facilities which would normally include a lounge, laundry, guest room and hairdressing/general utility room.

In the warden-assisted schemes, a warden service is available but communal facilities are not provided as an integral part of the scheme. A scheme in South Shields is linked to the local authority community alarm system but a warden is not resident on site.

The Trust also manages 162 purpose-designed properties for wheelchair users, and all ground floor flats of sheltered housing schemes are built to mobility standard. Adaptations to properties will also be carried out where they have been recommended by an occupational therapist. The Trust carries out internal decorations in properties purpose-designed for elderly residents, and will also assist elderly tenants in other properties with internal decorations.

Home from Home schemes

These schemes offer an alternative to conventional residential care. Older people who have to give up their own homes because they can no longer look after themselves are matched with host families who will welcome them into their homes, and give care and attention as if the elderly person were a member of their family. Hopefully a close and satisfying relationship will develop. The basic aims of such schemes are twofold:

1. To extend the current range of services offered to elderly people, by creating a new resource and thereby introducing an element of consumer choice.
2. To provide a service of high quality that gives a completely tailored form of care and attention, designed to meet individual needs.

Home from Home started in Liverpool and Leeds about ten years ago and has grown enormously over the last few years. There are now about 230 schemes operating around the country.

For further details contact: Ann Collins, Secretary, Special Interest Group–Adult Placement Schemes, Solihull Social Services, The Council House, Solihull, West Midlands B91 3QY (Tel: 021-704 6743).

Residential and nursing homes

We think that we scarcely need to urge caution when it comes to considering whether to move into, and actually choosing, residential accommodation. For the great majority of us, even if we are able to find a well run home with high standards, it is likely to be an unwanted, last resort. Though they offer basic care, which may have become essential, we know that residential home fees are expensive, that we will have to leave our own home, and that we may have to give up treasured possessions, almost certainly our pets and, even worse, at least some of our independence. Moreover, there have been sufficient critical reports for us to be aware that the way some homes are run leaves a great deal to be desired; at their worst they can be, as one writer put it, concentration camps for the old.

A survey published in March 1992 by the Elderly Accommodation Counsel (EAC – *see* below), revealed that about 100,000 of the 300,000 people in residential care would not need to be there if they were given proper community care. Before contemplating residential care, therefore, we think that you will wish to consider, with your family and friends, your doctor and your local social services department, whether you could continue to manage in your own home with extra help and, perhaps, some adaptations and special equipment. Alternatively, one of the housing options described above may be sufficient to meet your needs. Your local Age Concern group may well be able to offer you support and advice in these critical deliberations. Above all, save in the most exceptional circumstances, it should be *your* decision.

Should you decide that you really cannot go on without the care and support of a residential or nursing home, or that the burden on others has become too great, you will need to consider very carefully where you would like to live. Residential homes in the voluntary and private sectors, and all nursing homes, have to be registered under the Registered Homes Act 1984 (with a simplified procedure for small homes caring for three or fewer people). Standards of care are the subject of a code of practice, and homes are inspected at least twice a year. In the private sector, many homes belong to a representative organisation which also safeguards at least basic standards of care. The crucial consideration is whether those who run the home do so with imagination and sensitivity for the *feelings* of the residents, seeking not merely to make them comfortable, but also to accord them dignity, privacy and freedom of choice, so that the home is managed for the widest possible benefit of the people who live there rather than the convenience of the care staff. You need to have a personal checklist of life-style requirements which are most important to you. You may have to compromise, but hopefully as little as possible. No.29 of Age Concern England's free fact sheets, *Finding Residential and Nursing Home Accommodation* (*see* below), contains a list of questions to ask when choosing a home. There is plenty of more detailed guidance on the subject, and we would urge anyone faced with moving into a home, and their relatives and carers, to take time to read at least some of the literature which is described below.

There are about 13,500 residential care homes in Britain, about three-quarters of which are run by voluntary or private organisations, and the remainder by local authorities. Local authority homes are provided under Part III of the National Assistance Act 1948, and are often known as 'Part III accommodation'. Increasingly, however, local authorities are relying upon taking up places in homes run by charitable or private organisations. Local authority accommodation is not free: indeed, the charges are likely to be much the same as for private accommodation. However, people in poor circumstances, with little capital, are not charged the full fees.

In the private sector, where homes are run for profit, fees vary considerably. It is a matter of concern that although total social security support has risen to £1.6 billion, many elderly people find that their benefits do not fully meet the fees charged. These difficulties are particularly acute in the area around Greater London, where income support is pegged to the national rate, but charges tend to be high. We think that it is imperative, before committing yourself to taking up residence in a particular home, that you should have a clear written statement setting out all the fees, whether there are extra charges for any services, and an indication of how fees might increase year by year. It should also be possible to go for a trial period before making any final decision.

Facilities in homes in all categories vary greatly. The EAC survey showed in particular that although most homes have more than one storey, over half do not have lifts, and about a quarter do not have wheelchair access.

Bridging the gap between benefits and fees

'Topping-up' on a regular basis can be a huge financial commitment, whether from the savings of the individuals concerned or from a charitable fund. The problem can only be made worse by unrealistic fees or fee increases. If you need help in meeting fees, it is important to be aware that the Association of Charity Officers recommends to its members' funds ceilings above which it suggests that no top-up should be given.

General information about grants from charities is given in Section 1. Advice specifically concerning possible help with residential homes fees is available from any of the following organisations:

▸ *The Association of Charity Officers*
c/o RICS Benevolent Fund Ltd, 1st floor, Tavistock House North, Tavistock Square, London WC1H 9RJ (Tel: 071-383 5557).

▸ *Counsel and Care for the Elderly*
Twyman House, 16 Bonny Street, London NW1 9PG (Tel: casework – Mondays to Thursdays, 10.30 a.m. to 3.00 p.m., 071-485 1566).

▸ *Elderly Accommodation Counsel*
46A Chiswick High Road, London W4 1SZ (Tel: 081-742 1182/081-995 8320).

Finding residential and nursing home accommodation

Social Services Departments will be able to provide the addresses of all registered private and voluntary residential homes in their locality. District Health Authorities will similarly have a list of local nursing homes.

It is worth remembering that some occupational groups have societies which care for elderly retired staff. The Civil Service Benevolent Fund, for example, owns and manages ten homes around the United Kingdom. Ex-service organisations, similarly, may be able to offer residential accommodation to veteran personnel and their dependants.

If you are disabled, relevant charities (*see* Section 14) should have information about homes which specialise in meeting special needs, either for severely disabled people generally or in respect of particular impairments.

▸ *British Federation of Care-Home Proprietors (BFCHP)*
852 Melton Road, Thurmaston, Leicester LE4 8BN (Tel: 0533-640095).

BFCHP's declared aims are 'to further the education and training of all those engaged or interested in the care of the elderly and/or the handicapped and the operation of homes for them in order to improve the standard of care given and to establish professional standards in providing such care'.

BFCHP currently represents more than 1,200 homes. Membership is subject to confirmation that each home owned by an applicant meets Federation standards based on the national code of practice. Subsequently, standards are professionally monitored, each member being required to make his or her homes available for inspection every three years.

Caresearch
c/o United Response, 162-4 Upper Richmond Road, London SW15 2SL (Tel: 081-780 9596)

The Caresearch database contains information on residential care throughout Britain for mentally handicapped people. The clients' needs are matched with the database and the appropriate residential establishments are produced by the computer and sent to the enquirer. The fee for a search is £25.

Counsel and Care for the Elderly
Twyman House, 16 Bonny Street, London NW1 9PG (Tel: casework – Mondays to Thursdays, 10.30 a.m. to 3.00 p.m., 071-485 1566).

CCE caseworkers visit annually all the private and voluntary nursing and residential care homes in Greater London and therefore have information on the facilities provided in each home. Caseworkers are thus able to suggest suitable homes to meet the individual needs and preferences of each enquirer. For people seeking care outside the London area, CCE is able to put them in touch with other organisations that can help.

The Directory of Independent Hospitals and Health Services
(Longman Group UK Limited, 4th Avenue, Harlow, Essex CM19 5AA (Tel: 0279-429655), 1991), price £85 including postage and packing.

This directory, as well as giving details of independent hospitals and health services, also details voluntary and private rest homes, nursing homes, and private bed accommodation in NHS hospitals. The directory should be available in reference libraries.

Elderly Accommodation Counsel
46A Chiswick High Road, London W4 1SZ (Tel: 081-742 1182/081-995 8320).

EAC has a database (see page 102) which includes information on residential homes and nursing homes. A search fee of £5 is normally charged.

Finding Residential and Nursing Home Accommodation
Age Concern England fact sheet No.29 (see page 103)

Gives information to older people who are considering going to live permanently in either a residential or a nursing home. It poses some of the questions which need to be asked before the decision about going to live in a home is made and also gives details of sources of help. The fact sheet also discusses alternatives to going into a home.

National Care Homes Association
5 Bloomsbury Place, London WC1A 2QA (Tel: 071-436 1871).

NCHA was formed in 1982 by a group of care home owners whose main aim was to raise standards throughout the care sector for the benefit of residents. Since 1987, nursing homes have also been admitted to membership and NCHA now claims to be the largest and fastest growing representative body of care home owners in the United Kingdom.

NCHA offers advice and guidance to people who are seeking accommodation.

=► *Registered Nursing Homes Association*
Calthorpe House, Hagley Road, Edgbaston, Birmingham B16 8QY
(Tel: 021-454 2511).

More than 1,200 registered nursing homes are members of this Association. The sign of the Blue Cross indicates that homes have achieved and are maintaining standards set by the Association. All of the premises are inspected and membership is terminated if standards are not maintained to an acceptable level. The Association will provide information on these homes and publishes a directory of them.

Further information

=► *At Home in a Home*
By Pat Young (Age Concern England, 1988), available from Central Books, 99 Wallis Road, London E9 5LN, price £3.95.

The questions asked by older people when they are considering moving into residential accommodation are answered in this practical guide. The topics covered include fees, financial support and standards of care.

=► *But Can I Bring My Cat?*
(Scottish Consumer Council, 314 St Vincent Street, Glasgow G3 8XW, 1987), price £2.

This is an analysis of brochures produced for old people entering residential and nursing homes in Scotland. The Scottish Consumer Council is dissatisfied with many of the brochures they have seen and are making strong recommendations, for example that all those who run homes for elderly people should be required by law to produce informative handbooks. This book could be useful reading for anyone considering going into a home because it sets out the issues to be considered and the sort of information needed, while at the same time assessing the sort of written information the homes give out, or unfortunately, often do not give out.

=► *Help for People Who Live in Residential Care Homes or Nursing Homes*
(DSS leaflet, IS 50), free. Available from DSS offices.

=► *Living in Homes*
By Leonie Kellaher, Sheila Peace and Dianne Willcocks (BASE in association with CESSA, available from either). BASE, 119 Hassell Street, Newcastle under Lyme,

Staffordshire ST5 1AX. CESSA, Dept of Applied Social Studies, Polytechnic of North London, Ladbroke House, Highbury Grove, London N5 2AD. Price £3 including postage. Cheques should be made payable to BASE.

The British Association for Service to the Elderly (BASE) and the Centre for Environmental and Social Studies in Ageing (CESSA) have published jointly this consumer guide to residential homes – particularly those run by local authorities. The guide is based on information gained from 1,000 elderly people who were living in 100 local authority homes. The book aims first to inform older people and their relatives about the kind of life-style they may expect within their local authority residential homes, and second to encourage all potential residents to ask questions, so that they have as much information as possible on which to base their decisions.

This well-written guide describes very clearly the implications of moving into a home and thoughtfully discusses the very difficult decisions that have to be made. Many older people may choose to go into a home because they are lonely, but then there are residents who say they are lonely living in a home. There may be little privacy and staff may expect them to live a completely communal life, which may feel as unnatural as living alone.

The book disturbingly points out that two-thirds of those interviewed had not viewed the home before they went in. Although this may be partly accounted for through the need for emergency admissions, it is clearly a very unsatisfactory process. An additional source of estrangement was the policy of homes not to allow incoming residents to bring in any possessions other than small items and clothing. All furniture had to be discarded.

Residential routines also came in for criticism. While a home might claim to be flexible, in practice strict routines were mostly observed.

While the homes were not identified and therefore the comments were general, nevertheless the book is very helpful in helping older people to make decisions about where they are going to live, what expectations they can have if they decide to go into a home, and what demands they can make.

Residential Care: Is it for me?
By Rosemary Bland (1987), with cartoons by Donald Gunn, for Age Concern Scotland, published by HMSO but also available from Age Concern Scotland, 54A Fountainbridge, Edinburgh EH3 9PT (Tel: 031-228 5656), price £2.95.

The information in this booklet is presented in a very lively style with questions and answers and cartoon illustrations. It attempts to answer some of the very difficult questions to be considered when trying to decide whether to move into a home. First, it asks why you should consider going into a home and what the alternatives are, who runs homes, how to get into one, and what the costs are likely to be – and then goes on to discuss in detail life inside homes.

'Can I take a bath when I wish?' 'Can I have visitors when I want?' are the kinds of questions older residents advised Age Concern to deal with in the book. Questions on medical care, privacy, meals and illness or death in the home are answered clearly and simply. Throughout, the emphasis is on advising elderly people and their carers to take nothing for granted, but to ask about aspects of residential care that concern them.

This book provides an excellent and much-needed guide to the sorts of questions you should ask before making such a fundamental decision.

Television licence concessions

Concessions are available to retired people of pensionable age (60 for women and 65 for men) and disabled, mentally handicapped or mentally ill people who live in certain types of accommodation. This includes residential homes as defined by the National Assistance Act 1948 and residential homes and nursing homes as defined by the Registered Homes Act 1984, almshouses established on or before 1 November 1949, and sheltered housing estates which are comparable to residential homes in that they:

— are specially provided or managed by a local authority or a housing association solely for pensioners or disabled people;
— form a cohesive group of at least four dwellings, within a common and exclusive boundary;
— have a resident warden, or one who works solely on the scheme for at least 30 hours each week.

The fee for the special Accommodation for Residential Care Licence is £5 per unit of accommodation, but the use of sets in communal rooms or by staff (including resident wardens in their private accommodation) must be licensed at the standard rate.

Registered blind people (irrespective of where they live) can obtain a TV licence for £1.25 below the standard fee.

Further information

Further information and application forms are available from: ARC Section, National TV Licence Records Office, Bristol BS98 1TL (Tel: 0272-230130).

A more detailed explanation of the concessions is given in Age Concern England's Fact Sheet No.3, available from 1268 London Road, London SW16 4ER (Tel: 081-679 8000) (*see* page 103).

Household insurance

Special insurance facilities for people over 60

Age Concern Insurance Services
Garrod House, Chaldon Road, Caterham, Surrey CR3 5YZ (Tel: 0883-346964).

Age Concern operates a home contents and buildings insurance scheme for older people, from the above address.

Helpful organisations 101

▣▶ *Saga Services Ltd*
The Saga Building, Middelburg Square, Folkestone, Kent CT20 1AZ (Freephone: 0800-414525).

Saga offers a Homecare Plan for buildings and contents, restricted to people aged 55 or more. Premiums are said to reflect Saga's experience that because people of this age group are more conscious of the need for security and safety they represent a much reduced insurance risk.

Further information

▣▶ *Association of British Insurers (ABI)*
51 Gresham Street, London EC2V 7HO (Tel: 071-600 3333)

ABI has a free guide, *Buildings Insurance for Home Owners*, which aims to help you to arrange insurance protection for your home. It describes the property a policy covers and the types of risk insured. It also gives helpful advice on working out how much cover you should have according to the size and type of your property and its location. ABI point out that the information is of a general nature and that insurers may differ in the cover they provide and in their terms and conditions.

▣▶ *The Office of Fair Trading*
Field House, 15–25 Bream's Buidings, London EC4A 1PR (Tel: 071-242 2858).

OFT, with the Association of British Insurers, has produced a free brief guide to household insurance. It includes advice on how and where to complain.

Helpful organisations

▣▶ *Age Concern*
(for addresses *see* Section 14)

Almost all Age Concern groups take an active role to ensure that local elderly people are made aware of any relevant schemes offering financial or practical help with housing matters.
  Age Concern England issues a range of free fact sheets which provide brief, but accurate, impartial information and advice to people who want to move to other forms of accommodation as well as to those wanting to stay put. It has also produced a number of indispensable publications on housing issues.
  Age Concern Scotland has a Housing Policy and Projects Department which answers enquiries on housing matters, campaigns on housing issues and runs several Care and Repair projects.

102 House and home

▶ *The Almshouse Association (The National Association of Almshouses)*
Billingbear Lodge, Wokingham, Berkshire RG11 5RU (Tel: 0344-52922).

This Association is a charity which aims to assist and advise trustees of almshouses. There are over 1,750 almshouse charities in membership of the Association throughout the United Kingdom, about 80 per cent of the total. The Association can tell you whether there are any such charities in a particular location.

▶ *Centre for Accessible Environments*
35 Great Smith Street, London SW1P 3BJ (Tel: 071-222 7980).

The Centre for Accessible Environments, established in 1969, is the national voluntary organisation concerned with improving the design of the built environment to accommodate the needs of all users, including elderly and disabled people.

The Centre offers an information and advisory service on design and technical matters, including application of the building regulations; publishes design guidance and a journal; administers a national register of architects with experience of designing for disabled people; and runs an extensive seminar training programme for the professions involved in building provision.

▶ *Elderly Accommodation Counsel*
46A Chiswick High Road, London W4 1SZ (Tel: 081-995 8320 or 081-742 1182).

EAC is a charity service to aid retired or elderly people obtain detailed information on suitable types of accommodation available to them throughout the United Kingdom. It has created a central, national register of information, on computer, of all types of accommodation in the charity, voluntary and private sectors. This register includes sheltered housing in the private sector, voluntary sector sheltered housing through housing associations, sheltered accommodation (mainly in the voluntary sector), residential care homes and nursing homes, and hospices for those who are terminally ill.

Public sector sheltered housing and residential care homes are not included, as admission to these is at the discretion of the appropriate local authority.

On completion of a questionnaire you will be supplied with computer printouts which give details of: type of accommodation; who it is owned and run by – private individual, company, voluntary organisation, charity; the person to contact, with a telephone number; what it consists of, that is, numbers and types of rooms; what it offers in terms of facilities and amenities; the range of prices; type of location; and accessibility. Should any of the places given in the computer printouts appear suitable, you must then make contact direct to discuss vacancies and to arrange a visit.

A search fee of £5 is payable, although for anyone on a limited income this fee may be waived.

▶ *The Federation of Private Residents' Associations Ltd*
11 Dartmouth Street, London SW1H 9BL (Tel: 071-222 0037).

A co-ordinating body for tenants' and residents' associations in England and Wales. It provides a pack on how to form a tenants' or leaseholders' association in a block of flats/maisonettes or a conversion. It also advises member associations on the rights of tenants and obligations of landlords under various housing legislation.

> *The National Association of Estate Agents*
> Arbon House, 21 Jury Street, Warwick CV34 4EH (Tel: 0926-496800).

The NAEA has established a National Homelink Service which offers a free referral service to anyone wishing to buy or sell a property in another town or district. The scheme operates through local Homelink members, all of whom are governed by the NAEA Code of Conduct. For further information, telephone the Homelink Administrator on 0926-410785 or 0926-496800.

> *SHAC (The London Housing Aid Centre)*
> 189a Old Brompton Road, London SW5 0AR (Tel: 071-373 7276).

SHAC is a registered charity and provides a broad range of help and advice on housing matters throughout London. SHAC aims to be a place to which a person with any housing problem can go for help. Among other activities it has a legal unit. The work undertaken includes: legal advice to caseworkers, legal representation of clients, and participation in SHAC's training courses. SHAC's publications include guides on buying a home, housing rights, housing benefit, rights to repair and renovation grants.

> *Shelter – National Campaign for Homeless People*
> 88 Old Street, London EC1V 9HU (Tel: 071-253 0202).

Shelter provides free and confidential advice through a network of Housing Aid Centres to anyone experiencing housing problems. Details of your nearest centre can be obtained from the address above. Shelter also produces publications, runs training courses, and campaigns on homelessness and housing issues. In the Greater London area, Shelter Nightline (0800-446441) offers free telephone advice overnight and at weekends for people with housing problems.

Books and publications

Publications about aids and equipment for use in the home are referred to in Section 4.

> *Age Concern England*
> 1268 London Road, London SW16 4ER (Tel: 081-679 8000).

Age Concern's publications include the following fact sheets and books about housing for older people.

104 House and home

Fact sheets:
No. 2 *Sheltered Housing for Sale*
No. 6 *Finding Help at Home*
No. 8 *Rented Accommodation for Older People*
No. 9 *Rented Accommodation for Older People in Greater London*
No. 10 *Local Authorities and Residential Care*
No. 13 *Older Home Owners: Financial help with repairs*
No. 24 *Housing Schemes for Older People Where a Capital Sum is Required*
No. 29 *Finding Residential and Nursing Home Accommodation*

Single copies of these fact sheets are available free of charge in response to a request accompanied by a 9" × 6" stamped addressed envelope.

Books:
Available by mail order from Central Books, 99 Wallis Road, London E9 5LN (Tel: 081-986 4854). All prices include postage and packing.

Buying a Home
By John Smythe (SHAC, 189a Old Brompton Road, London SW5 0AR (Tel: 071-373 7276), 1991), price £4.95 including postage and packing.

This guide explores the various ways of financing house purchase and the pitfalls which await the unwary.

Counsel and Care for the Elderly Publications
Twyman House, 16 Bonny Street, London NW1 9LR (Tel: 071-485 1550).

Counsel and Care have a range of publications, including an Information Sheet *Accommodation for People Over Retirement Age*, and fact sheets: *What to Look For in a Private or Voluntary Home; Help at Home* – a guide to getting care or assistance at home to enable a disabled or frail person to cope with everyday living; and *Special Accommodation For Elderly People*. Fact sheets are free of charge, but please send a s.a.e.

Good Retirement Guide
By Rosemary Brown (Kogan Page Ltd, 120 Pentonville Road, London N1 9JN, 1992), price £12.99.

This excellent guide, which is described on page 356, includes a section *Your Home*, which briefly covers housing options, improvements and repairs, safety and security, using your home to raise money, housing benefit and the community charge.

Housing Options For Older People
By David Bookbinder (1991), price £4.95.

This book carefully considers all the options open to retired people and their practical implications.

Books and publications

◻▶ *Housing Rights Guide*
By Geoffrey Randall (SHAC, 189a Old Brompton Road, London SW5 0AR (Tel: 071-373 7276), 4th edition, 1991), price £6.95 including postage and packing.

A guide for all tenants and leaseholders, which has established itself as the leading publication in the field.

◻▶ *Housing Year Book 1992*
(Longman UK Limited, Consumer Services Department, 4th Avenue, Harlow, Essex CM19 5AA, December 1991), price £57.50 including postage and packing.

This directory includes information on local authority housing agencies and related departments in the United Kingdom, details of major British housing associations, advice centres and co-ordinating voluntary organisations. The *Year Book* should be available in public libraries.

◻▶ *Living and Retiring Abroad*
(See page 359 for details.)

Part 3 of this *Daily Telegraph* guide, now in its fifth edition, gives information on all aspects of seeking and securing a home overseas.

◻▶ *An Owner's Guide: Your home in retirement* (1990), price £2.50.

This book sets out to show how a home can be made more comfortable and easy to manage in retirement. Information on subjects such as repairs and maintenance, heating and insulation, home security (including alarm schemes) and fixtures and adaptations for disabled people are included.

◻▶ *Owning Your Flat – A practical guide to problems with your lease and landlord*
By Ed Jankowski and Perri (SHAC, 189a Old Brompton Road, London SW5 0AR (Tel: 071-373 7276), 3rd edition, 1991), price £3.95 including postage and packing.

This guide, written by two solicitors with extensive experience of such cases, outlines the problems of owning your own flat and provides guidance to help you avoid some of the pitfalls that await the unwary or inexperienced purchaser.

◻▶ *Retirement Homes and Finance*
A two-monthly retirement property magazine. Subscription £6.00 to: Subscription Department, Retirement Homes, Selwood Press Ltd, Suite 83/84, 12/13 Henrietta Street, London WC2B 8LH (Tel: 071-379 0249).

This magazine is packed with profiles of retirement developments at a range of prices and details of investments. It also has a retirement property index at the end of each edition. It is available on bookstalls.

Rights Guide for Homeowners
By Jan Luba and Derek McConnell (SHAC, 189a Old Brompton Road, London SW5 0AR (Tel: 071-373 7276), 8th edition, 1991), price £5.50 including postage and packing.

Aimed at home owners on a tight budget, and their advisers, this guide gives practical advice on negotiating with lenders, meeting repair bills, the problems associated with relationship breakdown and the welfare benefits to which home owners may be entitled.

Rights to Repair: A guide for council tenants

Rights to Repair: A guide for private tenants

Rights to Repair: A guide for housing association tenants
By John Gallagher (SHAC, 189a Old Brompton Road, London SW5 0AR (Tel: 071-373 7276), 1991), each £3.95 including postage and packing.

Warm Toes Burnt Fingers?
(Age Concern Scotland, 54A Fountainbridge, Edinburgh EH3 9PT (Tel: 031-228 5656).

A report on private sheltered housing reflecting the views of both developers and residents. It looks at the growing market for retirement housing and examines the problems experienced by some residents.

SECTION FOUR

Equipment for daily living

As we get older so our strength lessens and we lose some of our agility and dexterity. Routine household tasks and other daily living activities become harder to manage. Many of us are reluctant to admit that we need extra help, and we go on struggling to cope in the ways to which we have become accustomed. It does not make a lot of sense. Equipment to help with particular tasks is a perfectly normal feature of everyday living, either to extend the range of our activities or to compensate for some limitation. In virtually every aspect of living, equipment has been developed to help us with physical and sensory problems: from simple devices like bottle openers to sophisticated computer technology. A vast range of equipment is now available which can make life a lot easier and safer: such things as alarm systems, clothing to keep out the cold, mobility equipment, lifts of various kinds, adjustable chairs and beds, equipment to help in getting in and out of the bath, and tools which take the effort out of gardening.

Because the range of equipment is so wide, however, it can be difficult to find information on just what is available and is best suited to meet personal needs. It is easy to waste money on a product which you have seen advertised only to find that it is not right for you. If there is one thing worse than an unmet need, it is a need which is met inappropriately. Unfortunately, in practice, many items of equipment are acquired which are found to be unsuitable, difficult to use, or unnecessarily expensive. The best advice is to go somewhere where you can see a range of equipment and try it out. Although you may not think of yourself as disabled, the most convenient opportunity of seeing just what is available is to visit one of the increasing number of Disabled Living Centres. You will find details of these on page 116. By appointment, you can see a range of equipment and enlist the advice of a trained adviser. The great advantage of these centres is that you can get unbiased advice, so that you choose wisely. If you cannot visit a centre, much helpful guidance as to the many items of special equipment which are available and how they can be used can be gained from one of the specialist information services (*see* page 115), from books (*see* from page 117 onwards), from your doctor, or from social service departments of local authorities.

Categories

It is impracticable in this short section to list and describe all the special equipment currently available. The choice is vast, and the following paragraphs provide only a brief description of some of the more widely used aids.

Bathroom and personal hygiene equipment

With the right equipment and good design, a bathroom can be made a welcoming and safe place. Problems of getting in and out of a bath can be overcome, though some people will find showering much easier, particularly if a shower chair is used. Equipment includes handrails; bathlifters and hoists; rubber bath mats; lavatory backrests; and lever-operated taps.

Shallow baths are much easier to get in and out of than conventional designs; some have a slip resistant finish. Baths with built-in seating are also available. Alternatively, there are several kinds of shaped bath inserts, sometimes incorporating a seat, which can be fitted inside an existing bath and removed after use.

Another kind of sit-in bath is simply a shortened bath with a raised part to sit in. In some of these, mainly for the use of people in wheelchairs, the side lifts away to allow easy access direct from a chair.

Bath supports can make relaxing in the bath much more comfortable. A vacuum-controlled support, comprising a back cushion with two arms, is filled with polystyrene beads which take up the shape of the user. When the air is removed by a simple vacuum pump, the moulded shape becomes firm.

Specialised personal toilet accessories include nail brushes with suction pads which do not need to be held in the hand; long- or short-handled lambswool pads to enable you to reach difficult parts of your body; a nail clipper that fits on to your cutting hand with finger-retaining mounts; and wall-mounted dispensers for toothpaste, hand cream, etc.

If you find that the toilet seat is a little too low for comfort, a raised seat can be fitted. There are also toilet rising seats, some with backrest and arm supports, which help the user to be raised or lowered at the touch of a button. If self-cleansing has become a problem, there are automatic WCs which provide flushing, warm water washing and hot-air drying all in one simple operation.

Bedroom equipment

We spend a great deal of time in bed, so should be comfortable there, especially during periods of ill health. Good beds are expensive and it is therefore important to take advice to ensure that you buy the bed which is right for you. Adjustable beds can provide a great deal of flexible comfort and will have one or more of the following features: 'knees up', raising the upper part of the body, raising the feet, adjustable height. Alternatively, you can buy inflatable sub-mattresses, operated by low pressure air supplied by a small power unit, which angle the head of the regular mattress and slightly raise the lower section beneath the knees.

Back rests, with wooden or metal frames, can make sitting up in bed more comfortable. Once there, you may want an overbed table. There is a fairly wide range available, most having adjustable height and castors. A few models have book stops and book supports which can be set at various angles – though these usually come separately. If you want to do extensive work in bed, you can buy an overbed work centre strong enough to support heavy typewriters, etc. This has a square metal frame on four castors. The height of the table and its angle are adjustable. There is also a side table which can be swung away as required.

Comfortable chairs for the living room

Rising seats are particularly helpful if you find it difficult to get up from the depths of an easy chair! Quite a number of firms produce chairs of this kind. In some of them, the electrically powered seat, staying in a horizontal plane, raises the sitter to an almost standing position. In others, the seat or tilt-riser tips up. Seat lifting mechanisms which may be fitted to suitable chairs are also available.

Gardening tools

Many lightweight tools are now available which are specially designed to take the strain out of gardening. The considerable range of long-handled tools is an example. Weeding and planting can be made easier by the use of a kneeling stool, or an electric weeder which breaks up the ground. If you have trouble bending, or are in a wheelchair, raised beds can bring gardening within your reach. These can be supplied made from fibreglass or from fibre-reinforced concrete; some have exteriors attractively constructed with preserved and finished timber sections, others are cast in York stone.

Specialist information is available from a number of organisations, but the best, in our opinion, is the Society for Horticultural Therapy, Goulds Ground, Vallis Way, Frome, Somerset BA11 3DW (Tel: 0373-64782), which runs a service for gardeners with special needs. Its lively magazine *Growth Point* provides a wealth of information, along with *Come Gardening*, a quarterly magazine on tape or in braille for blind gardeners. The Society will provide a list of tools and equipment and will be glad to answer specific queries (please send a s.a.e.).

Hearing impairment

Hearing loss is one of the commonest problems of older people. It is, of course, something about which you will need medical advice. If you need a hearing aid, you will normally be referred to a hearing aid centre by your doctor. NHS hearing aids are nowadays much more cosmetically acceptable and unobtrusive. There are a considerable number of hearing aids which are commercially available, but many of these are expensive, and there has been some evidence of exploitation in this area. Watch out for false, exaggerated claims (and exaggerated prices) and take impartial advice before purchase. There is a British Standard for hearing aids, BS 6083.

Many other devices have been developed for people with hearing impairment. These include induction loops, visual 'doorbells', special alarm clocks, sound activated visual alarms, TV listening devices, telephone bells and amplifiers, and telephone keyboard communication systems.

≡▶ *The Royal National Institute for Deaf People*
105 Gower Street, London WC1E 6AH [Tel: 071-387 8033 (voice), 071-388 6038 (Qwerty), 071-383 3154 (Minicom), 071-388 2346 (Fax)] publishes a range of helpful publications.

≡▶ British Telecom (Freephone: voice 0800-800 150; text 0800-243 123) has a free guide, *The BT Guide For People Who Are Disabled Or Elderly 1992: The latest products and services to help you use the phone.*

Household equipment

This includes key turners and levers; hot water bottle stands to assist filling; easy-grip handles for electric plugs (better still if they are raised to a convenient height); and non-slip trays; some of which are designed to be carried in one hand.

Kitchen/eating equipment

Many specialised devices are produced to help older people to manage basic domestic tasks. Some of them are simple labour-saving utensils which are readily available in local shops. If your sight is failing, the Royal National Institute for the Blind (*see* page 345) lists and stocks many relevant items.

Kitchen utensils include cutting boxes or guides to help with bread cutting and buttering; kettle and saucepan stabilisers with magnetic feet; special peelers and scrapers, some for use with one hand; long tongs, grips and reachers; lever operated taps, some of which can be extended for use by hand or elbow; and wall-mounted can openers. There is even a device which lifts eggs out of the boiling water into cups with suction bases. For people who have particular functional difficulties, kitchens can now be designed and fitted to suit individual needs. A number of firms provide such a service, taking into account the needs of elderly people.

Eating and drinking utensils include a range of dishes with deep and curved walls, some of which can be heated with hot water in the base to keep food warm for slow eaters; non-slip mats; specially designed beakers and cups for those who find conventional cups difficult to hold or balance; cutlery which is easy to grip, including carving and bread knives with push–pull action.

The Disabled Living Foundation (*see* page 118) has a number of helpful books in this subject area.

Mobility equipment

If you need a walking frame or walking stick it will normally be medically prescribed. There are, however, many different types available, with a wide variety of grips, and you may wish to have something better than the standard hospital issue. Some walking frames have shopping basket attachments or incorporate seats. Relevant British Standards are BS 5104 (adjustable height walking frames), BS 5205 (adjustable metal walking sticks), BS 4922 (metal tripod and tetrapod walking sticks) and BS 5181 (wooden walking sticks). Walking sticks are available with lights, reflectors and alarms, as well as in stick seat versions. A huge range of ferrules and tips can be chosen.

Low speed pavement vehicles can be a boon to people with walking difficulties who want to travel relatively short distances for shopping etc. Brief guidance of their selection is given in Section 11, Getting Around and About.

Those whose mobility problems are caused by sight loss will find a new In Touch booklet, *Getting About Safely*, helpful in providing details of the various types of white sticks and how they should be used, as well as giving information about more sophisticated equipment such as sonic aids; available in large print or braille from Broadcasting Support Services, PO Box 7, London W3 6XJ or on audio cassette from RNIB, PO Box 173, Peterborough PE2 0WS, price £1.75.

Pressure relief

Prolonged periods of immobility can cause very painful pressure sores which are difficult to clear up. There is a considerable range of beds specially designed to reduce susceptibility to this problem and to provide greater comfort. These include air beds, some with a 'ripple' air supply, ribbed foam mattresses, suspended net beds and water beds. Also helpful are bed fleeces, pads for vulnerable parts of the body and special cushions and rings. This is most certainly an area in which you need to make careful enquiries and to seek advice.

Purpose-made equipment

Problems which arise as we get older may require equipment purpose-made to overcome particular disabilities. In such cases, the specialist organisation REMAP GB Technical Equipment for Disabled People offers engineering help, advice and research. It brings together engineers who, advised appropriately by members of the medical and paramedical professions, design and make items of equipment to suit the special needs of handicapped individuals.

REMAP GB operates through over 90 local panels which will make every attempt to solve problems which have not been overcome by standard equipment. By taking a fresh look at difficult problems, these panels are often able to devise ingenious solutions. The number of panels continues to grow.

Although donations to the charity are welcome, REMAP GB's work is voluntary. Details of local REMAPs are available from 'Hazeldene', Ightham, Sevenoaks, Kent TN15 9AD (Tel: 0732-883818).

See also page 120 for information about *The REMAP Yearbook*.

Stairlifts and lifts

If you have difficulty in climbing stairs, a stairlift or a home lift can make life a great deal easier, and may allow you to stay put in a house which would otherwise be unsuitable.

Detailed safety standards as to the design, construction, installation, operation and maintenance of stairlifts are set out in British Standard 5776 (1979), for powered home lifts in BS 5900 (1980), and for manually driven balanced personal home lifts in BS 5965 (1980), but the adoption of these standards by manufacturers is voluntary. They become binding only if a claim of compliance is made or invoked in a contract.

In the case of stairlifts, if space allows, safe transfer is assisted (and the staircase left clear) if the stairlift run can be extended at top and bottom. Alternatively, a swivel seat is helpful. Design features vary, most significantly between models in which the motor is housed within the chair or platform unit and those which have an external motor (usually at the top of or under the stairs). There are lifts for straight or curved staircases, and a number which will carry a person in a wheelchair.

Vertical powered home lifts are also available in a number of different designs. You can choose a lift which is enclosed on both the upper and lower floors and travels in a shaft, or one which is enclosed only on the upper floor and is carried on guide rails bolted to a sound wall. If space is very limited, or if cost needs to be kept to a minimum, you can obtain a home lift with no enclosures at all. In these, a compact open-top car designed to carry a seated passenger opens a ceiling trapdoor as the lift ascends, which returns to the closed position on descent. Various vertical wheelchair lifts are also available.

Before committing yourself to purchase. you would be well advised to seek expert advice (e.g. from your local Social Services Department) as to the suitability of particular lifts to your needs.

Visual handicap

Failing sight is a problem faced by many older people. Up to a point, of course, this can be corrected by suitable glasses and (something often neglected) good lighting as close as possible to your field of vision. If the problems are more serious, you will in the first instance wish to seek expert medical advice. There are also a number of organisations which will provide information, guidance and a variety of services relating to visual difficulties and low-vision aids. These include:

▶ *Royal National Institute for the Blind*
224 Great Portland Street, London W1N 6AA (Tel: 071-388 1266).

▶ *Optical Information Council*
57A Old Woking Road, West Byfleet, Weybridge, Surrey KT14 6LF (Tel: 0932-353283).

▶ *Partially Sighted Society*
62 Salusbury Road, London NW6 6NS (Tel: 071-372 1551).

A useful guide to basic equipment is *Articles Specially Designed Or Adapted For Blind People and Sold by RNIB*, available from the above RNIB address. For wider and more detailed advice, Thena Heshel and Margaret Ford's *In Touch Handbook* (Broadcasting Support Services) is invaluable. The print version can be obtained by post for £15 inclusive, from In Touch Handbook, PO Box 7, London W3 6XJ. Cheques should be made out to Broadcasting Support Services. A tape version costs £15 from RNIB, PO Box 173, Peterborough PE2 0WS. A braille version is available at a discounted price of £15 from Broadcasting Support Services, 252 Western Avenue, London W3 6XJ (Tel: 081-992 5522). Also helpful is the BBC's quarterly *In Touch Bulletin* (contact In Touch, BBC, Broadcasting House, London W1A 4WW for details).

In Touch has also produced a simple Care Guide, *Coping with Sight Loss at 80+*, available in large print or braille from Broadcasting Support Services, PO Box 7, London W3 6XJ or on audio cassette from RNIB, PO Box 173, Peterborough PE2 0WS, price £1.75.

Sources of supply

Statutory provision of equipment by local authorities

Many items of equipment are, of course, available commercially. But if you are disabled, you can ask your local social services department to provide necessary equipment or home adaptations. Local authorities also have the power to provide, or help to obtain, special aids to hearing for deaf people. These are known as environmental aids, for example flashing doorbells, vibrator pillows and induction loop systems. There is also special help for people who are visually impaired.

Statutory provision of equipment by the National Health Service

In general, equipment required in connection with medical and nursing care at home is supplied through the NHS. This can include ripple beds, cushions, hoists, and incontinence protection. General practitioners have lists of equipment which may be prescribed where necessary. They can also recommend to the Department of Health that large items be prescribed, even though they may not be on the regular list.

In the case of hearing aids, a wide range of modern devices is now available through the NHS. Doctors can refer their patients to a special clinic at a local hospital for examination. If a hearing aid is found to be necessary, patients are then referred to a hearing aid centre, where the appliance will be fitted and supplied. Hearing aids are also available on free loan. NHS hearing aids are serviced, maintained and supplied with batteries free of charge.

Not all equipment supplied under prescription is free, but where it is for the personal or domestic use of a disabled person, it normally carries the zero rate of value added tax.

Advice on the problems of incontinence should be sought from health visitors, district nurses or social workers. Both District Health Authorities (DHAs) and local authority social services departments can supply incontinence pads to people who live in their own homes. However, while DHAs may not charge for them, local authorities may do so, according to local policy. They cannot be prescribed by GPs, nor dispensed by chemists under the NHS, and it is left to the discretion of the supplying authority to decide the type of pad to be provided, to whom they will be supplied, and how they are delivered.

Equipment available on mail-order

See Books and Publications at the end of this section.

Equipment available on loan

▶ *British Red Cross Society*
9 Grosvenor Crescent, London SW1X 7EJ (Tel: 071-235 5454).

British Red Cross maintains 1,000 loan depots throughout the United Kingdom, each stocked to supply equipment such as wheelchairs, walking frames and commodes on short-term loan to members of the local community to meet urgent needs, for use at home or on holiday. Charges are very modest and can be waived in cases of hardship. Some depots operate a system of voluntary donations.

Information services

The principal national services specialising in the provision of information about equipment are as follows:

⇒ *Disabled Living Foundation Information Service*
380–4 Harrow Road, London W9 2HU (Tel: 071-289 6111; also available on Telecom Gold 84; DD P002).

The DLF information service and database offers a comprehensive service to disabled people and others requiring information on equipment and services. Information is available in the form of regularly updated product lists (*see* page 118) and/or on-line from DLF-DATA, a computerised database. This system is the most advanced in Europe and compares favourably with any other in this area worldwide. Benefits include fast accurate recall of information and a comprehensive range of help screens and search prompts. The DLF's services are normally supplied on subscription, but specific information in response to enquiries is free to disabled people.

The DLF also provides advisory services on clothing, footwear and incontinence. All these advisory services can give information and guidance in response to enquiries from people with disabilities and their families. The Information Service is open 10.00 a.m. to 4.00 p.m., Mondays to Fridays.

Send s.a.e. for catalogue of Resource Papers and Advice Notes.

⇒ *Northern Ireland Information Service for Disabled People*
2 Annadale Avenue, Belfast BT7 3JR (Tel: 0232-491011).

Information is available about the supply of equipment and housing adaptations. A subscription service based on the Disabled Living Foundation service is available, with regular dispatch of updating materials.

⇒ *Disability Scotland Information Service*
5 Shandwick Place, Edinburgh EH2 4RG (Tel: 031-229 8632).

With the most comprehensive bank of literature, contacts and computer databases in Scotland, enquiries can be answered on all aspects of disability (except the purely medical). Information directories in various subject areas are published and regularly updated. A mobile advice centre tours Scotland during the summer months.

⇒ *Wales Council for the Disabled (Cyngor Cymru I'r Anabl)*
'Llys Ifor', Crescent Road, Caerphilly, Mid Glamorgan CF8 1XL (Tel: 0222-887325)

Provides a wide-ranging information service on disability issues, both centrally and through a mobile disability advice and information unit.

Equipment centres

Disabled living centres

These Centres provide an equipment exhibition/demonstration and information service. Most centres cover wider aspects of daily living; some also have specialist advisory/support services. Centres employ trained staff who offer impartial advice. Further detailed information is available from:

The Disabled Living Centres Council (DLCC)
286 Camden Road, London N7 0BJ (Tel: 071-700 1707).

At the time of writing, there are centres in the following places (addresses from telephone directories or contact the DLCC in any case of difficulty): Aberdeen; Aylesbury; Belfast; Birmingham; Blackpool; Bodelwyddan; Braintree; Caerphilly; Cardiff; Colchester; Edinburgh; Exeter; Huddersfield; Hull; Inverness; Leeds; Leicester; Liverpool; London (DLF); Macclesfield; Manchester; Middlesbrough; Newcastle upon Tyne; Nottingham; Paisley; Portsmouth; Semington (Wiltshire); Southampton; Stockport; Swansea; Swindon; Welwyn Garden City.

Communication aids centres

These Centres, which usually operate in a hospital setting, offer assessment, advice and training in the use of communication aids. Access to such services will normally be by referral from a speech therapist.

Centres for blind and partially sighted people

Disabled Living Centres and Communication Aids Centres have a range of equipment for blind and partially sighted people (though this may be limited at the DLCs).

The Partially Sighted Society has a National Low Vision Advice Centre at Dean Clarke House, Southernhay East, Exeter EX1 1PE (Tel: 0392-210656).

The Royal National Institute for the Blind, 224 Great Portland Street, London W1N 6AA (Tel: 071-388 1266) displays and sells a wide range of equipment, both sophisticated and simple, to help visually handicapped people in their everyday lives. Many games such as chess, backgammon and ludo have also been specially adapted. There are also a large number of resource centres in other localities. These vary considerably in size and format. Some are large centres maintaining a sizeable range of literature and equipment, including training kitchens and hi-tech displays. Others are small information and advice points, with a limited selection of items of interest to visually handicapped people. The RNIB will advise on facilities in any particular area.

Centres for deaf and hearing impaired people

We know of the following Centres:

▶ *National Deaf Children's Society,*
Technology Information Centre, 4 Church Road, Birmingham B15 3TD
(Tel: voice and text 021-454 5151).

This Centre provides information on environmental aids, radio aids and other equipment for deaf people. An exhibition room is full of equipment in working order, giving deaf people the opportunity to compare similar products. Please make a prior appointment.

▶ *Breakthrough Deaf–Hearing Integration,*
Birmingham Centre, Charles W.Gillett Centre, 998 Bristol Road, Selly Oak, Birmingham B29 6LE (Tel: 021-472 6447; Text: 021-471 1001; Fax: 021-471 4368).

Breakthrough's reference and loans library has an extensive range of books and literature concerned with deafness. Information is available on environmental aids which enable deaf people to live independent lives. An electronic mail service is in operation for deaf and deaf-blind subscribers, by means of which advice is given on the use of telecommunications equipment now available to deaf people.

▶ *Sound Advantage PLC,*
1 Metro Centre, Welbeck Way, Peterborough PE2 7UH (Tel: 0733-361199; Text 0733-238020).

This is a company set up by the Royal National Institute for Deaf People to market products for people with impaired hearing. All profits go to the RNID. The aim is to maintain in one place the most comprehensive stock of relevant products in the United Kingdom together with first-class customer service. A fully illustrated mail-order catalogue is also available. It should be remembered, of course, that many items may alternatively be available through the NHS (*see* page 114).

Books and publications

▶ *Designed for Living*
Arthritis Care, 18 Stephenson Way, London NW1 2HD (Tel: 071-916 1500).

A free catalogue which features 75 products specially chosen for people with arthritis, supplied by Keep Able Ltd.

Equipment for daily living

► *The DLF Information Service Handbook*
The Disabled Living Foundation Information Service, 380-34 Harrow Road, London W9 2HU (Tel: 071-289 6111).

This wide-ranging handbook about equipment is made up of loose-leaf sections which are updated annually. They include brief descriptions of items of equipment, addresses of manufacturers and/or suppliers, details of relevant publications and, if relevant, notes on supply. Section 12, Notes on Incontinence, has line drawings, and several others have comparative product tables. The numbered sections cost £10 each. The Handbook is also available on subscription. Similar lists are available from the Northern Ireland Information Service for Disabled People and Disability Scotland Information Services (*see* page 115). The relevant subject headings on the DLF list are:

- Beds and bed accessories
- Chairs and chair accessories
- Children's equipment (general)
- Children's equipment (mobility and support)
- Children's equipment (development and play)
- Clothing
- Communication (in two parts)
- Eating and drinking equipment
- Footwear
- Hoists, lifts and lifting equipment
- Household equipment
- Household and environmental fittings
- Notes on incontinence
- Leisure activities
- Office furniture and equipment (except computers)
- Personal toilet
- Personal care
- Powered wheelchairs, scooters and buggies
- Pressure relief
- Sport and physical recreation
- Telephones, alarms and intercoms
- Transport
- Equipment for standing and walking
- Wheelchairs (manual)

The DLF also publishes many books. Send s.a.e. for publications list.

► *Equipment for Disabled People*
The Disability Information Trust, Mary Marlborough Lodge, Nuffield Orthopaedic Centre, Windmill Road, Headington, Oxford OX3 7LD (Tel: 0865-750103).

This is a fully illustrated series of books presenting facts and comment on hundreds of products and ideas to help with daily living. They include specially manufactured

Books and publications

equipment, everyday consumer goods and do-it-yourself ideas, with details of manufacturers and distributors. Most of the items have been assessed and tested prior to inclusion. There is also guidance on points to consider before any purchase is made.

The books are not produced simultaneously, and, as will be seen from the publication dates given below, some are more up to date than others. Most of them, however, are revised and republished regularly. The full list of titles and prices is as follows:

— *Arthritis: An equipment guide* (1st edn, 1991), £12.50
— *Clothing and Dressing* (6th edn, 1989), £8.50
— *Communication* (7th edn, 1990), £12.50
— *Disabled Child* (5th edn, 1986), £7.00
— *Furniture* (replacing *Housing and Furniture* in 1992), £12.00
— *Gardening* (1st edn, 1987), £8.50
— *Hoists and Lifts* (2nd edn, 1990), £11.50
— *Home Management* (6th edn, 1987), £8.50
— *Incontinence and Stoma Care* (1st edn, 1984), £7.00
— *Outdoor Transport* (6th edn, 1987), £8.50
— *Parents with Disabilities* (1st edn, 1989), £8.50
— *Personal Care* (6th edn, 1990), £11.50
— *Walking Aids* (2nd edn, 1991), £9.00
— *Wheelchairs* (6th edn, 1988), £9.50

Binding case for complete set, £6.00.

Everyday Aids and Appliances

More Everyday Aids and Appliances
(British Medical Journal Books, BMA House, Tavistock Square, London WC1H 9JR (Tel: 071-383 6184, 1989 and 1991)), price £6.95 and £8.95 including postage and packing.

Critical evaluation of some of the various kinds of equipment available.

Help with Daily Living
Chester-care, Low Moor Estate, Kirkby-in-Ashfield, Nottinghamshire NG17 7JZ (Tel: 0623-755585).

This free mail-order catalogue is very clearly set out and particularly helpful in illustrating a wide range of basic equipment, with prices, and a useful product index.

The Keep Able Catalogue
Keep Able, 2 Capital Interchange Way, Brentford, Middlesex TW8 0EX (Tel: 081-742 2181).

Keep Able is a store specialising in aids and equipment for disabled people. Its mail-order catalogue provides a helpful, copiously illustrated guide to many everyday aids.

New Design for Old: Function, style and older people
By Eric Midwinter, Centre for Policy on Ageing, 25-31 Ironmonger Row, London EC1V 3QP, 1988, price £7.80 plus postage and packing.

This is a report designed to encourage the application of good design to homes, clothing and articles in daily use intended to make life easier for older people. It argues that designers should take a more careful look at this sizeable but often ignored sector, and that design should be improved to help people to cope with the impairments associated with old age (here as distinct from the problems of outright disability). Current developments are reviewed and the reader is taken through a 'day in the life' of an older person, and shown how design affects every aspect of living. Practical design solutions are described and illustrated. The view is stressed throughout that older people have as much right to a stylish as well as a practical life-style as any other sector of society, and the report concludes with recommendations to promote further work.

The REMAP Yearbook
REMAP GB – Technical Equipment for Disabled People, 'Hazeldene', Ightham, Sevenoaks, Kent TN15 9AD (Tel: 0732-883818), price £3 including postage and packing.

This *Yearbook* is inspiring, encouraging and worth every penny of its cover price. It gives examples of all kinds of equipment, shows exactly what REMAP is about and describes how others can help its work.

Simple Solutions
Age Concern England, Astral House, 1268 London Road, London SW16 4ER (Tel: 081-679 8000).

A 32-page, full colour mail-order catalogue produced in association with Chester-care Ltd. It contains details of over 600 products designed to facilitate independent daily living. The emphasis is on small gadgets, but a selection of larger products is included.

SECTION FIVE

Keeping warm

Keeping warm in our climate is no easy matter, and however we try there will be many times when we are not as warm as we would wish for comfort. When we are retired and spending more time at home, and perhaps not as active as we have been, we notice the temperature of our home much more. Comfort and a pleasant atmosphere to live in are impossible to achieve if we are cold, but paying for the high cost of heating can be a constant problem. Cold can seriously threaten our health, aiding and abetting a range of illnesses including strokes and respiratory diseases. Having a warm home in winter is more than a simple human pleasure: to many older people it can make all the difference between life and death.

Somehow, we need to look at every way possible of keeping warm, including wearing the most suitable clothing, eating warming and nourishing food and keeping active. At the same time we need to heat our homes in the most economical way and, most importantly, look at ways of insulating and improving our homes so that they retain heat.

In Section 3 we describe 'Care and Repair' and 'Staying Put' schemes which enable older people to look at ways in which their homes can be made more comfortable if they have decided they would like to stay put. Ways of financing these improvements are looked at, including any financial grants.

Energy projects are described on page 133.

In this Section we look at the ways in which it is possible to keep warm, and give information on the agencies who will help. First, we look at hypothermia and ways in which this may be avoided. While a number of initiatives are under way to help individuals avoid hypothermia, it is a shocking indictment of our society that any old person should suffer and die in this way.

Financial help

If you are on Income Support you may be able to get an extra £6 for each very cold week. For details see Section 1. You may also be able to get grants for draughtproofing and insulation. For details, if you live in England, Scotland or Wales ring (free call) 0800-181 667, where you will find information about who is eligible and how you apply. If you live in Northern Ireland and would like information on home insulation grants ring Energy Action Northern Ireland, 128 Great Victoria Street, Belfast BT2 7BG (Tel: 0232-333790).

Winter warmth lines

Winter warmth lines are there for any older person to use or for anyone who is concerned about an older person or anybody else who may be in danger from the cold, such as people with chronic illness or young children. The calls are free of charge. The staff will be glad to advise you about any aspect of keeping warm. They can put you in touch with local Community Insulation Projects and other groups who will be able to give practical help locally.

They will also send you a copy of the free *Keep Warm, Keep Well* campaign booklet. This booklet is available in English, Welsh, Chinese, Greek, Polish, Turkish, Bengali, Gujarati, Hindi, Punjabi and Urdu. Copies of the booklet are also available from: Keep Warm, Keep Well, FREEPOST, London SE5 7BP.

England and Wales:
 0800-289 404; text only Minicom for deaf people:
 0800-26 96 26.

Scotland:
 0800-838 587.

Northern Ireland:
 the combined Winter Warmth Line and the Social Security Benefit Line number is 0800-616 757.

Hypothermia

Hypothermia is a condition of very low deep body temperature resulting in serious illness. It happens when the inner body temperature falls too low to keep the body functioning normally. It is possible for hypothermia to set in without an elderly person realising what is happening. You may not feel cold but may feel muzzy in the head, weak and unable to control limbs. Walking and balance may become difficult. As we get older our bodies often find it more difficult to maintain a constant temperature, so when we are exposed to cold our body temperature may fall too. Older people have a lower metabolic rate than young people which means that they are producing less heat. The mechanisms controlling the body temperature may be further impaired by disease or by some of the drugs prescribed for illness or for other problems such as anxiety or insomnia.

Hypothermia sets in when our body temperature falls below 35 degrees C (95 degrees

F). (The normal body temperature of a healthy person is 98.4 degrees F (36.9 degrees C).) However, it is clearly important to take action well before the body temperature falls as low as 35 degrees. Because this temperature is often mentioned as the danger mark, it may be thought that all is well if that low temperature has not been reached, but this is not so. The further the temperature drops the more dangerous the situation. In addition, it needs to be remembered that the body is reacting to, and suffering from, the effects of cold long before the temperature has dropped far enough for hypothermia to be present.

Because our body temperatures are higher than the environment, human beings are constantly losing heat to the surroundings, but this is usually balanced by the heat produced by the body itself plus any extra heat being added, for instance from a hot water bottle. However, when the amount of heat being lost by the body is greater than the heat being produced by the body, the body will start to cool, and if this continues hypothermia will eventually develop.

Older people themselves may not always be aware of the dangers because, as we have said above, they may not realise how cold they are. It is important, therefore, for visitors to be aware of this. It is a sign of hypothermia if someone has a very cold skin or if no complaints of feeling cold are made in a bitterly cold room. Other danger signals are: drowsiness, slurred speech, unsteady movement, pale and puffy complexion, mental confusion, slow responses, slow pulse and breathing, and blue coloured lips. It is important to take action if the living room has a temperature of 16 degrees C (61 degrees F) or less. If a living room has a temperature of 12 degrees C (54 degrees F) or less there exists a crisis, and it is important to call for immediate medical help.

In these circumstances you should never give alcohol, encourage movement or exercise, make the bedcovers too heavy or apply direct heat to the body, for example a hot water bottle. Rather, you should move the person into warmer surroundings if possible, wrap the person in a light layer of blankets or a duvet to avoid further loss of body heat, give warm nourishing drinks and call a doctor or nurse.

It is generally agreed that living rooms should average 21 degrees C (70 degrees F) and bedrooms 16 degrees (61 degrees F) to 18 degrees C (64 degrees F). Throughout this Section we describe ways to keep warm and give information on agencies who will be glad to help, so that you can keep warm and, at all costs, avoid hypothermia.

Age Concern Scotland has produced a very useful book *Dangerous Cold*, subtitled *Hypothermia and cold related illness in older people*. This describes very clearly and in detail the state of hypothermia and how this is caused. It also makes recommendations on sensible precautions. It is available from Age Concern Scotland, 54A Fountainbridge, Edinburgh EH3 9PT, price: £1.50.

Warm clothing

In the daytime

Wearing several layers of lighter clothing is much warmer than wearing one heavy layer, and covering as much of the body as possible minimises heat loss. It is worth bearing in mind that clothes made from natural fibres – wool, cotton or silk – will keep you warmer than clothes made from nylon, acrylic and other synthetics. A great deal of body heat is lost through our heads, particularly when our hair is thinning, and it is important to wear hats when going out. It might also be advisable to wear a shawl and a comfortable woolly hat indoors and very wise to wear one in bed. While we are sitting a rug can be warm and comforting – not so comforting that we sit for too long! Keeping on the move is important. Those nice leg warmers are lovely to wear and very warming.

Wearing thermal underwear can make a considerable difference to our warmth. Such clothing, which may have been considered 'old fashioned' at one time, has made a comeback and is now worn by many people. Consequently, there is a wide variety of this clothing available.

Even if you are warm indoors it is still very important to wrap up warmly when going outside. Several light warm layers, a hat, gloves and scarf are essential to keep out the cold. It is also important to wear strong, warm shoes or boots when you go outside. A warm insole can be added to insulate your feet against cold ground underfoot, and if your boots are roomy enough you can put on an extra pair of socks as well.

It is advisable to dress and undress in an area which is warm. You could create a warm area if you have screens to cut out draughts. Clothing and nightwear should be warmed before being put on. You can speed up dressing and undressing by choosing clothes which are easy to put on and take off – raglan sleeves, long zips, large buttons and velcro closures all help.

In the night-time

Light bedclothing which is not constricting, like duvets, can provide the warmth we need while we sleep. Electric blankets can be a boon, but it is important not to keep electric underblankets on while you are in bed. If you do not have an electric blanket, hot water bottles can be a great comfort and, of course, you can keep them in bed to cuddle and to keep your feet warm. It is very important not to use an electric blanket together with a hot water bottle. Rubber hot water bottles should be filled with water that is not too hot, and should be covered to avoid any risk of scalds through leakage. As well as being dangerous to handle, boiling or very hot water will perish the rubber. Rubber hot water bottles can be difficult to fill. There are special holders you can buy which make this much easier. The Disabled Living Foundation (DLF) (address at the end of this Section) will be glad to send you, free of charge, details of firms producing these useful devices. The DLF will also be glad to send you details of electric blankets and pads.

Electric blankets, while being much safer than they used to be, still need to be treated with care. Underblankets must usually be switched off before you get into bed, unless the instructions specifically state it is safe to leave the blanket switched on. The Inventum low voltage electric underblanket is described as being safe to sleep on while it remains switched on, even if it becomes wet. It is also washable. Details are available from: Invent-Heat, PO Box 890, Templecombe, Somerset BA8 0RR. Another waterproof electric underblanket is available from: RC Heated Products, 202-4 Burrs Road, Clacton-on-Sea CO15 4LN. Tel: 0255-421784. Overblankets tend to be more expensive. These usually have a variable heat switch and many have to be turned down before getting into bed. RC Heated Products also have an electrical heating pad covered with fire-retardant, waterproof cover for use on top of the bed with side flaps for tucking under the mattress. A number of firms produce electric pads or cushions which are useful to place against aching or painful areas of the body either in bed or when sitting in a chair.

Wearing a woolly hat in bed can save a great deal of heat loss through your head which, of course, is above the bedclothes. We often do not realise just how much heat is lost through our heads. In fact, it is said we lose a third of body heat that way if our heads are uncovered. As well as a woolly hat, a woolly shawl and bedsocks will help to keep you warm in bed and provide a feeling of comfort. Keeping a hot drink in a flask by the bedside in case you wake feeling cold can be a good idea. It is always wise to keep a warm dressing gown and slippers beside the bed in case you need to get up during the night. You may feel it is a good idea to consider sleeping in the living room for the winter if your bedroom is very cold and is too expensive to warm.

Living and sleeping in one room in winter

While living and perhaps sleeping in one room can be a very good idea it is important not to overheat this one room. In a very warm room the body needs to produce less heat and the body's heat preserving machanisms relax. Then when you leave the overheated room, the relaxed heat preserving mechanisms cause you to lose a lot of heat before the heat preserving systems can restart, and there will be a similar delay before the body starts to produce more heat. You may, therefore, become quite severely chilled. There is another danger, in that repeated changes from overheated to very cold temperatures put a great strain on many functions of the body which may lead to breakdown. If you are going to sleep in the same room, it is best to avoid sleeping overnight in an easy chair; it is much better to have your bed moved if you can. A commode by the bed may save you from leaving a warm room at night.

The Health Education Board for Scotland has a very useful resource pack, *Keep Warm This Winter*. For details *see* page 140.

Eating and drinking for warmth

The right food and drink are vitally important to keeping you warm and healthy in the long winter months. Aim to eat hot meals rather than cold food and drink plenty of hot drinks between meals. It is a good idea to start the day with a hot breakfast. Soups, preferably home-made, can provide warmth and nourishment and, with the addition of lentils, brown rice or pearl barley, can be a meal as well. In addition, a warm drink before going to bed may help to keep you warm. Also it might be a good idea to keep a vacuum flask filled with a hot drink by your bedside in case you wake up in the night feeling cold.

It is essential not to skimp on food, because not only is food the source of energy for activity and for producing heat, but the act of eating and digesting food generates body heat. It is important to remember that energy requirements are increased in cold weather. Adequate feeding will maintain the minimal heat production of the body at a satisfactory level – even eating a single meal raises the minimal heat production for several hours.

The book *Dangerous Cold* (*see* page 138) says that because 'fat produces more energy per unit of weight than any other food', therefore 'old people in winter should not discard the fat off the meat, and fried food may be of particular value'. 'The worry that saturated (animal) fat in the diet will increase the risk of a heart attack should be ignored by old people. The risk of heart attack is much greater if the body temperature is low, and the danger of hypothermia through inadequate food intake is much greater than the risk of a heart attack from eating fat.'

We are often told that alcoholic drinks will warm us up, but in fact, alcohol speeds up the loss of body heat and so drinking may increase the risk of hypothermia. *See* Section 7, page 159, where food for keeping warm is mentioned as well as suggestions about a winter store cupboard.

Keeping active to keep warm

Exercise produces heat and it is very important to keep active and moving for a lot of the day. Regular exercise helps the muscles get fitter. If you are fit you are less likely to be tired or exhausted. It is not only a great advantage for the quality of life to be fit but an exhausted person is more likely to become hypothermic. It seems to be true that regular exercise for older people improves the mechanisms in the body which regulate the body temperature.

It can be a good idea to spread the chores and jobs to be done throughout the day. It can sometimes be a temptation to get them out of the way, but doing tasks in between periods of sitting will ensure you do not stay still for too long. Physical activity improves the circulation and is a way of keeping warm in itself. Laura Mitchell, author and broadcaster, suggests exercising to music: 'While sitting, whenever you hear music on the radio, lift your arms above your head several times; clap above your head and look up at your hands keeping time to the music.' Arm swinging can be very good for the circulation.

Getting out and about as much as possible, provided you are well wrapped up, is both enjoyable, healthy and a way to keep warm by keeping the circulation going. While it is a good idea to resist the temptation to stay indoors when we are fit enough to go out, nevertheless, when it is very cold and icy it is better to take some form of indoor exercise rather than going outdoors. On the days when you do not go out, breathing fresh air from outside is good for the lungs.

In Section 7 we describe ways of taking part in activities and exercises.

Keeping warm and safe

It can be a temptation to sit close to fires, but this can be dangerous. It is important to put guards on all open fires.

Drying clothes in winter can be a problem, but it is important not to put wet clothes on or close to heaters. Apart from the fire risk involved, this could allow the spread of moist air to the rest of the house, and might lead to condensation problems.

If you are worried about the safety of any gas or electrical appliances, you can contact British Gas, who will do free safety checks for older people, and some electricity boards will visit your home and advise you.

Heating your home

Are you wasting energy in your home?

You can have your home checked for its Home Energy Rating. The Rating is a number on a scale of 0–10 which tells you how your home rates in the energy stakes. Ten is the best and means that your home should have very low running costs for its size, but there are only a handful of homes that score as high as ten. The average for the United Kingdom is between 4 and 5.

A National Home Energy Rating carried out by a qualified person known as an 'Assessor' will give you: a certificate showing your home's score; a breakdown of your total annual running costs; a bar chart diagram showing which parts of your home are the most inefficient; suggestions about how to make your home warmer and save money; and estimates of how much it would cost.

Helpline for further information: 0908-672787.

Gas services

Every region of British Gas has a team of Home Service Advisers. They can visit you in your own home to give advice on the use or choice of a gas appliance, or on using gas economically. If you have any difficulty in using the controls on appliances, the Home Service Adviser will be glad to discuss having special adaptors fitted *free* of charge. All calls are free and you can arrange one through the local British Gas showroom or office (found under 'Gas' in the telephone book). Remember to check the identity of anyone calling before letting them in. All British Gas employees carry identity cards, which they will willingly show if you ask them.

British Gas employees rarely make calls without an appointment except to read your meter. If you are blind or partially sighted British Gas has a special 'password scheme' to let you make sure the caller is genuine. You choose the password and it is known only to British Gas. You then ask the meter reader for it when he or she calls.

Complaints

If you have a complaint about any aspect of the services provided by British Gas first contact the local offices/showroom (*see* under 'Gas' in the telephone book). If you are not satisfied with their actions in response to your complaint, you can contact the Gas Consumers Council (*see* page 140).

Free gas safety checks

On request, British Gas will carry out a free gas safety check on your appliances and installations if:

(a) you are over 60 years of age and live alone or with someone who qualifies;
(b) you are a registered disabled person of any age and you live alone or with someone who qualifies; or
(c) you receive a state disability benefit and you live alone or with someone who also qualifies.

The check will show whether your gas appliances and installation are safe to use and includes the cost of any necessary adjustments and materials up to £2.50 plus VAT. You can have one free check in any period of 12 months. If any additional work needs to be done an official estimate can be given of any costs involved which you would have to pay yourself. You may be able to get help towards this cost. Ask your local Social Services Department to see if you are entitled to help before ordering any work to be done.

Paying electricity and gas bills

Often the biggest problem about heating is paying the bills. There are ways of paying bills in instalments so that you can pay as you go along and do not get the shock of a big bill all in one go. If the credit meter reader has not been able to get into your house to read the meter then you may get an estimated bill. To check this, look under the column headed 'Present'. If there is a letter 'E' next to the four numbers it has been estimated. If you think the estimate is wrong there is space on the back of the bill for you to enter the actual meter reading and instructions on how to take the reading. Once you know how much fuel you have used, you can return the bill and ask for an amended amount. The Gas Consumers Council (*see* address on page 140) has produced a handy little guide *Meter Beater*, described as 'The easy way to work out your gas bills'. It shows you, step by step, how to read your meter and leaves space for you to fill in the figures. Your local British Gas showroom will have copies.

If you receive a bill, and you cannot pay it all at once, it is important to act quickly and not to wait for the red Reminder notice. You need to go to the showroom or to telephone the number on your bill and explain that you cannot pay the bill all at once. Someone will then arrange for you to pay off the bill weekly before the next one becomes due. You need to tell them what you can really afford to pay off. For the future, there are various pay-as-you-go schemes and we describe these below. Gas Boards have a booklet *How To Get Help If You Can't Pay Your Gas Bill*, available from any showroom. This is usually sent to customers who are in arrears with payments, together with a leaflet about disconnection.

Electricity companies are required, under the Code of Practice (see below), to offer customers in difficulty special payment plans which take account of the individual's particular circumstances.

If you have any difficulties in making these arrangements, you can contact the Citizens Advice Bureau, who will be glad to help you, or you could contact a social worker at your local social services office. While you are having these discussions it is still a good idea to pay off whatever you can from the bill – and keep receipts of any payments you make. Also it is important to keep the fuel boards informed that you have contacted the social services or CAB.

Prepayment meters

British Gas has two types of prepayment meter; one takes tokens, the other takes coins. You must put your tokens or coins into the meter before gas can be used. You can buy tokens from some British Gas showrooms and some Post Offices. You can ask for a prepayment meter to be installed, but the charge for gas will be slightly higher than when using a credit meter.

If you already have a British Gas or electricity prepayment meter and find it difficult to reach, it can be repositioned at a more convenient height up to one metre (about 3 feet) *free* of charge. If the coin mechanism is difficult to operate, a special attachment handle is available, free of charge, to make this easier. Meters can also be 'adjusted' to help you pay back arrears.

The companies have to offer a prepayment meter (where it is safe and practical to do so) before taking any steps to disconnect the customer for debt.

Budget accounts

Electricity and gas suppliers offer monthly budget payment schemes by cash, bank Giro, or monthly standing order. These payments are the same each month, thus evening out the payments for winter and summer months. A settlement is made annually and then the level of monthly payments is also reviewed. Quarterly accounts advise the consumer of the amount of electricity that has been used, enabling the consumer to check that all payments have been credited to the account. Interim payment schemes are similar but settlement is made quarterly.

Most suppliers also offer payment schemes at their shops, where the customer can pay an amount and collect a personal card or book of payment receipts. A gas savings stamp scheme is available, with stamps of £1 value available from British Gas showrooms.

Some sub-Post Offices also sell stamps. Gas savings stamps can also be used to pay electricity accounts at Electricity Board shops.

Codes of practice

Electricity suppliers

Under their public electricity licences the companies are each required to produce:
– a code of practice on the payment of bills;
– methods for dealing with domestic tariff customers in default;
– a code of practice covering the services to the elderly and disabled;
– a code of practice and statements concerning the efficient use of electricity; and
– a complaint handling procedure.

These five documents are known collectively as the Codes of Practice.

It is said that any consumer in genuine difficulty can expect sympathetic treatment, but the customer should make the supplier aware of any problems at the earliest opportunity. In the event of complaint, you should contact the electricity supplier in the first instance – details on your electricity bill. If your approach to the company fails to sort out the problem you should get in touch with the nearest Offer Regional Office and Consumers' Committee. Offer's Regional Office will investigate the complaint. If they are unable to resolve the problem straight away it may be considered by the local Electricity Consumers' Committee. The Director General of Offer, the Office of Electricity Regulation, will be involved where it may be necessary for him to exercise his enforcement powers. For details of Offer see page 141.

British Gas

A Code of Practice is available from British Gas showrooms which provides special help and services for older or disabled consumers. For instance, the Code of Practice states that households where everyone is a pensioner will not be disconnected between 1 October and 31 March. However, the Code also states that this will not apply if pensioners 'can pay but haven't', and 'in such cases the supply may not be reconnected for the following winter'. If you are having difficulties ask for the leaflet *How To Get Help If You Can't Pay Your Gas Bill* ..., issued by the Gas Industry.

See 'Helpful Organisations' at the end of this Section.

Publications

▶ *The Fuel Rights Handbook* (8th edition, 1992–3) is principally intended for those who advise consumers, but could also be of use to individual consumers. It aims, as far as possible, to be a comprehensive guide to fuel supply, payment and disconnection. It includes coverage of the impact of electricity and gas privatisation and details the procedures for taking up complaints against the electricity and gas industries.

Price: £6.95 including postage. Available from: Child Poverty Action Group Ltd, 1–5 Bath Street, London EC1V 9PY.

Electricity publications

The Electricity Association produces a range of helpful booklets and leaflets including the following:

- *Making Life Easier for the Disabled*, describing a range of appliances and how they may be used by people with limited dexterity or strength or with other difficulties.

- *Advice for Elderly People*. This 12-page booklet contains a great deal of helpful advice and tips on keeping warm, electrical appliances, safety, and easy ways to pay. Useful addresses are also given.

- *Warmth Without Waste*
- *Using Energy Wisely*
- *A Guide to Running Costs*
- *Safety in Your Home*
- *Lighting and Low Vision*
- *Plugs and Fuses*

The publications are available from some electricity shops and libraries. Single copies may be obtained by writing to Electricity Publications, Robert Guy Services Ltd, 54–62 Raymouth Road, London SE16 2DF.

Gas publications

Publications from the Gas Consumers Council, Abford House, 15 Wilton Road, London SW1V 1LT. Available from gas showrooms.

- *Meter Beater: The easy way to work out your gas bills*
- *Annual Report*
- *Choosing and Using a New Gas Fire*

- *Choosing and Using a New Gas Cooker*

In addition, the following publications are available from British Gas showrooms:

- *Advice for Older People*
- *Our Commitment to Older or Disabled Customers*
- *Our Commitment to Your Safety*
- *How To Get Help If You Can't Pay Your Gas Bill.*
  This is a leaflet describing a Code of Practice for domestic customers.
- *Advice for Disabled People*
- *Commitment to our customers: A guide to the standards and quality of service we aim to give all our customers*
- *Choosing and Using Your Gas Appliances*
- *Our Commitment to Energy Efficiency*

Insulating your home

Most of us could cut down sharply on heating costs if our homes were properly insulated, and we would still be warm and comfortable. This is all the more likely if we live in an old house. It is estimated that some homes lose around 75 per cent of their heating through badly insulated walls, doors and windows, not to mention the heat just rushing out of the roof through an uninsulated loft – probably as much as 25 per cent. Heat will also escape up the chimney and through the floor. As a result we are putting up with unnecessary cold and paying for the privilege. Of course, when we do start looking at how we can insulate our homes better we do have to be careful to maintain a reasonable flow of air or we will suffer the problems of condensation and dampness. Wherever possible, it is always best to seek advice before setting about insulating our homes.

In the meantime, there are some simple things we can do to improve the warmth. It is worth remembering to draw curtains at dusk (even in rooms not in use) to stop heat escaping and to prevent draughts. Fully lined curtains can make quite a big difference. A heavy curtain over the front door can make the hall warmer. Remember too not to have curtains or furniture in front of radiators. Sausage shaped cushions can really help to prevent draughts under doors and stop the cold around our feet. A more long lasting remedy against draughts would be to fit brush or rubber draught excluders at the bottom of doors. Do not forget also to fit an internal flap over the letter box.

Energy projects

It is worth finding out if there is an energy project in your area. As there are several hundred of these projects there is a good chance that there is one not too far away. Energy projects are run by a wide variety of voluntary and other organisations. Local authorities run some projects, as do agencies which specialise in setting up Community Programme Schemes. Your local Citizens Advice Bureau would know if there was an energy project nearby.

Energy Action Scotland and Energy Action Northern Ireland have details of local projects, and Neighbourhood Energy Action have details of projects in England and Wales. *See* pages 139 and 141.

Energy projects exist to help people on low incomes who could not afford to employ a contractor to insulate their homes. Payment is usually a nominal sum at most. The projects can offer practical help with loft insulation and draughtproofing to pensioners and other people in need. If you are able to contact a local project you will usually first receive a visit by a survey assistant, who will see what insulation and draughtproofing materials need to be installed. The survey assistant will also explain which grants are available and will help to claim them on your behalf. An insulation team will call to fit the materials, once grants have been approved.

All of these workers have been trained to do a good job quickly and efficiently. They will understand about the dangers of over draughtproofing a house, leading to problems with condensation and dampness. They will also know about the need for adequate ventilation to ensure the safe use of heating appliances and to provide sufficient circulation of clean air.

See also information on Care and Repair agencies (in Section 3), which provide help with improving your home to make it more comfortable and easier to manage.

Help with paying for insulation in your home

⇒▶ *Energy Action Grants Agency*
Bank Chambers, 9-17 Collingwood Street, Newcastle upon Tyne NE1 1JL
(Freephone 0800-181 667).

The Department of Energy's Home Energy Efficiency Scheme (HEES) provides grants to people on low incomes for basic home insulation, whether they rent, own or are buying their own home. It is administered by the Energy Action Grants Agency.

If you are on Income Support, Community Charge Benefit, Disability Working Allowance, Housing Benefit or Family Credit, you can apply for a grant for draughtproofing your doors and windows, and insulating your hot water tank, loft, pipes and cold water tank. You must make a small contribution, but the main cost up to a prescribed maximum (1992: £289) will be covered by the HEES grant.

Work must be carried out only by 'network installers' and listed contractors who can meet certain stringent criteria.

If you wish to apply for a grant you will first have to get approval from the Energy Action Grants Agency.

If you live in England, Scotland or Wales, use the freephone number (0800-181 667) to get up-to-date information on your eligibility for a grant and how you can apply. If you live in Northern Ireland and want information on home insulation grants, contact: Energy Action Northern Ireland, 128 Great Victoria Street, Belfast BT2 7BG.

For further details of grants to improve or repair your home see Section 2.

Trade organisations

When employing a firm to carry out work for you it is important to try to ensure that the company is reputable and reliable. One way is to find out if the company is a member of a representative trade association, which may also have a code of practice for its members. These Trade Associations will be glad to send you names of members in your area and other information about their trade. So it is worth contacting them before employing a firm you don't know. However, if a local voluntary group is helping you because you have a low income (e.g. energy projects, Care and Repair agencies), it will ensure that any firms carrying out work in your home are reliable and will, if you wish, oversee the work.

The Cavity Foam Bureau
PO Box 79, Oldbury, Warley, West Midlands B69 4PW (Tel: 021-544 4949).

The Bureau is the trade association for the cavity foam insulation industry and has some 60 contracting member companies throughout the United Kingdom. A key requirement for Bureau membership is that contractors must be registered with the British Standards Institution. BSI registration means that contractors have the proper ability to install the insulation system. BSI inspectors undertake an inspection of the contractor before registration is granted to ensure that the company is operating to proper standards. After registration is given, BSI inspectors regularly visit the company, sometimes without prior warning, to check that standards are maintained.

The Bureau says: 'In the majority of homes the greatest heat loss is through the walls. Cavity foam reduces that loss by up to 65 per cent. The system is suitable for the majority of houses and bungalows built since the early 1930s when the cavity construction of outside walls became a standard building feature. It costs around £400 to install cavity foam in a semi-detached house and say £250 to £400 for a detached bungalow.' Cavity foam insulation works very simply. A free-flowing foam is injected through the outer wall till it fills the cavity. The foam then sets into a heat-retaining barrier which greatly slows the loss of heat through the walls. To quote the Bureau: 'This makes the rooms quicker to warm up in the morning, slower to cool during the night. Condensation is also considerably reduced, if not eliminated altogether.'

The Cavity Foam Bureau will be very glad to give you information on cavity foam and names and addresses of contractors in your area.

CORGI – The Council for Registered Gas Installers
4 Elmwood, Chineham Business Park, Crockford Lane, Basingstoke, Hampshire RG24 0WG (Tel: 0256-707060).

If you need to call in a firm which installs or services gas appliances it is important to establish whether they are on the register of CORGI. Before such individuals and firms are accepted on the register they are checked to see that they are providing a good service and they must agree to conform to a code of practice. CORGI would be glad to advise you of local gas installers who are registered with them.

Draught Proofing Advisory Association
PO Box 12, Haslemere, Surrey GU27 3AH (Tel: 0428-654011).

The aim of the Association is to promote the advantages of fitting high-quality draught excluders, together with the resulting good insulation. Technical literature is available, and also a list of members, including specialist contractors. The Association is working to ensure that the customer can be confident both of product and workmanship. It has adopted a new Code of Professional Practice, to which all members agree to abide.

Electrical Contractors Association
ESCA House, 34 Palace Court, London W2 4HY (Tel: 071-229 1266).

The ECA will be glad to give you the names of firms who are registered members of the Association and who work in your area. All work is covered by the ECA's Guarantees of Work and Contract Completion.

Eurisol UK Mineral Wool Association
39 High Street, Redbourn, Hertfordshire AL3 7LW (Tel: 0582-794624).

Eurisol is a Trade Association which represents the manufacturers of mineral wool insulation. They produce literature and give technical advice for the installation of insulation and the advantages to be gained. In the case of cavity wall insulation the material being used is mineral wool in granular form which is blown into the cavity. Under pressure it forms into a continuous layer of insulation.

Two leaflets are available, *The Eurisol Guide to Home Insulation* and *Insulate Against the Greenhouse Effect*.

External Wall Insulation Association
PO Box 12, Haslemere, Surrey GU27 3AH (Tel: 0428-654011).

The aims of the Association are to establish good technical, ethical and legal standards for the industry, to give impartial advice and to promote the concept and advantages of external wall insulation, as designed and applied by member companies. It will be glad to send you a list of members and a useful leaflet, *Why Insulate Externally?*, which describes very clearly the advantages of such insulation.

▪ *Heating and Ventilating Contractors' Association*
ESCA House, 34 Palace Court, Bayswater, London W2 4JG (Tel: 071-229 2488); 23 Heriot Row, Edinburgh EH3 6EW (Tel: 031-225 8212); 3 Castle Avenue, Belfast BT15 4GE (Tel: 0232-774706).

Home Heating Linkline Tel: 0345-581 158. If you ring this number you can leave your address and HVCA will send you details of your two nearest HVCA members and will also send you some free literature.

The HVCA is the officially recognised organisation representing central heating contractors. One of its main objects is to promote fair dealing and sound installation of heating systems.

Membership of the HVCA is restricted to contractors who have been trading on a sound basis for at least two years. They must also be insured against injury to you and damage to your property while carrying out the work. The rules of the association require a member to give frank and impartial advice about the choice of fuel and about the type of system and control most suitable for the customer. An estimate from an HVCA member will be free, with a fully detailed specification telling you precisely what you will get and what extras are available.

Every one-off central heating system supplied by an HVCA member direct to a domestic consumer is protected by a double guarantee. The member's own guarantee covers quality of design, quality of workmanship and quality of materials. This is backed for one year by HVCA's guarantee, which remains valid even if the contractor dies or ceases to trade for any other reason.

Prospective customers can call the Home Heating Linkline (0345-581 158) for the names of their two nearest HVCA members, or can contact HVCA direct.

HVCA will be glad to send you a copy of their leaflet *Your Guide To Central Heating* and details of their Code of Fair Trading.

▪ *National Association of Loft Insulation Contractors*
PO Box 12, Haslemere, Surrey GU27 3AH (Tel: 0428-654011).

A register of members is available. They will work to standards laid down by the Association, using only approved materials and processes. All members agree to abide by a Code of Practice which lays down technical, as well as ethical, guidelines. There are many different methods of loft insulation. Association members will recommend to customers the product or system best suited for their individual needs, and give advice on all aspects of loft insulation.

▪ *National Cavity Insulation Association*
PO Box 12, Haslemere, Surrey GU27 3AH (Tel: 0428-654011).

The aim of the Association is to raise and to maintain high standards of competence and conduct in the business of cavity wall insulation. The Association has its own Code of Practice and all companies applying for membership are closely vetted. A member of NCIA must be a British Standard Registered Firm or be British Board of Agreement approved. Materials used by members include u.f. foam, mineral fibre (rock and glass) and expanded polystyrene beads (loose and bonded). Technical and general literature and a register of members are available from the address above.

▶ *National Inspection Council for Electrical Installation Contracting (NICEIC)*
Vintage House, Albert Embankment, London SE1 7UJ (Tel: 071-582 7746).

The National Inspection Council for Electrical Installation Contracting keeps a list of approved electrical contractors. If you need electrical work done, you can ask NICEIC to send you the list of contractors in your locality.

Helpful organisations

▶ *Age Concern England*
Astral House, 1268 London Road, London SW16 4ER (Tel: 081-679 8000).

▶ *Age Concern Wales*
4th Floor, 1 Cathedral Road, Cardiff CF1 9SD (Tel: 0222-371566).

▶ *Age Concern Scotland*
54A Fountainbridge, Edinburgh EH3 9PT (Tel: 031-228 5656).

▶ *Age Concern Northern Ireland*
6 Lower Crescent, Belfast BT7 1NR (Tel: 0232-245729).

The Age Concern national organisations all have information on keeping warm in winter and will be glad to advise. At the same time, there are many local Age Concern groups throughout the United Kingdom which are active in many ways and will be involved with schemes to help older people keep fit and warm throughout the winter. Many local Age Concern groups stock up with supplies of blankets and thermos flasks at the beginning of winter. They co-ordinate their activities with other organisations to try to reach the most isolated and vulnerable elderly people. Most groups make sure that all their volunteers are alert to the dangers of low body temperatures among the people they visit or contact. Many Age Concern groups extend the opening hours of their day centres and pop-ins so that older people can be sure of a warm place to go. Your local group would be very glad to hear from you at any time. The address will be in the telephone book.

A few of the publications available from Age Concerns:

▶ From Age Concern Northern Ireland: *Cutting the Cost of Keeping Warm*, describing sources of help; *Your Heating in Retirement*, aimed at providing advice and information for elderly people on heating costs and fuel problems; and a useful chart/thermometer which shows the temperature in a room and advises on a suitable temperature.

⇒ From Age Concern England: *Coldwatch*, a very useful pack for local groups including: details of national action being taken by Age Concern together with other agencies; a national policy statement; a briefing on hypothermia; information on training of permanent staff and volunteers, and on bulk fuel purchasing. In addition, there is advice for elderly people including keeping an emergency food store cupboard, eating for warmth – some hints, safety of appliances, cold weather payments, burst pipes, and grants for insulation and draughtproofing. A fact sheet, *Help with Heating*, is available in the above pack and as a separate sheet. This provides information on financial benefits, insulation grants, easy ways to save energy, easier payment schemes for gas and electricity, and disconnection. Also available is a leaflet, *How to Cut the Cost of Keeping Warm*.

⇒ From Age Concern Scotland: *Dangerous Cold*, a booklet describing hypothermia and age-related illness in older people. Price: £1.50. They also have free copies of a booklet *Keep Warm This Winter*. This booklet gives specific advice on clothing, heating, exercise, dampness and food. For further information you can phone *Keep Warm* free of charge: 0800 83 85 87.

⇒ *Age Concern Insurance Services ACIS*
Garrod House, Chaldon Road, Caterham CR3 5YZ (Tel: 0883-346964).

ACIS can provide low cost, specialist insurance cover which includes access to Helplines, the most important kind of which in periods of cold weather is the Domestic Helpline. This Helpline provides practical help with emergencies in the home from competent and authorised repairers in the client's local area. The client will be responsible for paying the repair bills/call out charge (which are described as fair and reasonable) and these may be recoverable under the client's home insurance. The ACIS client simply phones a 24-hour control room for immediate assistance in the event of any domestic problems including:

– total failure of central heating or water heating system
– major electrical or gas supply faults within the property
– burst pipes or blocked drains causing flooding
– serious storm damage.

⇒ *Care and Repair*
22a The Ropewalk, Nottingham NG1 5DT (Tel: 0602-799091).

In Section 3 we discuss Care and Repair agencies. There are now 180 of these in the United Kingdom. They are run by housing associations, voluntary organisations or local authorities. These schemes will help older people to carry out repairs and improvements including insulation and more efficient heating systems. They will provide advice and help and will also help you to find ways to pay for any improvements you need through grants, etc. Energy projects work in a similar way but concentrate particularly on making your home warm by concentrating on insulation and draughtproofing. Care and Repair will tell you if there is an agency in your area.

Citizens Advice Bureau

The Citizens Advice Bureau may be able to help you in a number of ways. As well as looking at a means of paying particular bills it may be able to suggest ways in which you could budget to relieve some of the problems. It will be concerned to help you as an individual and will therefore want to try to help you improve any circumstances you find unsatisfactory. It will help you claim any financial benefits to which you may be entitled. Details of these are given in Section 1. In addition, you may be entitled to Cold Weather Payments. You will find the address and telephone number of your nearest CAB in your telephone book.

Domestic Coal Consumers' Council
Freepost, London SW1P 2YZ (Tel: 071-233 0583).

The DCCC is an independent body which represents all consumers who burn solid fuel in their home. The Council is especially concerned with the supply, quality and price of solid fuel and safety matters.

If you cannot resolve a dispute with your supplier or coal merchant, contact the Approved Coal Merchants Scheme (in the telephone book) or, if this fails, you can send your complaint to the Council.

Free leaflets are available, including *What You Need To Know If You Burn Solid Fuel* and *The Solid Fuel Safety Code*, which provides tips on safety, complaints and where to go for help.

The Council recommends that if you are concerned about which fuel to use, whether your fire is safe, and need advice as to who to install it you should contact the Smokeless Fuels Federation. It can provide you with free advice on a wide range of fuels and appliances, can tell you about Approved Coal Merchants and can help you to find someone to install your appliance safely. It can also tell you where to find a chimney sweep. You can find the nearest address in the telephone directory under 'S', or ask a Citizens Advice Bureau, or write to the Domestic Coal Consumers' Council as above.

Energy Action Northern Ireland
128 Great Victoria Street, Belfast BT2 7BG (Tel: 0232-333790).

This is a new charity set up in November 1991 to assist and co-ordinate the work of the nine independently-sponsored energy projects currently covering Northern Ireland.

Energy Action Scotland
21 West Nile Street, Glasgow G1 2PJ (Tel: 041-226 3064).

Energy Action Scotland is an independent charity which promotes and supports community-based initiatives to tackle fuel poverty and create jobs. It will be glad to inform you whether you are eligible for special help and tell you whom to contact locally.

Gas Consumers Council
6th Floor, Abford House, 15 Wilton Road, London SW1V 1LT (Tel: 071-931 0977); 86 George Street, Edinburgh EH2 3BU (Tel: 031-226 6523).

The Gas Consumers Council has twelve branch offices, one to each region of British Gas. It represents the interests of the consumer to British Gas, and is completely free and independent. Each office has its own guardian; a Councillor who, though a member of the main Council, is specifically appointed for his or her local knowledge and contacts. Two Councillors have particular responsibility for services to disabled and elderly people and also to people in ethnic minorities. There is a range of leaflets, which has been described on page 131.

General Consumer Council for Northern Ireland
Elizabeth House, 116 Holywood Road, Belfast BT4 1NY (Tel: 0232-672488).

If you have a problem to do with electricity and have not been able to sort it out with the Northern Ireland Electricity Service yourself, you can refer it to the General Consumer Council or your advice centre. The Council will investigate, but you must have given the Electricity Service a chance to put matters right first before going to the Council.

Health Education Board for Scotland
Woodburn House, Canaan Lane, Edinburgh EH10 4SG (Tel: 031-447 8044).

The Board offers advice on health and heat-related problems. It has a resource pack *Keep Warm This Winter*, which is available to enquirers. It includes information on cold-related information and hypothermia, and how these can be prevented; sources of financial help; improving energy efficiency; clothing; heating; food; exercise. There is also a contact and resource list. Included in the pack is a hypothermia thermometer as well as a leaflet about the Home Energy Efficiency Scheme which describes grants which are available for those on low incomes who would like to improve the insulation in their homes.

Help the Aged
St James's Walk, London EC1R 0BE (Tel: 071-253 0253).

Help the Aged operates the Winter Warmth Line (freephone 0800-289 404) as part of the government's Keep Warm, Keep Well campaign, in association with the charities Neighbourhood Energy Action and Age Concern. Advice workers can give advice on a range of winter warmth topics including making the most of body heat, insulation and draughtproofing, and coping with winter fuel bills. A *Keep Warm, Keep Well* booklet is available by calling the line; it is also available on audio cassette.

Helpful organisations 141

=▶ *National Debtline*
The Birmingham Settlement, 318 Summer Lane, Birmingham B19 3RL
(Tel: 021-359 8501).

If you need advice on mortgage arrears, rent arrears or other debts, including fuel debts, contact the National Debtline telephone number above. National Debtline also has a range of leaflets including one entitled *Dealing With Your Debts*. This provides practical advice on how to cope with debts in a realistic way. This is clearly described in stages, and figures and budgets are set out in a simple way. A section specifically discusses how to cope with gas and electricity arrears. (*See also* p.56.)

=▶ *Neighbourhood Energy Action*
2/4 Bigg Market, Newcastle upon Tyne NE1 1UW (Tel: 091-261 5677).

Neighbourhood Energy Action (NEA) is a national charity which seeks to resolve the heating and insulation problems of elderly and disabled people, single parents and other low-income households. Among other work, it supports a national network of local agencies which provide insulation, draughtproofing and energy advice services in the homes of people who have low incomes. NEA works in partnership with Energy Action Scotland and Energy Action Northern Ireland.

=▶ *Office of Electricity Regulation (Offer)*
Hagley House, Hagley Road, Edgbaston, Birmingham B16 8QG
(Tel: 021-456 6208).

Offer is the Government department responsible for the regulation of the electricity supply industry. There are 14 regional Offer offices throughout England, Scotland and Wales – one for each area where there is a Regional Electricity Company (formerly area boards).

Some of the areas in which Offer can help are: disconnections; payment of bills; difficulty in getting an electricity supply; and problems with meters. Offer cannot deal with problems relating to electrical goods and appliances.

Customers who have a problem should first contact their Regional Electricity Company. If they are not satisfied with the result, they should telephone or write to their regional Offer office. The address can be found on the back of your electricity bill, or by contacting Offer headquarters.

Offer has produced an audio tape, *Consumer Matters*, and a video, *Electricity: A new generation*, which describe how it has agreed Codes of Practice with Public Electricity Suppliers, and show how some customers have had their electricity bills reduced thanks to help from Offer, its 14 regional offices, and Electricity Consumers' Committees.

=▶ *The Office of Gas Supply (Ofgas)*
Southside, 105 Victoria Street, London SW1E 6QT (Tel: 071-828 0898).

Ofgas is an independent body, set up to keep a check on the activities of British Gas since its privatisation. Ofgas is concerned to ensure that British Gas has the interests of its customers in mind at all times, checking on both the price and supply of gas. If British Gas fails to meet certain obligations to its customers, the Director General of Ofgas has legal powers to safeguard consumers' rights, and the responsibility to investigate complaints where legal action may be necessary.

One of Ofgas's main concerns is the provision of a number of ways of paying gas bills and that customers facing hardship or difficulties are treated sympathetically. We describe some of the ways in which gas bills may be paid on page 128. Arrangements which have been discussed with British Gas to help people pay their debts are explained in the leaflet *Principles for the Collection of Domestic Gas Debt*, and in the Code of Practice available from British Gas head offices.

SECTION SIX

Keeping safe

Throughout our lives we have to take care and, in our everyday lives, balance the risks which we inevitably take. Living is, after all, a risky business in itself. When we are older, dangers are not so easy to overcome, so we do have to be more careful and live within our capabilities. However, while we can seek to avoid obvious dangers and to take reasonable precautions, if we become unreasonably safety conscious this could limit our activities too much. There is a fine balance between taking necessary care and becoming so worried about safety that we are constantly fearful.

As older people we have, after all, had a good deal of experience in looking after ourselves, and to have survived beyond retirement age means we have been quite good at it. We have, throughout our lives, faced all manner of dangers and somehow we have come through.

We tend to gain the impression from newspapers that older people are in considerable danger of being mugged. However, the actual danger is a lot less than is suggested. Police figures show that the people most in danger from assault are young men and that comparatively few older people suffer this sort of harassment. A booklet issued by the Home Office, *Practical Ways To Crack Crime*, says, 'Any crime against an elderly person is disturbing but, in fact, crimes against the elderly are still rare.' (For details of the booklet see under the heading 'Help from the Police' at the end of this Section.)

In this Section we describe things you can do which will make your home a safer place as well as ideas for protecting yourself, either at home or outside.

Community alarm systems – calling for help

Community alarms are designed to enable people in their own homes to call for help even if they cannot reach a telephone. All that is needed to connect one is a telephone line with a modern plug-in socket and a 13 amp power point within 6 to 12 feet of the socket. If you do not have a telephone, don't worry, contact Help the Aged (see below) for help.

However, community alarms are not there to be used only in an emergency. The monitoring services usually also provide friendly advice and assistance when needed, and they can be a useful point of contact with other services of help to elderly or disabled people.

There is now a wide range of monitored alarm systems throughout the country where older people, by setting the alarm off, can summon help. Some of the alarms will automatically summon help in the event of an accident, without being activated by the person concerned. Alarms which can summon help so easily can be a great boon to older people living alone, giving them security and peace of mind, since they know that if they have an accident in the home help will soon be on its way. It can also be a great comfort to relatives and friends to know that the person is safe unless they hear otherwise, but it is important that an alarm is not used as an excuse to avoid visiting as often as possible.

People who live in sheltered housing schemes will usually have either a resident warden or a mobile warden on whom they can call for help. This may be by telephone or by contact points in various places. However, when the warden is off-duty there is often a link with an emergency centre.

How do community alarms work?

The alarms approved by Help the Aged work as a normal telephone, with the additional feature that they can automatically dial a control centre when triggered by pressing a button on the telephone or on a pendant that is worn at all times. The pendant has a range of at least 25 yards. This will usually cover every room in the house. There is also a loudspeaker and a tiny microphone built into the unit so that control centre staff can talk to the user even if the caller cannot reach the telephone. They find out what the problem is and send whatever help is needed. If the operator cannot hear a reply, he or she will assume that it is an emergency and send the emergency services or a warden.

When an emergency call is received the details of the caller will either appear on a computer screen or, on older systems, a reference number indicates the caller's file. This contains information which the client has previously supplied, including name and address, brief medical details (so that special precautions can be taken if necessary) and information on people to contact. These include the doctor and local friends and relatives who have keys to the property so that emergency services do not have to break in.

Most alarm units are set up to dial an emergency centre. These are run by manufacturers, commercial firms, housing associations, charities and local authorities. The main advantage of emergency centres is that they are nearly all staffed 365 days a year and 24 hours a day. So you need never worry about disturbing them at night.

Who provides alarms?

Alarm systems are provided by local authorities, charities, housing associations and commercial firms. Availability will depend on where you live. *Before you make any decisions we strongly recommend you contact Help the Aged, who run a national alarms scheme and will gladly advise you.* For details, *see* below.

Local authorities

Many alarm systems are run by local authority housing or social service departments. Some have mobile wardens who respond to calls; others will contact friends and relatives who you have nominated – and who you are happy to give your front door key to. In certain areas, schemes include regular telephoning or visits to check on how you are. The authority will supply, install and may maintain the alarm equipment.

Even if you are considered eligible to join the scheme by reason of your age, health or because you live alone, you may have to wait a time to join the scheme, as there is often a waiting list.

Charities

A few charities sell or rent alarm units and arrange for monitoring. Help the Aged is the main charity involved in providing advice and helping older people obtain alarms which are linked into a monitoring system. For details, *see* below.

Housing associations

Housing associations will usually provide an alarm system for their tenants, while some will also supply and monitor alarms for non-tenants. Depending on the association, you will either buy, rent or wait for an alarm to be donated.

Commercial firms

A number of firms sell direct to the public. A few run their own emergency centre; others will put you in touch with organisations which supply their alarms and run emergency centres. Before considering contacting a commercial firm, we would recommend you contact Help the Aged, who can give you impartial advice.

What will the equipment and the monitoring system cost?

Local authorities – charges vary. Alarms are provided free by some local authorities, although this may be limited to council tenants and people receiving Income Support or other benefits. Where charges are made, they may be between about £2 and £3.50 a week to cover renting the equipment and the costs of the monitoring service. Some authorities sell alarms.

Housing associations – depending on the association, you will either buy, rent or wait for an alarm to be donated. Monitoring costs may be around £2 a week.

Commercial firms – you will need to buy the equipment, which may cost between £200 and £300. Monitoring charges vary, but may be around £2 a week. With many firms you have to sign on for a minimum period – usually from three months to a year.

Help the Aged's community alarm programme

Help the Aged
Community Alarms Department, St James's Walk, London EC1R OBE.
Tel: 071-253 0253; SeniorLine freephone: 0800-289 404 (10 a.m.–4 p.m., Mondays to Fridays).

Help the Aged maintains information on the supply of alarm units and monitoring services throughout Great Britain and Northern Ireland. It can advise you on whether your local authority has an alarm scheme, what it will cost and whom to contact. You can contact Help the Aged free of charge through its SeniorLine number shown above.

If you cannot afford a unit, Help the Aged may be able to help. If you are able to contribute you will be asked to make a donation of £230 to cover the cost. Help the Aged, where necessary, may also be able to help with costs such as the conversion of an old British Telecom socket to the new plug-in type or the installation of a new 13 amp socket. It is able to help only people of pensionable age who need an alarm, are willing to have one and are able to use it. You can apply to Help the Aged for help with funding, and it may then seek this funding on your behalf. You will be asked to fill in a yellow 'application for assistance' form. In addition to funding the unit, Help the Aged may also pay the charge levied by the control centre for one year. In subsequent years this charge will be the responsibility of the recipient of the unit. This is usually £35–60.

Help the Aged works very closely with local authorities. It negotiates with the authorities, using approved equipment on the type of service it offers elderly people and the price it charges for this. If Help the Aged considers the service is good and the price fair, it encourages the local authority to sign an agreement to allow the charity to link elderly people who have received an alarm from Help the Aged to their centre.

Help the Aged recommends that, where possible, you link in with a local authority system. It prefers equipment where there is a two-way speech system. It says too that it is better to be linked into a 24-hour monitoring centre than to relatives who may be out or may be reluctant to help on all occasions. Finally, it prefers systems where the monitoring centre is in the local area.

To find out whether your local authority is running a scheme in your area contact the Housing or Social Services Department (Social Work Department in Scotland). You can find it in your telephone book under the name of your local authority. You can then find out if you would be eligible to join its scheme. Local authorities differ in their rules about who they will supply alarms to, how they run the service, the type of alarm they provide and their charges.

Keeping safe out of doors

As we said at the beginning of this Section, newspaper stories give the impression that older people are at serious risk of being mugged while they are out in the street. While any attack on any one person is one too many and, for the person concerned, a horrific experience, fortunately, according to the police, comparatively few older people suffer this sort of harassment. However, we do have to be careful, and try to avoid areas which are deserted, and where there might be trouble.

While our physical strength may be limited when we are older, there are some tricks to be learnt. For instance the British Judo Association tells us that most local judo clubs offer self-defence judo for older people. Judo does not depend so much on the strength of an individual but on techniques for getting the better of another person in a tricky situation. Surprise moves can throw any aggressor off guard and may deter him altogether. Many women, trained in judo, have learnt to get the better of stronger men.

Then again, some people feel more comfortable if they are carrying around a personal alarm. The sudden noise can both attract help and put off any potential aggressor.

Personal alarms to carry around

A number of small alarms are available which you can carry around. When you press the top of the alarm it gives off a loud, screeching noise. Some also have a torchlight. The Talisman SOS screech alarm contains a gas cartridge which is sufficient to emit about 30 screeches. You then have to obtain a replacement cartridge. SOS Talisman alarms are available from Talman Ltd, 21 Grays Inn Corner, Ley Street, Ilford, Essex IG2 7RQ (Tel: 081-554 5579). Alarms are also available from hardware shops. Price: about £4.60.

Before you buy an alarm you have to consider how easy it would be to use in an emergency. If you carry it in a handbag, it could be difficult to retrieve in time. A pocket might be better. The alarms can be sold with a holster. In the end, it might be easier to rely on your own voice unless you feel you might be struck screamless.

A word of warning: some personal alarms have been found not to be very effective. The aerosol alarms have sometimes failed on testing, while battery powered alarms do not always give very loud sounds. It would be worth it, before buying, to have the alarms tried out in front of you. The police would always be glad to advise you about effective alarms. It would be unwise to place too much faith in a particular alarm unless you could be sure it would work well.

Walking in wintry conditions

Winter weather can be very hazardous. It's not only that we need to keep warm but also that icy conditions can be very treacherous. It is important to choose boots or shoes that will grip the ground as well as possible. Some seem meant to send you toppling!

Microcellular rubber or PU soles are recommended as being the best to get a grip on treacherous surfaces, followed by crêpe rubber. Leather (especially new) and PVC soles can prove very slippery in ice and snow and also on wet or leafy pavements.

Even if you do not usually use a walking stick maybe you would find it useful to take one with you when there is ice and snow about. It is possible to buy special gadgets which can be fitted on to the end of the stick which will help the stick to grip the ice and snow. Some sticks have retractable tungsten carbide tips which can be extended through the rubber tip of the stick to produce a positive grip on ice or other dangerous surfaces.

Not being seen in the dark can be another hazard. It is essential to wear at least some light coloured clothing when you are out walking in the dark, particularly on the upper part of the body. In addition, you could buy reflective strips to attach to your walking stick. Bicycle shops may be able to advise.

Keeping safe indoors

Help the Aged has produced a useful booklet, *Safety in Your Home*. This very briefly discusses the benefits of staying active, being careful with medicines, taking care in the kitchen and in the bathroom, as well as being careful in the use of tools and of heating appliances.

Available free from: Help the Aged, St James's Walk, London EC1R OBE (Tel: 071-253 0253).

Dealing with unknown callers

People will arrive on our doorsteps with all sorts of stories to gain admission. Very often they say they are from the Council or they may say they are doing a survey. Sometimes they say they have noticed you have loose tiles and they will arrange to have these fixed for you. Then again they may tell you that they have picked your house as a showhouse. You may be flattered and then you will be offered something 'at a very special price': double glazing, fitted kitchens – it could be anything. Other reasons to call could be that they have come to advise on security or to check the water pressure or to trace a gas leak. Once in, they may find some reason for you to leave the room to get something they have asked for: then they will look around for money or valuables. These people know where to look, because they have learnt that many people put cash in particular places. So it is wise to do the following:

— Fit a doorchain and viewer and always use them. It would be useful to have an outside light so that you can identify callers.
— Before opening the door fully to an unexpected visitor, call out but keep the doorchain on and ask for a name and proof of identity. It is necessary to check their identity carefully – they may be flashing any card at you thinking you will not look carefully – and do not be embarrassed about keeping them waiting until you are

satisfied they are genuine. After all, if they are genuine they will understand why you are taking precautions. Until you are satisfied be sure not to let them in, even if it is a woman or child. Sadly, children can make good thieves and there could be an adult in the background.
- It is wise to remember that *all* public service employees carry identity cards and are required to show them. Do not be taken in by someone who says he has left his identification behind. It is possible he has done so, in which case he will have to come back another time – that is his problem, not yours.
- If a salesperson calls you can always ask him or her to return later. In the meantime you can ring the company he says he represents to check him out. *See* details of the leaflet *Be Sure Who's At the Door* below.
- If you are at all suspicious about anyone call the police at once by dialling 999. They won't mind if it turns out to be a false alarm.
- If you are selling your home, try not to show people around on your own. You may be able to arrange for a relative or neighbour to come in. Agents always make appointments for prospective buyers and you should never show anyone around who does not have an appointment. Agents will often arrange for one of their staff to accompany anyone who has arranged with them to see your home. You could especially request this.
- Never leave door keys in 'safe' places such as under doormats or flowerpots or on a string which can be reached through the letter box. An unwelcome visitor, on finding you were out, would try all those places. Never give your keys to workpeople or tradespeople – it is easy to make a copy.

▶ *Be Sure Who's At the Door*

This is an advice leaflet from Help the Aged and the Office of Fair Trading about doorstep trading. It recommends that you never sign anything on the spot or make up your mind without making further enquiries. The leaflet describes how salespeople can put pressure on you, and how important it is to resist this. It points out that if you have signed a contract in response to a call you have not requested, you have seven days in which you can cancel and get back any money you have paid.

The leaflet is available free from Help the Aged, 16–18 St James's Walk, London EC1R OBE (Tel: 071-253 0253). Please send a s.a.e.

The Office of Fair Trading (OFT) also has a free booklet *How To Cope With Doorstep Salesmen*. The OFT says 'Most [doorstep salesmen] are reputable, and you may find their service useful – but some are rogues who can bring misery if you don't know how to spot them'. The booklet is available from the OFT at Field House, 15–25 Bream's Buildings, London EC4A 1PR.

Protecting yourself from fire

Fire is an ever-present danger, so we have to be constantly careful with electrical and gas appliances as well as open fires. Cigarettes are probably one of the single most common causes of fires. If you do smoke, never smoke in bed. Make sure you put ashtrays where they cannot be knocked over and never knock ash into wastepaper baskets.

When you are cooking never leave the cooker unattended. Particular care should be taken when cooking with fats and oils. All food cooked in this way should be dried with a kitchen towel before being placed in the pan to prevent the fat splashing. Never put cloths on top of the cooker. For some reason this is a temptation for all of us, but it is very dangerous.

Heaters need to be very carefully placed, not too near any bedclothes, furniture or curtains and not in a position where they can be knocked over. Open fires should have a guard placed in front of them to prevent sparks flying out. Some electric blankets are designed so that they can be left on all night but underblankets must be turned off before you get into bed. We say more about electric blankets on page 124.

You may like to consider getting a smoke detector to improve the safety of your home. Battery powered detectors can be fitted by a competent DIY person. The detector will indicate when the batteries need changing. Buy detectors bearing the British Standard number BS 5446 and the kite mark. They are available from hardware shops. They work by detecting and alerting you by means of an alarm to a build-up of smoke in your home, enabling you to make an early escape and to raise the alarm. Given good warning the Fire Brigade may be able to deal with the fire before it has done much damage.

Help the Aged has a very useful checklist in their leaflet *Fire*, which advises on the various precautions and actions you should take. It is very useful just to remind us to do all the little things that will save us from having a fire. So many fires start with a small carelessness. The checklist also gives advice about what to do if there is a fire in your home and what to do if you are unable to get out of your house. The leaflet including checklist is available free with a large s.a.e. from Help the Aged, St James's Walk, London EC1R OBE (Tel: 071-253 0253).

Information from your local Fire Brigade

Your local Fire Brigade will have a number of leaflets which you may find helpful when you are considering fire safety. Some of these leaflets will have been produced by the Central Office of Information (COI) and are likely to be widely available from fire brigades around the country, while others will be produced locally. It is worth asking what is available. COI leaflets include: *Safe Frying at Home*; *How To Use and Choose Fire Extinguishers for the Home*; *Fire: How safe is your home?*; *Smoke Detectors in the Home*; and *Electrical Safety Leads to Fire Safety*.

Protecting yourself against burglary

We can do quite a lot to protect ourselves from break-ins. Unless we are obviously wealthy, professional burglars are usually not interested in us. We are more likely to suffer from petty thieves and then only if we have not taken the precaution to protect our homes. Petty thieves do not like to bother with 'difficult' homes. They prefer open or easy-to-open doors and windows. Window locks can be an effective deterrent. Breaking windows is not favoured because the noise of tinkling glass causes attention and it is not easy to climb through broken glass. If there are too many problems, they will move on to somewhere easier.

If you are not sure how to best go about securing your home, it would be a good idea to contact your local police station and ask to speak to the Crime Prevention Officer who will be glad to come round to advise you on home security.

Bogus Callers: The knock code

Is a leaflet available free from: Association of British Insurers, 51 Gresham Street, London EC2V 7HQ
(Tel: 071-600 3333). Knock stands for:
Know your caller
Never allow entry without identification
Open the door only when you are satisfied that the caller is genuine
Call the police if you are suspicious
Keep an eye on any caller while he or she is in the house.

Going out for a while

When you go out you will, of course, lock all the outside doors and check that all the windows are closed, and it is important to do this even if you are just popping out for a few minutes. If you are going out for the evening, you can leave a light on in the front of the house; not the hall though – that's an old trick, and nobody takes any notice. You can buy time switches to turn on lights at different times even when you are away. Burglars know that householders often put keys under mats and flower pots or hang them on string through the letter box – so be warned! At all times keep ladders locked away.

Going away

If you are going away, do not forget to cancel the milk or newspapers personally – do not leave notes. Leave the curtains half open. Closed curtains all day are a giveaway. Ask a neighbour to remove circulars from your letterbox, and if possible to call in from time to time to see that all is well.

Looking after your home while you are away

There are some organisations who will provide a 'home sitter' service. We give brief details of two of these below.

⊫ *Homesitters*
The Old Bakery, Western Road, Tring, Hertfordshire HP23 4BB
(Tel: 0442-891188).

Homesitters has been established to provide a live-in caretaking service to allow home owners to leave their homes in safe keeping, knowing that any pets will be well cared for, and minimising the fuss and bother of 'shutting up the house'.

⊫ *Housewatch Limited*
Little London, Berden, Bishop's Stortford, Hertfordshire CM23 1BE
(Tel: 0279-777412).

Housewatch is a home security service offering you the reassurance of having a responsible person in permanent attendance at your property during your absence. The service may also include feeding, exercising and caring for any animals, mowing your lawn, and watering your plants.

Marking your possessions

It is quite simple to mark your valuables so that they may be more easily found by the police. This can be done by etching, die-stamping or using a security marker which can only be read under an ultra-violet light. When you have marked your property you can put a sticker in the window to warn thieves that your things are marked. This will act as a deterrent.

You simply put your post code and your house or flat number (or the first two letters of the name) on items you are concerned about. You can buy a fine drill for engraving or a hammer and a set of punches bearing marking information for punching on heavy metal items such as bicycles, mowers, etc. from DIY shops. If you do not want to have a visible mark on the item or if it would devalue it to be marked in this way, then you can use an invisible ultra-violet marker. These are available from most DIY stores and stationers for about £2. This marking will have to be renewed from time to time as it fades.

You can protect your car by using a special window etching kit, which can also be used on glassware such as decanters.

Intruder alarms

An intruder alarm system can be tailor-made to your needs, and having one professionally installed could reduce your insurance premium, particularly if the installer is a member of NACOSS (*see* below).

Having a burglar alarm system can in itself act as a deterrent to petty thieves as well as to burglars. It is easier to burgle a home which is not protected in this way. However, it is important to employ a reputable firm. You want the alarm to work efficiently and you want to be able to call the firm back if it needs attention. Your local Crime Prevention Officer at the police station will be glad to advise you as to the best system for your needs. You need to check that the system you buy meets British Standard (BS) 4737 (professionally installed) or BS 6707 (DIY fitted).

You would be wise to choose an installer who is approved by the National Approval Council for Security Systems (NACOSS). An approved installer is entitled to issue a NACOSS Certificate of Compliance for each security system it completes. This certificate is a guarantee that the customer's installation has been completed in accordance with established codes of practice and British Standards. It would be as well to get estimates from several firms (approved by NACOSS), so that you can compare prices.

A list of NACOSS Approved Installers is available free of charge from:
The National Approval Council for Security Systems, Queensgate House, 14 Cookham Road, Maidenhead, Berkshire SL6 8AJ (Tel: 0628-37512).

Publications on home security

Your local police should have a variety of publications on personal and home security. Some have special information for women. They may have leaflets on marking property and other practical ways to protect yourself, your possessions and your home.

▻ *Security in Your Home*

This free Help the Aged leaflet advises on locking up, with information on the most appropriate locks for doors and windows. Please send a s.a.e. to Help the Aged, St James's Walk, London EC1R OBE (Tel: 071-253 0253).

▻ *Beat the Burglar*

This is a free leaflet produced by the Association of British Insurers. It briefly describes the most suitable types of locks for doors and windows and provides general advice. Please send a s.a.e. to Association of British Insurers, 51 Gresham Street, London EC2V 7HQ (Tel: 071-600 3333).

Further information

Insurance

It is always wise to have good insurance cover. Some insurance companies offer reduced premiums for people with burglar alarms. It would be worth having a word with your insurance company to see if it prefers a particular system. Apart from all the upset a break-in causes, if you have insurance you are at least spared the financial worry. It is worth shopping around for a good package at a reasonable price. For details see Section 3.

First aid and other courses

▸ *St John Ambulance*
Headquarters, 1 Grosvenor Crescent, London SW1X 7EF (Tel: 071-235 5231).

The St John Ambulance Association holds first-aid training courses at locations throughout the country. Some of these are specifically for older members of the community. One course is entitled 'Home Care for the Elderly'. This is a three module presentation covering: (a) personal care; (b) safety in the home; and (c) first aid. An informal approach is used, based on discussion, demonstration and audience participation. Details of all courses may be obtained from local St John Ambulance Headquarters.

▸ *Victim Support*
National Office, Cranmer House, 39 Brixton Road, London SW9 6DZ (Tel: 071-735 9166).

While it is, fortunately, only a very small number of older people who are attacked or otherwise become victims of crime, nevertheless, if it happens to you or someone you know you will be glad to have an organisation to turn to which really understands what you are going through and can give you positive support.

Many local Victim Support schemes exist and work through a network of over 7,000 volunteer visitors. They provide very practical support as well as being very understanding of the emotional effects of a crime. In one particular instance they were able to help a family suffering harassment from their neighbours. The whole family was able to discuss their fears and the victim support scheme was able to support them in their application to be rehoused. Other people may be helped to strengthen their locks to avoid another break-in and to build up their confidence. Others may be helped to obtain Criminal Injuries Compensation. For most victims, helping them to feel safe again is an important goal.

Local Victim Support schemes are listed in the phone book and can also be contacted through the police, Citizens Advice Bureaux or Age Concern group. Failing that the national office above would be able to let you know if there was a local group.

Details of training to be a Victims Support volunteer are given on page 223.

▸ *Victim Support Scotland*
7A Royal Terrace, Edinburgh EH7 5AB (Tel: 031-558 1380).

A community-based, independent voluntary organisation which offers a free confidential service to victims of crime. Victim Support is run by local people through local Victim Support schemes and is supported by all police forces and social work departments in Scotland. Trained volunteers offer practical help, emotional support, advice and information to crime victims.

Help from the police

Your local police force may have booklets and leaflets which make helpful suggestions about how you can protect yourself inside and outside your home. You can ask your local police Crime Prevention Officer for a free home security survey. She or he will be glad to visit (usually in plain clothes) and will advise you on the best locks and bolts to use for doors and windows. If you have a car, they will advise on protecting that as well. Door locks should conform with British Standard 3621 and this will be marked on the package.

You could also ask at your local police station what publications they have. The Metropolitan Police in London have a number of publications including *Positive Steps: Help and advice for women on personal safety* and *Practical Ways to Crack Crime*. Other police forces will have different publications.

Women are recommended never to advertise that they are female. For telephone directories it is best just to give an initial and surname and not a female first name. The same would apply to nameplates at the door.

▶ *Practical Ways to Crack Crime*

This useful booklet is produced by the Home Office. It has practical advice on how to help members of a family – particularly women, children and elderly people – feel safer and more secure in their everyday lives. Advice is given on how to make your home more secure, and how to take more care when you are out and about.

The booklet is available free from: Public Relations Branch, Home Office, 50 Queen Anne's Gate, London SW1H 9AT (Tel: 071-273 2193).

▶ *Criminal Injuries Compensation Board*

Blythswood House, 200 West Regent Street, Glasgow G2 4SW (Tel: 041-221 0945).

If you have been injured as a direct result of a crime of violence you may be eligible to receive compensation. CICB will be glad to send you *A Guide to the Criminal Injuries Compensation Scheme* which sets out who can apply and what injuries qualify. You can also ask for a copy of the Scheme itself. It is explained in the guide that while the guide should enable most applications to be made without assistance, there will be some cases in which applicants may have to think carefully whether to obtain the services of a solicitor or other adviser first. However, the Board does not pay for the cost of legal advice or representation.

SECTION SEVEN

Healthy living

We have heard so much about the dos and don'ts of keeping healthy in recent years, some of it contradictory, that it can be difficult to know exactly what we should do, especially with regard to eating. Then again, while it is only sensible to eat a balanced diet and avoid eating too much of those foods which are really not very good for us in order to preserve and improve our health, we may also wish to avoid just being faddy. Those of us over a certain age can remember enjoying dripping sandwiches, and smoking without feeling guilty. However, we do not have to make martyrs of ourselves to live as healthy lives as possible, and even if we now realise we have to give up certain pleasures to protect our health, the rewards of feeling fitter can far outweigh any sacrifices. The shops are now selling a very much wider range of Health foods, so that we now have a great deal more choice than before.

We describe below some of the organisations which have useful information to help you decide how to plan your healthy living. 'Eating for Health' need not be as complicated as it sometimes sounds. 'Not Smoking for Health', which follows, can be more difficult, but it is now clear that it is never too late to stop, and you will reap the benefit in terms of feeling healthier. We talk about exercise of the gentle kind as well as the more rigorous. Then we describe organisations which will help you with specific areas of health such as keeping your heart healthy. The Patient's Charter now requires that Regional Health Authorities provide health information which you can obtain for the price of a local telephone call.

Each Regional Health Authority in England now has a Health Information Centre having a Linkline telephone number. In addition, some areas are setting up local health information points. The information you can obtain on the Linkline covers the following:

— common illnesses and treatments (including self-help groups)
— maintaining personal health
— waiting times
— NHS services
— complaints procedures
— local Patient's Charter standards.

Linkline telephone numbers for each Region are:
  Northern: 0345-678 100   Yorkshire: 0345-678 200
  Trent: 0345-678 300   East Anglia: 0345-678 333
  N.W. Thames: 0345-678 400   N.E. Thames: 0345-678 444
  S.E. Thames: 0345-678 500   S.W. Thames: 0345-678 555
  Wessex: 0345-678 679   Oxford: 0345-678 700
  S. Western: 0345-678 777   W. Midlands: 0345-678 800
  N. Western: 0345-678 888   Mersey: 0800-838 909

All calls will be charged at the local rate for those telephoning within a particular regional area to the appropriate number.

Eating for health

It really does matter what we eat. A balanced, varied diet is essential to give us energy and to keep our bodies strong and working as well as possible. Eating well really will keep us alive in body, mind and spirit as well as giving us the best protection against illness. It is important to enjoy food so it is worth shopping carefully and cooking imaginatively so that mealtimes can be really pleasurable occasions. The fun element of eating is important in adding to our zest for life.

As we get older, it becomes more important to look carefully at exactly what we are eating and to vary our diet: as our metabolic rate tends to slow down, so we put on weight more easily. It is all too easy to take a succession of easy snacks of biscuits and cakes which are at hand but which do not give our bodies the essential nutrients. Instead, these foods can add to weight problems and lead to ill health.

Variety in our diet, lots of different foodstuffs, will ensure we get the right balance. It can be fun to be adventurous and to try different flavours to tempt the tastebuds.

The British Nutrition Foundation (for details *see* page 184) has a range of materials, including popular leaflets. One of these, *How To Eat a Healthy Diet*, describes the nutrients we need in our diet in a clear straightforward way.

The Health Education Board for Scotland, under the encouraging title *Eat To Your Heart's Content*, has produced a very well illustrated booklet showing mouth watering as well as healthy recipes. These are well set out and very easy to follow and show how easy it is to produce a wide variety of meals, including 'scrumptious breakfasts', which are satisfying and nutritious. The aim of the booklet is to show how healthier eating can improve your health. It clearly describes the types of foods we should cut down on and those we should largely avoid. Snacks are described which are filling and are high in fibre and low in fat. *Eat To Your Heart's Content* is available from the Health Education Board for Scotland, Woodburn House, Canaan Lane, Edinburgh EH10 4SG (Tel: 031-447 8044).

The British Heart Foundation, among its range of free literature, has a booklet *Food Should Be Fun*, containing advice an recipes for healthy eating. Available from the British Heart Foundation, 14 Fitzhardinge Street, London W1H 4DH (Tel: 071-935 0185).

A properly balanced diet should include: proteins (for growth and repair of tissue and also for the maintenance of normal everyday body functions), carbohydrates and fats (for energy), roughage/fibre (for digestion) and vitamins and minerals (for health).

Enjoy Healthy Eating is an informative and well-illustrated booklet from the Health Education Authority. For details *see* page 192.

Eat as much as you like of ...

Vegetables, salads and fruit are good for you. The latest scientific research confirms this common sense. What is news is just how vital these foods are for all round health. We need to eat a minimum of 400 grams (around a pound) of fruit, salads and vegetables a day, not including potatoes. This means eating at least five portions of fruit or vegetables every day. Tinned, frozen or fresh ... they all count. But when you buy tinned foods choose those which are lower in salt or canned in natural juice.

Pulses (beans), nuts and seeds are also included in the recommended amount for fruit and vegetables. Eat at least 30 grams (about an ounce) a day.

So for good health, eat vegetables, salad or fruit with every meal. Snack on fresh fruit and remember you can eat as much of these foods as you like. Also eat lots of wholegrain bread, potatoes and cereals, as well as low-fat meat and dairy products if you like, and lots of all sorts of fish.

The above information has been taken, with permission, from the booklet *Eat Well ... Live Well*, available from the Coronary Prevention Group. For details, *see* page 184.

The importance of fibre in our diet

We now know that we need to eat more foods rich in starch and fibre, or roughage as it is sometimes called. But what is dietary fibre? There are different sorts of starch and fibre, and these are only found in plants or food made from plants. It is best to base most of your meals around staple foods like bread, potatoes, rice, pasta, maize and yams. They are rich in starch and useful sources of fibre. Fibre is contained in the cell walls of plants and is the substance which provides structural support without which plants would not be able to stand upright. The greatest concentration of fibre is generally obtained from the external surface of the food, for instance apple peel, potato skin and the outer layer of brown rice or cereal grain (e.g. wheat bran). Fibre values of foods are often reduced by cooking, processing or refining. At an early stage the milling of white flour removes the outer bran coating and, immediately, this depletes the grain of some of its natural fibre, which remains in wholegrain or wholemeal flour.

We need plenty of fibre in our diet because it keeps our gut and bowels healthy and working well – no need to be constipated on a balanced diet with plenty of roughage. And, an added bonus, fibre (roughage) gives a feeling of fullness without too many calories, so you feel well satisfied and are not left feeling hungry. For instance, two ounces of wholemeal bread would be far more filling than the same amount of white bread.

Good sources of fibre are: wholemeal, wholegrain and unrefined produces, dried fruits, fibrous fruit and vegetables, leafy vegetables, peas, beans, lentils and nuts. A good way to increase the fibre you eat is to boil and then eat potatoes in their scrubbed skins. Baked potatoes can also be eaten in their skins.

While there are differences of opinion regarding exactly the right diets to keep us healthy it is generally agreed that we should eat less fat (particularly animal fat – *see* below for a description of fats), less sugar, less salt, and more fibre.

Eating well in winter

Eating well in winter is particularly important. Food is our body's fuel, and the right food not only keeps you warm, it also helps you fight off any bugs or illnesses that might be around. Poor nutrition can mean that your body does not have the strength to fight off the infections that would normally be easy to throw off. Not only is food the source of energy for activity and for producing heat, but the act of eating and digesting food generates body heat. It is important to remember that the energy requirements of the body are increased in the cold.

An emergency winter store cupboard

In case you get stuck indoors due to bad weather or if you have a period of illness, it is important to have a well stocked store cupboard having a range of foods providing you with plenty of choice and variety.

Good staples to keep in stock are: tinned sardines or tuna fish; baked beans; tinned vegetables (with no added salt); tinned fruit (with no added sugar); tins of evaporated milk; tins of soup; sultanas; lentils; dried onions; packet, tinned or condensed soups; long-life carton fruit juices; canned juices; cereals (porridge oats, pudding cereals, flour, brown rice, pasta); butter; margarine; cooking oil; instant potatoes (with added vitamin C).

Cutting down on sugar

Once you have got used to much less added sugar it is surprising how attractive foods can become when you are getting the real, sometimes tangy, taste. Sugar can so easily cover up other tastes. Cereals which can seem rather dull without sugar can taste very different with the addition of fruit, particularly dates and dried fruits which have their own natural sweetness. It is important to remember that sugar is naturally present in fruits and vegetables. It is the processed sugars (from sugar cane and sugar beet) we need to cut down on. Processed sugars cause tooth decay. They can also cause obesity. It is important to choose wholefoods, without added sugar, to look after your health.

Sugars in manufactured foods are listed in the ingredients as 'sugar, sucrose, syrup, glucose, dextrose, fructose, invert sugar'. All are processed sugars. Caramel is a form of sugar. The Coronary Prevention Group explain: 'White sugar sold in packets, and all the sugars listed above, are best avoided because they have no nutritional value other than providing a source of calories.' They go on to say: 'Brown sugars are no healthier than white. Honey and molasses contain more minerals than white and brown sugars, and have distinctive flavours. But use them sparingly, like sugar, because minerals are much better obtained from fresh, whole foods.'

Do You Take Sugar? provides suggestions on cutting down on sugar. For details *see* Health Education Authority publications on page 192.

Cutting down on salt

It really is important for us to cut down on salt. The trouble is, cooked vegetables can seem dull at first. However, the addition of herbs can make all the difference. Mashed potatoes with pepper and a variety of herbs can taste wonderful. No need to be mystified by herbs either – it is a case of try them and see. Some shops are starting to sell tinned vegetables without added salt, but you have to check the labels carefully. There are several salt substitutes on the market. Ordinary salt is sodium chloride and these substitutes are usually potassium chloride alone or a mixture of sodium chloride and potassium chloride. Potassium chloride tastes like salt, but it does have a slightly bitter aftertaste, particularly when cooked. It can also be expensive. While these substitutes are useful to the hardened salt eater, a simpler solution is just to use less salt. In time your taste buds adapt and foods begin to have a better flavour – in fact you find flavours you didn't know existed because they have been lost under the salt.

Cutting down on animal fats

The Coronary Prevention Group (for details *see* 'Looking after your Heart' later in this Section) has given us the following information.

The most harmful fats are found in dairy foods (fat on top of milk, cream, butter, hard cheeses), meats (particularly beef, lamb, and pork) and processed fats (hardened margarines, fats, and cooking fats). It suggests using more fresh skimmed and semi-skimmed milk, cooking with good oils (sunflower, soya, corn (maize), olive, safflower), eating less butter, choosing margarine labelled 'high in polyunsaturates', and eating fewer cakes and biscuits. Fats are solid at room temperature – oils are liquid. Oils can be processed ('hydrogenated') to make them hard – for example, to make margarines. Many people think that all oils are 'healthy' and all solid fats 'unhealthy', but that is not strictly true. What is important is the *type* of fat – not whether it is solid or liquid.

Saturated fats

These fats tend to be hard, solid at room temperature and to keep well. Eaten in large amounts, they encourage the liver to produce *cholesterol*. This cholesterol is released into the blood and deposited on the walls of the arteries. Saturated fats also make the blood thicker and more prone to clot. For these reasons, saturated fat is an important cause of heart attacks and other blood disorders.

Polyunsaturated fats

These fats have several important jobs to do in the human body. They are essential for the brain and nerves to grow and develop properly, and for their maintenance. They also help to keep the walls of arteries (blood vessels) clear, by making blood less sticky and less likely to clot.

Trans fats

These are fats which you may hear more about in the next few years. When polyunsaturated oils and fats are hardened and processed, a proportion of them change their chemistry to make 'trans' fats: these are best described as a sort of saturated fat.

Cholesterol

Cholesterol is a sort of fat, a cousin to the family of fats and oils. All human cells contain some cholesterol, which is made in the liver. While the liver makes quite enough – the human body is 'self-sufficient' in cholesterol manufacture – extra cholesterol is found in animal foods (dairy fats, eggs, meats). And saturated fats in food stimulate the liver to make more cholesterol than is needed. So the food we eat can make the cholesterol level in the blood high, which results in deposits forming on the artery walls. These can block the artery so blood cannot travel through. That is why cholesterol in blood is important.

Vegetarian and vegan diets

Vegetarians eat dairy foods and eggs but no meat. Vegans eat no animal foods at all. There is no reason why a properly balanced vegetarian diet should not be perfectly adequate for healthy adults. Fresh fruit and vegetables, beans, oils, different grains and cereals supply all the essential nutrients, with the exception of vitamin B12.

A vegan diet, containing no meat, milk, eggs, fish or any other animal foods can be healthy, providing it does not become restricted to any one food group and precautionary B12 supplements are taken regularly.

If you are thinking of becoming a vegetarian or vegan, it would be wise to get some advice from the Vegetarian Society or Vegan Society first. We give details at the end of this Section. The Societies have some very interesting and informative publications.

Drinking for health

While we are on the subject of diet, do not forget to drink plenty of liquids. Some people lose their sense of thirst as they get older and, of course, if you do not feel thirsty you may forget to drink. Lack of fluids (or too much alcohol) can lead to headaches, and feelings of confusion and unsteadiness. You need about two to four pints of fluid a day (about eight average-sized cupfuls), and more in the summer or after doing heavy work, when you will have lost extra fluid through perspiring more than usual. Otherwise it is necessary continually to replace regular loss of fluids through breath, urine and sweat. Water, tea, soup and fruit juices (without added sugar) can all be enjoyable drinks. A little beer, wine or sherry is fine but it is important to remember that alcoholic drinks do not give your body extra fluids, enjoyable as they may be, because the alcohol actually makes you lose water.

Going easy on alcohol for a healthy life

A little alcohol can be a great pleasure and can make a social occasion that much more enjoyable. However, we do have to be a bit more careful as we get older because quite small amounts of alcohol can have dramatic effects on us because our livers are less efficient at breaking it down. Also, as we get older we need to concentrate more on keeping our balance and not tripping up. A couple of drinks, though not serious in themselves, may quite well cause us to have an accident which could be serious. We cannot so easily allow our concentration to lapse and recovery may not be as quick as before.

It is easy to tip over into regularly drinking that much too much. We may not always like to admit we are drinking too much, even to ourselves. However, knowing there are organisations who understand and who will help can provide us with the necessary courage to face up to the problem. Excess drinking can be cured at any age. You can get help from your doctor or you could contact the local branch of Alcoholics Anonymous (for details *see* page 182), or you could contact Alcohol Concern, who can offer information by telephone or letter and who have published, in association with Age Concern, four booklets in a series *Safer Drinking for the Over 60s*. The titles are:

- *A DIY Guide for Older People*
- *A Guide for Relatives and Friends*
- *A Guide for Health and Social Services and Voluntary Group Workers*

=▶ *A Guide for Alcohol Agencies*

Single copies of the booklets are free of charge and are available from Age Concern or from Alcohol Concern, 305 Gray's Inn Road, London WC1X 8QF (Tel: 071-833 3471).

The Health Education Authority has a useful booklet, *That's the Limit: A guide to sensible drinking*. This describes, very wittily and with lots of illustrations, the facts about alcoholic drinks and how these add up, shows ways of working out just how much you drink and talks about sensible limits. It also describes the effects of too much alcohol. It finishes on a positive note – the advantages of drinking within clear limits and saying that habits can be changed – and it is not as hard as it may seem. It is available free from: Distribution Department, Health Education Authority, Hamilton House, Mabledon Place, London WC1H 9TX.

The Scottish Council on Alcohol (for details see the end of this Section) has a useful range of publications, including a Drinkwise Pack and a self-help pack for the partners of problem drinkers. For details see 'Publications and resources' at the end of this Section.

AL-ANON is an organisation concerned with the relatives and close friends of problem drinkers. For details *see* the end of this Section.

Not smoking for health

Smoking is not only closely associated with heart disease and lung cancer, but also causes older people a great deal of discomfort by aiding the development of poor circulation in hands and feet. Nicotine narrows the blood vessels and reduces the blood supply to many parts of the body.

There is now no doubt that smoking not only seriously damages the smoker's health but also damages the health of anyone near a smoker (passive smoking), and that is really not acceptable. It is estimated that cigarette smoking causes the premature deaths each year of about 100,000 people in the United Kingdom. The Health Education Authority has a question-and-answer booklet *Passive Smoking*. For details *see* page 193.

However, we may know all this but it does not make it any easier to give up. We may be encouraged to know that it is never too late to give up. Studies have shown that ex-smokers have a much lower risk of having coronary disease than those who continue to smoke. In fact, within just a year or two the risk is said to be greatly reduced, and after five years, it approaches that of the non-smoker. There are organisations who will send you information which may help you. These include ASH, QUIT! (the National Society of Non-Smokers), the Ulster Cancer Foundation (the Stop Smoking Group and Advice Centre) and the Coronary Prevention Group. Their addresses and details of publications, and more information on how they can help you give up smoking yourself or join in the campaign against smoking, are all at the end of this Section under 'Helpful Organisations'.

The Coronary Prevention Group has a useful leaflet *Smoking and Your Heart*, and the following suggestions for giving up smoking are taken from this:

- First make up your mind – This is the most important step. You must convince yourself that you really want to give up smoking and that you are going to be successful.
- When to give up – Choose the time carefully. It does not matter whether it is tomorrow, next weekend or in three weeks' time as long as you stick to it.
- Throw away all temptation – Make sure that you throw away any cigarettes that you may have left. Do not leave them lying around to tempt you.
- Tablets may help – Some people benefit from nicotine-containing chewing gum, tablets that make cigarettes taste nasty, or dummy cigarettes. You may be one of these people – ask your doctor.
- Be a 'non-smoker' – When you are offered cigarettes make a point of saying that you do not smoke. Tell everyone that you have given up, it will be much more difficult for you to go back on your decision.
- Put your savings aside – Work out how much you are saving by not smoking and put that money aside; for your holiday perhaps.
- 'No-Smoking' – Travel in the non-smoking areas of trains, tubes, buses and planes where you will not be tempted.
- Give up with a friend – Get together with a friend and give up together, in this way you can monitor each other's progress.
- Change your eating habits – For some reason, eating and drinking seem to trigger the craving for a cigarette. For the first few days at least, try to do without the drinks and snacks that would normally be accompanied by a cigarette. Also make a very firm effort not to smoke after meals.

Moving and exercising for health

Keeping active is the best way to keep on enjoying life and taking part in those interests which we have built up over the years. Of course, many older people, finding they have more time on their hands, take up entirely new activities, discovering that this provides a completely new lease of life. Even if we are restricted in our movements due to increasing disabilities, we still need to keep as active as we can, however limited this may be. Exercise is now recommended at a stage in life when in earlier times we might have been confined to a very quiet life. Doctors suggest that exercise in moderation, even for people who have undergone heart surgery, is beneficial so long as it causes no pain, shortness of breath or other adverse symptoms.

Alongside a healthy diet, which in itself will help us to be more active, exercise, whether in formal classes or at home, or simply making the effort to move around and walk wherever possible, provides the best means for keeping us going. Breathing fresh air for a few minutes every day, even just through an open window, can be beneficial and it will help you to breathe more easily and sleep better. A very simple exercise is to swing your arms – this can be good for circulation.

In Section 12 on 'Arts, Sport and Leisure' we describe a range of sporting activities such as swimming which, in themselves, provide excellent exercise as well as a great deal of fun and a sense of achievement.

Keep Fit classes for older people are held during the week in most towns and some villages throughout the country. There is no need to worry about ability: classes cater for all standards and aptitudes, combining fitness with fun. It can be very pleasurable joining in with others in exercising to music in a happy and relaxed atmosphere. Joining in Keep Fit classes will improve circulation and respiration, maintain full body movement, tone up muscles, restore vitality, give extra energy, help to release tension, stress, and strain, aid relaxation and sleep while, at the same time, providing a source of interest, enjoyment and friendship. Exercise is also very helpful for those who have osteoporosis (the weak bone disease). Details of the National Osteoporosis Society are given in Section 14. For details of Keep Fit classes in your area, enquire at your local Adult Education College or at the library.

You may be concerned about what clothes to wear. Anything in which you can do a knees bend, a stretch or twist will do. Regular class members usually wear leotards and footless tights though a loose tracksuit is perfectly fine. Participants are advised to work with bare feet or to wear no-slip slipperettes. If there are no sports or dance shops locally, your teacher would be able to advise you of a suitable mail order firm from whom you could buy leotards or tights, if you wanted to buy these things.

Two books by Laura Mitchell, who has often appeared on television, are very good reads, and discuss exercise and relaxation in a practical and encouraging way. The books are described at the end of this Section and are called *Simple Relaxation* and *The Magic of Movement*.

Helpful publications on exercise

Exercise. Why Bother?
For details of this Health Education Authority booklet *see* page 192.

The following two books are by Margaret Graham and are available from the British Wheel of Yoga, 1 Hamilton Place, Boston Road, Sleaford, Lincolnshire NG34 7ES (Tel: 0529 306851).

Keep Moving, Keep Young gives details of gentle Yoga exercises for elderly people. The author is a qualified yoga teacher and she has drawn on her extensive experience of working with older people to develop an exercise programme specifically for people from 70 to 100 years. The approach is positive, with the accent on what you can achieve. No special equipment or clothing is needed; all the basic exercises are performed seated or standing with a chair for support. The book can be dipped into for help with specific problems – an aching back, arthritic hands – or it can be followed progressively to work out routines for individuals or groups. Price: £3.65 including postage and packing.

=▶ *It's Never Too Late*. Though it was originally written for yoga teachers working with older people we are assured that this book is being used by many individual people who are older and also by those who are caring for older people. In the first seven pages of this book, which is only 32 pages long, the author describes how she and her colleagues initiated the practice of modified yoga in a home for elderly people, and the response to it. The main section of the book describes the exercises, with clear illustrations followed by suggestions for four typical class programmes. These are done sitting in a dining chair (or wheelchair even), while some exercises are for standing while holding a chair for support. No special clothing or equipment is needed. There is no mystique involved and these gentle exercises are suitable for any elderly person, regardless of age or limitations. Price: £1.45 including postage and packing.

Healthy living holidays

Saga arranges Healthy Living holidays. You can choose between a wide variety of walking holidays throughout the United Kingdom, cycling holidays in Holland, and tennis holidays, as well as its 'Keep Fit – Feeling Good' holidays, held at the University of Dundee. These are hosted by members of the University's Department of Physiology and Physical Education. A complete programme of activities is organised by the fitness instructors, and the food is selected by a dietician. Also included is a physiology test.

For details of Saga holidays see Section 13.

=▶ *Health and Beauty Exercise (The Women's League of Health and Beauty)*
Walter House, 418/422 The Strand, London WC2R OPT (Tel: 071-240 8456).

There are 280 centres in the UK having 20,000 members as well as branches in other countries. The classes cater for women of all ages, being graded to take into account the needs of every individual. Membership costs a minimum of £5 a year plus the costs of classes.

=▶ *EXTEND – Exercise Training Ltd*
1A North Street, Sheringham, Norfolk NR26 8LJ (Tel: 0263-822479).

EXTEND runs Movement to Music classes for people who are over 60 as well as for disabled people of all ages. There are training courses for those wishing to train as teachers. Exercise booklets and musical cassette tapes are available from Head Office. Please enclose a s.a.e. with your enquiry.

=▶ *The Medau Society* (Movement and exercise for people with special needs)
8b Robson House, East Street, Epsom, Surrey KT17 1HH (Tel: 0372-729056).

The Medau Society promotes classes for all ages and abilities throughout the country in conjunction with local education authorities, sports and leisure centres, and other organisations. Recreational movement classes aim to provide well-balanced enjoyable lessons which improve posture, co-ordination and muscle-tone, while developing suppleness, strength and stamina. The use of small hand apparatus such as balls, hoops, clubs and scarves encourages class members to move more freely and without awkwardness, whatever their ages.

Looking after your body

Looking after your heart

▶ *The Coronary Prevention Group*
102 Gloucester Place, London W1H 3DA (Tel: 071-935 2889).

The CPG has a range of publications. For details *see* page 184.

One of the publications, *You and Your Heart*, describes very clearly how our hearts work, and what heart disease is, pointing out that the United Kingdom has the highest death rate from coronary disease in the world for both men and women. To reduce the risk of coronary heart disease you are recommended to eat a healthy diet, not to smoke, to get your blood pressure checked regularly, to take regular exercise, not to become overweight, and to relax and enjoy life. A healthy diet is described as eating more bread (wholemeal), potatoes, pasta, rice, noodles, fresh vegetables, fresh and dried fruit, nuts, beans, poultry and fish, while eating less of fatty meats, dairy products, sugar, salt and eggs. You are also recommended to drink only a little alcohol.

▶ *British Heart Foundation* publications – for details *see* page 183.

▶ *Preventing Heart Disease* – for details of this Consumers' Association book *see* page 195.

▶ *How to Take Care of Your Heart* – for details of this book *see* page 193.

▶ *Action on Coronary Heart Disease in Asians* and *Making a New Start* are Health Education Authority publications – for details *see* pages 192 and 193.

Looking after your teeth

More and more people are able to keep their natural teeth for all their lifetime. With better dentistry and the eating of less sugar, as well as care and persistence with oral hygiene, it is possible to keep teeth for far longer than before. However, some people still need to have dentures and for these people good dentistry means that their dentures fit better and are altogether more comfortable than they would have been only a few years back.

In order to keep our natural teeth it is important to clean our teeth, gums and mouth adequately. It is not quite as simple as it sounds and if you have never been shown it is worth asking your dentist. She or he will not be surprised as it is only fairly recently that we have learnt that cleaning means more than pushing the toothbrush backwards and forwards! A regular six-monthly visit to the dentist is, in any case, a good idea.

Neglected teeth or badly fitting dentures do not help anyone's appearance and make eating difficult. Not only that, but they can lead to infections. So visiting your dentist regularly is very important as well as being careful about oral hygiene. This is vital for maintaining healthy gums, for without healthy gums we will not retain our teeth. While developments in dental techniques have meant that it is now possible to fill and retain or crown almost any tooth, advanced gum disease is more difficult to treat and can lead to a loosening of the teeth so that they eventually fall out.

Age Concern England has a most useful fact sheet, *Dental Care in Retirement*, which looks at dental care for older people and provides information on improving dental fitness. It gives information on the prevention of dental ill health, finding a dentist, emergency treatment, NHS charges, how to claim free dental treatment, dental charges, private treatment, and problems with dentures. Send a s.a.e. to Age Concern England (*see* page 181).

Finding a dentist

Your local Family Health Services Authority (which used to be called the Family Practitioner Committee) keeps a list of NHS dentists in the area. All dentists treating patients under the NHS have to be registered with the Family Health Services Authority. Lists of dentists are also held in libraries.

All dentists are now required to produce patient information leaflets about their practices, and you may find it useful to read a few before you make a decision on your choice of dentist. The leaflets must include such information as normal surgery hours, dentist's qualifications and when obtained, arrangements for home visits, and whether the premises, surgery and toilets are accessible to people using wheelchairs.

Dentists do not have to take on everyone who applies to be a patient. If you have difficulty finding a dentist who will treat you on the NHS, you could try contacting the following local organisations in case they can give you any further information: the Community Health Council, the nearest Age Concern or Old People's Welfare group, Citizens' Advice Bureau, or the District Dental Officer of the Local Community Dental Service.

For details of possible help with NHS dental charges, see Section 1.

Looking after your eyes

It is very important to have a regular check-up from a registered optometrist, preferably once a year. As we grow older, our eyes become more vulnerable to diseases and other disorders, but if you are having a regular check-up you will be able to get help quickly if the need arises. Unlike our teeth or our feet, our eyes are slow to let us know if something is wrong. Glaucoma (one of the most common causes of blindness) can be successfully treated if caught early enough, usually before any symptoms become obvious to us. Cataracts can also be successfully treated. In some cases, not only do our eyes show when they have a problem but it is also possible for an optometrist to see when there are other disorders in the body, for example diabetes. Many of these conditions do not cause pain and an annual eye test will detect changes early on. (For details of the International Glaucoma Association, *see* page 185.)

A great deal can now be done for eye problems if the diagnosis is made early enough.

If you need spectacles it is important to have regular eyesight tests to make sure you always have the best prescription for your sight. Some people struggle to see when all they need is a new pair of glasses. If you are having difficulty seeing to read even with spectacles there is a wide variety of low vision aids and magnifiers which can be very helpul and which will make all the difference to you. It is also important that you have good lighting concentrated on your reading or other close work. When we are over 60 our eyes need three times as much light as a normal eye needed at 20 years of age. A centre light in the room does not usually provide enough light to comfortably read by even for people whose eyesight is good.

Low vision aids

Your optometrist will help you with low vision aids. You could also contact the Partially Sighted Society for further information: *see* page 186.

In Touch, the Radio 4 programme for those who are blind or partially sighted, produces *The In Touch Handbook* packed full of information, including up-to-date details of low vision aids: *see* page 194. *In Touch* also has a bulletin that is a quarterly summary of all the information broadcast on the programme. It is available free in print, in braille or moon script, and on tape. For details write to: In Touch, Room 6114, Broadcasting House, London W1A 4WW. The In Touch kitchen is a permanent but changing exhibition of over 200 pieces of equipment selected for ease of use by blind people. It can be visited, by appointment, at the Disabled Living Foundation, 380/384 Harrow Road, London W9 2HU (Tel: 071-289 6111).

Cataracts

Operations for cataracts are now very simple procedures and mean only a short stay in hospital – either a few hours as a day patient or a bit longer if this is considered necessary. With the aid of spectacles or perhaps contact lenses you will find your sight restored. Sometimes older people have a plastic lens inserted into the eye. Your optometrist will discuss this with you and will be able to answer any worries you may have.

Further information on eye care

A useful advice leaflet, *Eye Care*, is available free from Help the Aged and the Optical Information Council, 57a Old Woking Road, West Byfleet, Surrey KT14 6LF (Tel: 09323-53283). The leaflet includes information on choosing a regular optometrist, cataracts, and the importance of lighting. For a copy of the leaflet please send a 9" × 6" s.a.e. to: Help the Aged, St James's Walk, London EC1R OBE.

Other leaflets in a series *Open Your Eyes to ...* available free from the Optical Information Council (*see* above) are: *Types of Lenses*, which describes bifocals, trifocals and multifocal lenses; *Contact Lenses*, which describes these lenses and also the differences between the various contact lenses; *Understanding Cataracts*, describing what a cataract is, what the operation involves, and aftercare; *The Look of Fashion*, which discusses choosing spectacles which are not only useful but may also enhance your appearance; *Sports and Pastimes*, showing that wearing spectacles need be no hindrance to sport or leisure activities; and *Driving*. This last leaflet reminds readers that 'with licences being issued which are valid to age 70, it should be remembered that, in law, the onus is on drivers to see that their vision is up to the required Department of Transport standard'. Information is given on the D.o.T. standard and then there are brief details of the various types of frames and lenses.

▶ *Royal National Institute for the Blind*
224 Great Portland Street, London W1N 6AA (Tel: 071-388 1266).

The RNIB has a series of leaflets about eye conditions available free of charge: *All About Cataracts*; *All About Glaucoma*; *All About Macular Degeneration*; *All About Diabetic Retinopathy*.

▶ *Eye Care Information Bureau*
PO Box 294, London SE1 8NE (Tel: 071-928 9435).

The Bureau will be glad to answer general questions about eye care and eye problems, visiting the optometrist and so on. If the Bureau cannot itself provide the information you need, it will be able to recommend where you may be further helped.

Among information available from the Bureau are useful booklets (individual copies available free). These have been produced by the Association of Optometrists.

There is a Family Doctor booklet called *Your Eyes* which explains how our eyes work and what can go wrong with vision, and discusses the causes and treatments of all the common eye problems. Price: £1.20 plus 22p postage. Available from: Family Doctor Booklets, British Medical Journal, PO Box 295, London WC1H 9JR (Tel: 071-387 4499).

Registration for blindness and partial sight

To be registered as blind does not necessarily mean total loss of sight. Registration as blind means, according to the National Assistance Act 1948, that a person is 'so blind as to be unable to perform any work for which sight is essential'.

Partial sight is the term covering those whose sight, though poor, is not bad enough for them to be registered as blind.

Registration for blind and partially sighted people is worthwhile because it is necessary to qualify for most financial benefits and for help from most voluntary agencies. Registration for a blind or partially sighted person can be arranged through a hospital or by contacting the local social services department or office. Town halls, libraries or Citizens Advice Bureaux have addresses and telephone numbers. For details of aids and equipment, *see* Section 4. Very full information is given in *The In Touch Handbook*. For details, *see* page 194. For details of the Royal National Institute for the Blind, see Section 14.

For details of possible help with NHS charges for sight tests and glasses, *see* Section 4.

Looking after your feet

Our feet work so hard for us all our lives, and we very often suffer in ill-fitting shoes. We need to take very good care of our feet if they are to help us to remain active. Sore and aching feet make us reluctant to walk, and we then do not get the exercise we need. When we have uncomfortable shoes but nevertheless have to walk, it can be a painful process and this shows in our face as well!

While some foot problems are the result of specific conditions such as arthritis and diabetes, the majority of complaints are the result of ill-fitting shoes. A very useful leaflet from Help the Aged, *Fitter Feet*, is available free in response to a s.a.e. The address is given on page 338. The leaflet describes how to buy suitable footwear and discusses basic hygiene. Common complaints, including aching heels, athlete's foot, bunions, chilblains, corns and callouses, in-growing toenails and verrucas, are all briefly described.

People with diabetes need to take very good care of their feet. The possible lack of sensation means that you may not always be aware of any damage and therefore you need to check your feet regularly and, if there is any damage, to seek help immediately. Poor circulation means that you will have a devitalised skin and a much slower healing time. Because of circulation problems and possible damage to nerve endings the feet of people with diabetes are more liable to infection. Footwear should be checked regularly. Rucks in the lining or nails coming through could cause wounds. Shoes and socks need to fit well. Ill-fitting footwear causes rubbing and consequent problems. It is probably better never to go barefoot, if you have diabetes. It is important that you should see a chiropodist regularly who can check your feet, cut toenails and deal with corns or callouses.

Keeping feet warm can be a problem for many people. It obviously helps to wear warm socks and perhaps fleecy in-soles. However it is important to remember to buy bigger shoes to accommodate these, otherwise your feet will suffer from too tight shoes and may be colder as a result.

Regular chiropody treatment could help you keep your feet in good order to make your walking much more comfortable. Your health centre, library or town hall will have a list of community chiropody services in your area. If it is difficult for you to visit a clinic, health centre or hospital it may be possible for you to have a home visit by a chiropodist. A chiropodist will also be able to advise on suitable footwear. If you are seeking private treatment always look for a State Registered Chiropodist with the letters S R Ch after his or her name. The titles State Registered Chiropodist, Registered Chiropodist and State Chiropodist are protected by law and may only be used by those whose name appears on the register which should be available in your public library. Their names may also be found in Yellow Pages.

Futher information on footcare

The Society of Chiropodists
53 Welbeck Street, London W1M 7HE (Tel: 071-486 3381).

The Society of Chiropodists will give you details of chiropodists in your area. They have a publication, *Care of Your Feet*, which describes basic foot care, care of feet in warm weather and cold weather, how to deal with sweaty feet, and help for disabled people. They also have a leaflet *Ageing Feet and Arthritic Feet*.

Disabled Living Foundation
380–4 Harrow Road, London W9 2HU (Tel: 071-289 6111).

Problems Afoot: Need and efficiency in footcare (price: £4.45). This book is written for professionals and laypeople alike. The DLF Clothing and Footwear Advisory Service is always glad to help anyone with particular problems. It has useful leaflets, including *Footwear for Swollen Feet* (price: £1.25), which describes types of footwear and also adaptations which can be made to shoes already purchased. A helpful list of addresses is also given, including particular shoe manufacturers. Other leaflets include: *Footwear for Odd Sized Feet* (£1.25); *Footwear for Cold Feet* (£2.00); *Footwear and Hosiery Dressing with Stiff Hips* (£2.00); and *Fastening Footwear: Methods, aids and adaptations* (£1.25).

British Footwear Manufacturers Federation
Royalty House, 72 Dean Street, London W1V 5HB (Tel: 071-437 5573).

The BFMF will be glad to send you details of firms who supply made-to-measure shoes and boots. Some will make home visits while others may use designated local retailers. (You may also find local made-to-measure firms in your Yellow Pages.) BFMF will also supply a list of manufacturers who are prepared to help people with different sized feet. They will either supply you direct themselves or recommend a local stockist, normally at an extra charge. Other lists supplied cover: narrow heels (shoes to fit narrow heels); men's footwear (extreme sizes); women's footwear (extreme sizes).

=▶ *The Foot Care Book: An A–Z of fitter feet.* A useful booklet of self-care described at the end of this Section under publications.

Looking after your legs

One of the problems so many people have with their legs is varicose veins. They may arise as a result of a great deal of standing in our working lives. Very often, the condition is not serious, although if you have any doubts about this you should see your doctor. A useful booklet, *Help and Advice on Leg Problems: Varicose veins, coping with long term conditions*, describes what varicose veins are, how they start, and how they can be treated. The leaflet is available from: The Health Education Board for Scotland, Woodburn House, Canaan Lane, Edinburgh EH10 4SG (Tel: 031-447 8044).

Looking after your ears

Most of us experience some loss of hearing as we get older. However, we should not accept it as an inevitable fact of ageing. As soon as you find it difficult to hear ordinary conversation you should visit your doctor. It may be simply that you have too much wax in your ears and this can easily be removed.

Hearing aids have greatly improved in recent years and they are now relatively unobtrusive to wear. There is no need to be shy about wearing one.

The Royal National Institute for Deaf People will be glad to supply information and also the British Association for the Hard of Hearing. For details see Section 14.

The British Tinnitus Association, which works for the relief and cure of permanent head noise, has an interesting newsletter, *Quiet*, and information leaflets about tinnitus. For details of the BTA *see* page 332.

=▶ *Coping With Ear Problems*
By David L Cowan. Published by W & R Chambers Ltd, 43–5 Annandale Street, Edinburgh EH7 4AZ (Tel: 031-557 4571).

This useful book is one in a series *Coping with* …. It describes how the ear works, possible causes of pain in the ear, why it sometimes discharges. There is information on tinnitus, including on treatment of the condition, as well as information on tinnitus maskers. A masker is a device that looks like a hearing aid but produces a noise below the level of the tinnitus, helping to obstruct and re-educate the brain. The book goes on to describe different kinds of deafness, and to look at hearing aids. Price: £3.95.

Looking after your bones

Many older people (one in four women and one in eight men) are likely to suffer from osteoporosis, a long term condition of the bones in the skeleton. The bones become thinner and less strong so there is a greater risk of them breaking. Prevention and management of the condition is important. Some doctors recommend Hormone Replacement Therapy, a treatment which is not a cure-all but which can benefit some of those at risk. Diet and exercise are important and are the main areas for prevention of osteoporosis. A leaflet, *Help and Advice on Osteoporosis: Coping with long term conditions*, provides information on the risk factors for osteoporosis and on preventing the condition. It also gives details of a recommended diet for prevention. The leaflet is available from: The Health Education Board for Scotland, Woodburn House, Canaan Lane, Edinburgh EH10 4SG (Tel: 031-447 8044).

For advice and information about osteoporosis contact: The National Osteoporosis Society. For details see Section 14.

Alternatives in health care

Most of us have cause to be grateful for what might be called conventional health care through the National Health Service. We usually take our health problems first to our family doctor. However, GPs often seem not to have the time to listen, and health problems which are bothering us just linger on even when we feel there has to be an answer. It is often as a result of such dissatisfaction that we may think of turning to an alternative way of treating our problem. Sometimes too, friends have had good experiences with alternative practitioners regarding their backaches, migraines and so on and this inspires us to have a try. There is one big snag – alternative health treatment is rarely available on the NHS and can be very costly. If you are thinking of looking for alternative remedies it is important to check what the costs may be.

There are very many forms of alternative therapy – far too many to describe here. We list below a few to give you a taster of what is available. You could also contact The Institute for Complementary Medicine: for details *see* below.

British Acupuncture Association and Register
34 Alderney Street, London SW1V 4EV (Tel: 071-834 1012).

Acupuncture is part of a system of medicine which originated in China several thousand years ago. The principal method of treatment is by the insertion of very fine needles into points which lie beneath the skin. Acupuncture is applied primarily to regulate body functions and promote the restoration of health. It is said to be a safe and effective form of treatment for a wide variety of conditions including: migraine, headaches, ulcers and digestive troubles, lumbago, arthritis, fibrositis, neuritis, sciatica, rheumatism, dermatitis, eczema, psoriasis and other skin conditions, high blood pressure, depressions and anxiety states, and asthma and bronchitis.

A list of members is available. All full members are also qualified in another form of medicine apart from acupuncture. Anyone can set up in practice in this country as an acupuncturist, even with little or no training, so it is wise to check with the

Association before seeking treatment to be sure you find someone who is suitably qualified. Registers are available, price £2.10 including postage.

British Chiropractic Association
Premier House, 10 Greycoat Place, London SW1P 1SB (Tel: 071-222 8866).

Chiropractors specialise in diagnosing and treating disorders of the spine, joints and muscles. Drugs and surgery are never used. Chiropractors treat people with back pain and they also treat a wide range of other common aches and pains including neck, shoulder and arm pain, and headaches. Migraine, it is said, can sometimes be helped by chiropractic treatment, as well as other conditions which at first sight may not seem to be related to the spine, like dizziness, 'pins and needles', and numbness. Sciatica and other leg pains are also described as responding to chiropractic treatment, as well as hip and knee problems. It is also said that some people diagnosed as having arthritis can be greatly helped by chiropractic in terms of pain control and improved function. Muscular aches and joint pains, for instance in the elbows, feet and ankles, can also be treated.

The British Chiropractic Association has a register of members who have all completed a four-year full-time course at a college of chiropractic recognised by the European Chiropractic Union, and who are required to subscribe to the Association's code of ethics and rules. It is important if you choose to visit a chiropractor that he or she is properly qualified. In Britain at the moment there is no official registration, which means that people with little or no proper training can call themselves chiropractors.

A set of leaflets is available to help people with specific problems. These are: *Backache and Leg Pain; Neck, Shoulder and Arm Pains; Headache and Migraine; Sports Injuries; Backpain Is An Overhead.*

To obtain copies of the register or leaflets, send a 9" × 6" s.a.e. with two first class stamps and £1 to the above address.

British Homoeopathic Association
27a Devonshire Street, London W1N 1RJ (Tel: 071-935 2163).

Homoeopathy is based on the recognition that like may be treated with like using the smallest effective dose. The medicines used are employed in treatment on data compiled clinically by human test, not animal trials. The suitability of any given medicine used orally and homoeopathically relates to an overview of its effect on the whole human system both in clinical evaluation and medicinal use.

Homoeopaths consider it better to treat the sick person rather than the disease, so the *patient* is treated rather than her disease. Because the patient is treated and not the disease, patients suffering from the same 'disease' will often require different remedies; while another group of patients with different 'diseases' may all benefit from the same remedy.

The treatment is available on the National Health Service, and there are clinics at hospitals in London, Glasgow, Liverpool, Bristol and Tunbridge Wells. The Information Service is open daily to deal with any enquiries by telephone or post. (The

BHA does not itself give medical advice but will direct enquiries appropriately.) There are General Practitioners in many parts of the United Kingdom who provide homoeopathic treatment – either privately or within the NHS. Names and addresses of GPs in different areas can be provided on request from the BHA.

Membership is open to all members of the public interested in the development of homoeopathy and to all qualified doctors. Members receive a bi-monthly journal and may use the extensive library. Annual subscription is £10. A publications list is available.

The Incorporated Society of Registered Naturopaths
328 Harrogate Road, Leeds LS17 6PR (Tel: 0532-685 992).

Naturopaths do not view the body as a battleground in which hostile germs and viruses must be vanquished by ever-more-powerful wonder drugs, but as an organism capable of curing itself if allowed to do so without outside interference. It follows from this that Nature Cure provides no quick and easy solutions. The Nature Cure practitioner does not dole out magic remedies: he or she may require the patient to adopt a completely new life-style. The fundamental tenet of Nature Cure is that a person who lives in accordance with the rules of nature is likely to be a healthy person.

So naturopaths will concentrate on diet, exercise, and on the psychological aspect so that the patient will begin to understand herself or himself a little better and to comprehend the reasons for a particular behaviour pattern. A publications list is available.

All members of the Register are fully qualified practitioners and have had a minimum of four years' full-time professional training. The Society does not supply lists of practitioners' addresses; to find the name of a local ISRN registered practitioner you should telephone Peter Fenton, Secretary, on the above telephone number.

The Institute for Complementary Medicine
4 Tavern Quay, Plough Way, Surrey Quay, London SE16 1QZ (Tel: 071-237 5165).

Complementary Medicine is the general name for a number of therapeutic techniques. It is a style of medical practice that regards health and disease in terms of the whole person. Thus conventional medicine and the natural therapies provide systems of medicine which complement each other.

The Institute is a charity, founded to increase public awareness of the natural therapies through education and research. It acts as a guide to the therapies, and will give you details of your nearest practitioner in the therapy of your choice. The Institute has established 72 volunteer-staffed Public Information Points (PIPs) for local referrals. They provide: information on the therapies; public classes and lectures on self-help and self-care; and at-home discussions. The Institute will be glad to give you the name of your nearest PIP. A directory, according to region, is held by all PIPs.

The Institute is also able to supply contacts with training organisations in many of the less formally organised disciplines, so that people can get in touch with others who have successfully completed their courses.

When writing to the Institute, please enclose a s.a.e. for a reply.

=▶ *The National Institute of Medical Herbalists*
9 Palace Gate, Exeter, EX1 1JA (Tel: 0392-426022; Scotland: 041-889 8416).

The practice of herbal medicine (phytotherapy) offers the sufferer not just relief from symptoms but an improved standard of general health and vitality. Diagnostic techniques of members of the Institute resemble those of general practitioners, using the same equipment; but as well as assessing presenting symptoms, the practitioner looks beyond these to evaluate the overall balance of the body's systems, musculo-skeletal, nervous, cardio-vascular, digestive, genito-urinary and endocrine, to discover underlying and predisposing disharmonies. Thus, entirely different remedies may successfully be given to treat two patients apparently suffering from the same complaint, For this reason the trained herbal practitioner cannot give herbal medicine without seeing the patient, for it is the whole person who is treated, not the diseases.

The Institute provides information leaflets and a regional directory of members.

=▶ *The Yoga for Health Foundation*
Ickwell Bury, Biggleswade, Bedfordshire SG18 9EF (Tel: 0767-27271).

The Yoga for Health Foundation is a charity, 'devoted to helping people discover within themselves the true health, mental and physical, which can be achieved through yoga'. The Foundation's brochure reads: 'Yoga is self-realisation: through yoga techniques it is possible to become aware of mind and body development, to establish a harmonious and peaceful basis to life and to help the body's immune system to overcome a wide range of illness. Health and happiness are inter-linked: so yoga activities are neither clinical – in the established medical sense – nor purely philosophical. They are a linking of mind and body to achieve both basic health and happiness, with that greatest boon of all – peace of mind.'

The Foundation runs and supervises local groups.

The Centre, which is open seven days a week, operates as a residential club with a General Membership fee of £11.50 p.a. and £16 per family (living at one address). All members of Yoga for Health Clubs are automatically members of the Centre. As a member you will have access to the Centre and its facilities, including specific advice, and you will receive copies of the Foundation's journal *Yoga and Life*. A mail order brochure is available including details of publications and of tapes which can be helpful in practising yoga sessions at home.

Disabled people are welcome at the Centre and, in addition, there is a special holiday for those with disablement and their families.

See also pages 165 and 166 for details of the books *It's Never Too Late* and *Keep Moving, Keep Young* on gentle yoga exercises for older people.

Continence management

Many people, both young and old, have minor urinary incontinence problems. It is a very common complaint, and one about which we often feel helpless and embarrassed.

Others may have faecal (bowel) incontinence. Some people are even afraid to leave the house for fear of having an accident. But this need not be so. There is a good deal of help available to manage the problem, even for those people for whom it has become severe. With proper diagnosis and management techniques, it has been found that only a small proportion of people need to use appliances on a long-term basis.

In seeking help, it is important to persist, even if the first doctor or nurse approached is not helpful. Your doctor should be prepared to help, while the local district nursing service can offer help on day-to-day management. It is worth noting that attached to some District General Hospitals are Incontinence Clinics to which you may wish to be referred. There are also a number of books you might find useful. The Disabled Living Foundation, 380–4 Harrow Road, London W9 2HU (Tel: 071-289 6111), has a Continence Advisor who is glad to answer personal questions by letter or telephone. There is also a Northern Region Continence Advisory Service Helpline: 091-213 0050. This is available 2 p.m. to 7 p.m. Monday to Friday.

Aids for continence management include special garments, pads, appliances and deodorants. Most people who need such equipment will have it prescribed for them. There is usually no need to buy such items for yourself, as it is the responsibility of the NHS to provide the most appropriate aids for the management of incontinence in each individual case.

Clothing

If you are struggling with difficult fastenings and awkward clothing this can make the management of continence all the more difficult. If you have little warning of the need to pass urine your clothing may need to be adjusted with speed. The Disabled Living Foundation (*see* below), as well as having a Continence Advisory Service (*see* below), has a clothing and footwear service. Three of its leaflets are particularly helpful in this matter: *Clothing for Continence: Women*; *Clothing for Women Who Are Incontinent*; and *Clothing for Men Who Are Incontinent*. These leaflets are well illustrated to show that just because you have incontinence problems you do not need to wear dowdy clothes.

Cleanliness and smell

Smell can cause embarrassment and difficulties and must be dealt with immediately and efficiently. Your District Nurse will advise you on coping with soiled clothing and bed linen. She may also arrange for you to have help from a laundry service which may be provided by either health or social services. Also a waste collection service for disposable items may be available.

A neutralising deodorant will also be of help in this respect. One example is Daydrop. A drop or two can be used in appliances, commode pans and urinals, and on protective padding, etc. It is available from most retail chemists. In case of difficulty, contact

Loxley Medical, Unit 5D, Carnaby Industrial Estate, Bridlington YO15 3QY (Tel: 0262-603979).

Further information on incontinence

▶ *Age Concern England*
Astral House, 1268 London Road, London SW16 4ER (Tel: 081-679 8000). Please send a large s.a.e. with your enquiry when you send for any of the fact sheets or leaflets.

Age Concern England has produced a set of ten leaflets about urinary and faecal incontinence, as well as a fact sheet.
   The leaflets are:
- *Steps to Prevent Incontinence*
- *What You Should Do If You Have Bowel Problems*
- *Why Men Suffer from Urinary Incontinence*
- *How To Manage a Catheter*
- *What Help Is Available*
- *Why People Have Bowel Problems*
- *Why Women Suffer from Urinary Incontinence*
- *How To Use Pad and Pant Systems*
- *What You Should Do If You Have Urinary Incontinence*
- *How To Use a Collection Device (Male)*

These leaflets are available from Age Concern England groups or from Age Concern England.
   The fact sheet *Help with Incontinence* describes different ways in which incontinence can affect you, what you can do about it, and what help may be available. There is also a list of advice services and telephone helplines.

▶ *In Control – Help with incontinence* by Penny Mares, produced by Age Concern. This book is written in a straightforward and sympathetic way and is full of information. Details are given about the nature and causes of incontinence and where you can get help. The book is illustrated throughout with diagrams and it also offers interesting case studies. Price £4.50.

▶ *Disabled Living Centres*: for details of these *see* p. 116. These centres will provide advice on managing incontinence, and on special clothing and equipment.

▶ *Disabled Living Foundation*
380–4 Harrow Road, London W9 2HU (Tel: 071-289 6111).

The DLF has a Continence Advisory Service which will be glad to answer queries and to provide advice. It has a number of publications (please send s.a.e. for the list) including:

- *Incontinence: Your problems answered*. Price: £3.50. This describes the various forms of incontinence and also has a section 'Urinary incontinence and the older generation'. Other information covers: commodes, aids in the lavatory, male and female urinals, pads and pants, catheters, odour control, and a list of suppliers.
- *Adult Bedwetting: Causes, sources of help, and suggested remedies*. Price: £1.50.
- *Your Prostate Operation: For professionals and public; and post prostatectomy incontinence*. Price: £2.00.
- *Stress Incontinence and Bladder Training*. Price: £1.50.
- *Notes on Bowel Problems*. Price: £3.00.

Understanding Incontinence
By Dorothy Mandelstam. Published for the Disabled Living Foundation by Chapman and Hall. Available from: Thompson International Publishing Services, North Way, Andover, Hampshire SP10 5BE (Tel: 0264-332424). Price: £9.95.

This well-illustrated book describes the nature of incontinence and how it can be managed, and gives information about the aids, equipment and services available to help those affected by this problem. There is also a list of the suppliers of protective equipment and aids to continence. In addition, there is a list of useful addresses of helpful organisations, as well as an appendix providing information on further reading. For laypeople there is a most helpful glossary.

Directory of Continence and Toiletting Aids (1988).
Available from: The Association of Continence Advisors, 4 St Pancras Way, London NW1 OPE. Price: £17.00.

This is a loose leaf binder so that the information can be updated. It is intended for professionals rather than for the general public. However, it can be useful to know about it so that you can refer professionals to it who perhaps may not know about it.

Incontinence and Stoma Care
Available from: The Disability Information Trust, Mary Marlborough Lodge, Nuffield Orthopaedic Centre, Headington, Oxford OX3 7LD. (Tel: 0865-750103). Price: £8 post free.

This is one in a series of books *Equipment for Disabled People* describing aids and equipment for anyone who has a disability.

The book gives information on: management of incontinence; provision of incontinence aids and stoma equipment; hand held urinals; odour control; pants and pads; body-worn urinals; condom drainage; drainage bags; drainage bag attachments; night drainage bags; drainage bag holders; stoma equipment; sources of help; and has a select bibliography.

=▶ *The Healthcall Directory* operate a Telephone Tape *Incontinence*. The telephone number is 0898-600835. The calls are charged at special rates – 36p per minute (off-peak rates), and 48p per minute (peak rates).

Operations

One of the biggest problems surrounding very many operations now is the long waiting lists. There are ways of hastening the process – for instance being prepared to be a stand-by patient, in which case you should tell your GP. You may then be able to have your operation earlier if someone else cannot keep their appointment. Or it may be possible to go to another district where the waiting list is shorter for that particular operation.

Regional Health Authorities have now set up Health Information Centres in every NHS Region in England. The information they provide includes waiting times. For details see the beginning of this Section. The College of Health also has a Waiting List Helpline for those living in the Thames Health Regions (Tel: 0345-678 1133).

The College of Health has also produced two booklets which, although they are rather old, nevertheless have useful information about operations. Each is priced at 75p. Available from: College of Health, St Margaret's House, 21 Old Ford Road, London E2 9PL.

- *Going Into Hospital*, describing the questions you should ask the consultant, and what to do if you want a second opinion; waiting for admission – diet, exercise, smoking, relaxation; admission – what to pack, what to do about valuables, visiting; waiting for your operation; operation day; recovery; going home; your rights; and what to do if you have a complaint.
- *Hip-Replacement Operation*, describing what the operation is, how you may feel after the operation, learning to walk again, aids to mobility, driving, and sex.

Helpful organisations

Many organisations are listed and described in Section 14. We list here some of those having a special concern with health.

=▶ *Age Concern England*
Astral House, 1268 London Road, London SW16 4ER (Tel: 081-679 8000).

=▶ *Age Concern Scotland*
54A Fountainbridge, Edinburgh EH3 9PT (Tel: 031-228 5656).

=▶ *Age Concern Wales*
4th Floor, 1 Cathedral Road, Cardiff, South Glamorgan CF1 9SD (Tel: 0222-371 566).

Age Concern Northern Ireland
6 Lower Crescent, Belfast BT7 1NR (Tel: 0232-245729).

AL-ANON Family Groups UK and Eire
61 Great Dover Street, London SE1 4YF (Tel: 071-403 0888 – a confidential 24-hour helpline).

AL-ANON is a worldwide fellowship providing understanding and support for the relatives and friends of problem drinkers, whether the alcoholic is still drinking or not.

ALATEEN is a part of AL-ANON specially for teenagers who are or have been affected by an alcoholic parent.

Over 1,000 groups meet in the United Kingdom and Eire. Everything is confidential and there are no dues and fees. AL-ANON is entirely self-supporting through the sale of its literature and members' voluntary contributions.

Contact as above for further information and for details of local meetings.

AL-ANON members are available to give talks to groups and professionals.

Alcoholics Anonymous
The General Service Office, PO Box 1, Stonebow House, Stonebow, York YO1 2NJ (Tel: 0904-644026).

Alcoholics Anonymous is a worldwide fellowship of men and women who help each other to stay sober. They offer the same help to anyone who has a drinking problem and wants to do something about it. Since they are all alcoholics themselves, they have a special understanding of each other. They know what the illness feels like – and they have learnt how to recover from it in AA.

Alcoholics Anonymous is made up of about 65,000 local groups, in 110 countries. In Great Britain and the Channel Islands there are more than 2,200 local groups. Newcomers do not pay any fees for membership. For the address of a local group look in the phone directory, but if you do not find a local group listed contact Alcoholics Anonymous.

ASH – Action on Smoking and Health
109 Gloucester Place, London W1H 3PH (Tel: 071-935 3519).

ASH aims to alert the public to the dangers of smoking, to prevent the death, disease and disability which it causes, and to make non-smoking the norm in society. ASH is a public information campaign; it gathers and disseminates information on all aspects of smoking by monitoring the national and local press, scientific and medical publications, and trade magazines. As a result ASH is able to provide up-to-date information about smoking issues, how to deal with smoking in the workplace and public places, and how individuals can give up smoking.

ASH has a range of fact sheets. These include:

– *Smoking Statistics*
– *The Constituents of Tobacco Smoke*

- *The Economics of Smoking*
- *Smoking and Lung Disease*
- *Tobacco and Cancer*
- *Children and Smoking*
- *Passive Smoking*
- *Smoking and Reproduction*
- *Women and Tobacco*
- *Smoking and Arterial Disease*
- *Smoking Cessation Aids*
- *Tobacco and Cancer*
- *Pipe and Cigar Smoking*.

The price of each fact sheet is 10p.

The ASH catalogue has some very interesting items. As well as publications there are a variety of posters and a great many imaginatively designed signs asking people not to smoke, suitable for work and even for home.

The Beth Johnson Foundation
Parkfield House, 64 Princes Road, Hartshill, Stoke-on-Trent ST4 7JL (Tel: 0782-44036).

The project in North Staffordshire provides a range of imaginative services and it is hoped that these may spread to other places. One of these services is *Self Health Care in Old Age Project*, including Peer Health Counselling where older volunteers help their peers towards positive health and well-being. It is always encouraging to be advised by others who are of a similar age to yourself. Peer Health Counsellors are retired people who have an interest in self-health and want to share their enthusiasm with their peer group in the form of satisfying voluntary work. They must be willing to undertake training and to attend monthly support meetings. Training courses for new Peer Health Counsellors are scheduled to take place each year. Subjects covered include mental, emotional and physical health; working with frail and infirm people; seeking out resource and information material; liaison with statutory and voluntary agencies; and communication skills.

The project also operates a telephone Care Line. Referrals are received from social workers, health visitors, nurses and carers who feel that a particular old person is at some risk and would appreciate a daily call. A Care Line volunteer visits to introduce the service and to check on the home situation. Useful information is then available to the volunteer telephonist.

In addition, there is a Senior Health Shop. A variety of courses are also run, including Look After Yourself; Stress Control; Weight Control; Yoga; and Keep Fit – these take place at a Senior Centre.

British Heart Foundation
14 Fitzhardinge Street, London W1H 4DH (Tel: 071-935 0185).

This is a research organisation which also provides publications free to the general public. The titles include: *Food Should Be Fun*, containing advice on recipes for healthy eating; and *A New Start for You and Your Heart*, for patients about to undergo a coronary artery by-pass, graft or valve surgery. There is also a Heart Information series of pamphlets which includes: *Back to Normal*; *What is Angina?*; *Food and Your Heart*; *Heart Surgery for Adults*; *Reducing the Risk of a Heart Attack*. In addition, there are leaflets and posters, and a sign 'No Smoking Please'.

The British Nutrition Foundation
15 Belgrave Square, London SW1X 8PS (Tel: 071-235 4904).

The BNF is an impartial scientific organisation which sets out to provide reliable information and scientifically-based advice on nutrition and related health matters, with the ultimate objective of helping individuals to understand how they may best match their diet with their life-style. The Foundation offers information and advice, arranges seminars, etc., and publishes a wide range of materials, including popular leaflets. Two of these are *How To Eat a Healthy Diet* and *Nutrition and the Elderly*.

BUPA Medicall
Provident House, Essex Street, London WC2R 3BR.

This is a 24-hour telephone service on family health information available to non-members of the BUPA private health insurance as well as to members. Subjects covered include: alcohol abuse; alternative medicine and therapies; back and neck problems; breathing problems; cancer; chiropody; ears and hearing problems; eye problems; heart and circulation; muscle, bone and joint disorder; older people; sleep; smoking; and surgical operations. Pre-recorded messages provide the information. For a list of subjects and telephone numbers and for details of the subjects contact the above address.

Coronary Prevention Group
102 Gloucester Place, London WC1N 3HR (Tel: 071-935 2889).

The Coronary Prevention Group (CPG) is the only UK charity whose entire work is devoted to the prevention of coronary heart disease (CHD). It provides information on the causes and prevention of CHD. It provides practical advice and support to the public, health professionals, schools, industry and voluntary organisations on issues such as smoking, diet, exercise and stress, and work for health-promoting public policies.

The CPG has a range of publications, including *Eat Well ... Live Well* on healthy eating. Full of colour pictures, it costs £1.95 including postage and packing. Copies of the CPG's leaflets, *You and Your Heart, Smoking and Your Heart, Blood Pressure and Your Heart, Stress and Your Heart, Blood Cholesterol and Your Heart* and *Exercise and Your Heart*, can be obtained for 50 pence each from the above address, or send a large s.a.e. for a free information pack, which includes a sample booklet.

The CPG has an Associate/Corporate membership through which interested individuals and organisations can keep in touch with their work. As a member you will be sent the Annual Report, details of publications, seminars and conferences, and a free copy of the quarterly newsletter. Associate/Corporate membership is £10/£50 p.a.

Health Education Board for Scotland
Health Education Centre, Woodburn House, Canaan Lane, Edinburgh EH10 4SG (Tel: 031-447 8044).

HEBS has a very interesting range of materials (including health education films and videos) covering many aspect of health including alcohol, smoking, dental health and mental health and it also has a particular concern for the health of older people. It will be glad to send you details of its information services.

Health Information Network
Algarve House, 1A The Colonnade, High Street, Maidenhead, Berkshire SL6 1QL (Tel: 0628-778744).

The Network has a range of information including a series of authoritative medical booklets written by medical experts in easy-to-understand plain English to provide the lay reader with reliable and trustworthy medical information. The information is continually updated as new ideas and treatments evolve. It will be glad to send you a catalogue of titles. Please send a large s.a.e.

Health Search Scotland
Woodburn House, Canaan Lane, Edinburgh EH10 4SG (Tel: 031-452 8666).

This is a free health information service for health care staff, the public, people caring for relatives and friends, and organisations concerned with health. The aim is to help people become more involved with their own health care by providing details of local and national self-help groups and supplying information on health matters. You can contact Health Search by telephone or letter or you can visit.

In addition, Health Search Scotland has an extensive collection of self-help leaflets and booklets. Leaflets on specific subjects can be given out free to individual enquirers.

International Glaucoma Association
King's College Hospital, Denmark Hill, London SE5 9RS (Tel: 071-737 3265).

The IGA is a charity and offers all patients, doctors, optometrists and those interested in preventing blindness from glaucoma a forum for the exchange of ideas on glaucoma as well as the opportunity to campaign actively for greater government recognition of the problem. Its aim is to prevent loss of sight from glaucoma throughout the world. Membership is open to all. The annual subscription is £7.50.

The IGA holds two discussion forum meetings each year and issues a twice yearly newsletter for members. The Association also supports glaucoma research and has a very active public awareness campaign, sending out more than 60,000 information booklets each year.

Questions of a general nature are answered by letter, and factual information is sent on request. The information booklet on glaucoma will be sent on receipt of a 7" × 9" s.a.e.. No charge is made for information, although donations are always welcomed.

Partially Sighted Society

This Society has a registered office, a National Low Vision Advice Centre and a Greater London office:

Registered office dealing with general administration, printing, enlarging, mail order, membership, *Oculus* distribution and free literature: Queen's Road, Doncaster DN1 2NX (Tel: 0302-368998).

Oculus is the magazine of the Partially Sighted Society and is produced in large clear print on a bi-monthly basis. Enquiries should be directed to the editor at the Doncaster address above.

National Low Vision Advice Centre and the South West Regional Office: Sight Centre, Dean Clarke House, Southernhay East, Exeter EX1 1PE (Tel: 0392-210656).

The NLVAC incorporates the South West Regional Office and houses a wide range of lenses, lighting, electronic equipment, literature and other vision enhancement as well as RNIB catalogue items and articles which are commercially available. The Centre also operates a low vision training project and the Society's Advisory Information and Counselling Service. Visitors are welcome at the Centre.

Greater London Office: 62 Salusbury Road, London NW6 6NS (Tel: 071-372 1551).

The Greater London Development Officer, based in the Greater London office, aims to develop the activities of the Society throughout Greater London, including the setting up of self-help groups throughout the region. The Development Officer welcomes enquiries on matters relating to visual impairment and vision enhancement. A limited range of aids, apparatus and literature is kept at the London office.

Information and advice is available free of charge by letter or telephone on any aspect of living or working with impaired vision.

Membership of the Society is open to anyone who wishes to support the work of the Society. Partially sighted members receive *Oculus*, which gives up-to-the minute information on appliances and services, news of events, reviews, and general interest items. Full membership (with voting rights) for individual members is £17.50 and Supporters membership (without voting rights) is £7.50 for individuals.

QUIT! National Society of Non-smokers
102 Gloucester Place, London W1H 3DA
(Tel: 071-487 2858 (office); 071-487 3000 (Helpline)).

QUIT! is the only UK charity specialising in offering practical help for smokers to quit. They started No Smoking Day, which helps 50,000 smokers to quit every year.

Quit runs a range of services including:

- *Quitline* – a 'live' helpline offering counselling, information packs and referral to local stop smoking groups.
- Publications including *Quit and Stay Slim!* and a *Consumer's Guide To Stop Smoking Methods.*
- *Quit In Practice* – a training programme to help GPs manage smoking more effectively with their practices.
- *Quit in the Workplace* – a range of programmes for employers wanting to help their staff to quit.

▶ *Relaxation for Living*
29 Burwood Park Road, Walton-on-Thames, Surrey KT12 5LH

This is a charity aiming to promote the teaching of physical relaxation to combat the stress, strain, anxiety and tension of modern life and to reduce fatigue.

Day and evening classes are in courses of six or seven at weekly intervals and group discussion is an important feature. Pupils have included women and men with ages ranging from 16 to the mid 80s. In some areas, courses are run in conjunction with the adult education or other services. For pupils unable to reach a teacher, a correspondence course is available. Leaflets and short practice tapes have been published to assist people to understand and help themselves better.

A newsletter is published four times a year and contains reports, articles, book and tape reviews, readers' letters, etc. The annual subscription is £6.

A list of authorised teachers is available. Further information can be obtained by sending a large s.a.e.

▶ *St John Ambulance Association*
1 Grosvenor Crescent, London SW1X 7EF (Tel: 071-235 5231).

The St John Ambulance Association holds First Aid Training courses at locations throughout the country, both during the day and in the evenings. St John teaches the practical skills needed to deal with emergencies in the home, in the street or at work, and gives the individual the confidence to act. The basic Emergency Aid Courses take two hours, *Save a Life* four hours, and the Public First Aid Course 15 hours. A charge is made to cover the cost of these courses. For details send for the leaflet *Emergency Aid and Public First Aid Training.*

▶ *Ulster Cancer Foundation*
40–2 Eglantine Avenue, Belfast BT9 6DX (Tel: 0232-663281).

This Smoking Withdrawal Centre operates as a free service to the community. It is open every Wednesday evening 7 to 9 p.m. (no appointment necessary). There is also a *Stop Smoking Tips* phone-in service. This operates 24 hours a day and by dialling Belfast 664926 you can get three minutes of pre-recorded helpful advice on giving up smoking.

The Centre will be glad to send you a leaflet describing its services with ideas on giving up smoking.

⇒ *The Vegan Society*
7 Battle Road, St Leonards-on-Sea, East Sussex TN37 7AA (Tel: 0424-427393).

The Vegan Society promotes a diet free of all animal products for the benefit of people, animals and the environment. It publishes a quarterly magazine *The Vegan* and the following books: *Animal Free Shopper*, *Vegan Nutrition* and *The Caring Cook*. For further information about these titles, the Vegan Society and the vegan diet send a large s.a.e.

⇒ *VMM*
Century House, 100 Nelson Road, London N8 9RT
(Tel: 081-348 5229 (London and South);
061-973 7500, office hours (North and Scotland)).

VMM encourages vegetarians and vegans to get together to make new contacts and new friends. Members meet at get-togethers, parties, on weekends away or by using the personalised confidential introduction service. There is also a newsletter, *VooMM*. All ages welcome.

⇒ *The Vegetarian Society (UK) Ltd*
Parkdale, Dunham Road, Altrincham, Cheshire WA14 4QG (Tel: 061-928 0793).

Membership of the Vegetarian Society entitles you to copies of *The Vegetarian*, a bi-monthly magazine, a host of discounts (a list will be sent to you on request if you send a s.a.e.), and a free copy of *The Vegetarian Handbook*. Cookery courses are held regularly and there are regional groups of members which you can join at no extra charge. Reduced membership subscription rates for Senior Citizens – £10. A range of leaflets and publications is available, including a leaflet *Healthy Nutrition in Later Life*. There is also a vegetarian catalogue showing an appetising range of food available on mail order as well as toilet and beauty products.

Health care professionals

In local communities, there are a number of health care professionals concerned with keeping everyone as healthy as possible. Besides your own doctor, there are others, such as district nurses, health visitors, and community psychiatric nurses, whom you can call upon. This would normally be arranged after consultation with your GP.

District Nurse/Community Nurse

The District Nurse may be able to help with bathing and with any incontinence problems. After you have had a period in hospital, the nurse may be needed to change a dressing or to ensure that medication and recommended diets are properly maintained. District Nurses will also put you in touch with other agencies who may be able to help.

Health Visitor

Health Visitors are particularly concerned to offer advice and support on matters which directly affect your health. It might be your diet, your smoking or drinking habits, or it might be about something that is worrying or depressing you.

Community Psychiatric Nurse

If you, or a relative that you are looking after, are suffering from mental stress or anxiety, the Community Psychiatric Nurse can offer support and practical help, This might take the form of regular home visits or it might involve helping you to deal with situations in the community which are difficult for you to handle.

Chiropodist

Chiropodists offer treatment in a clinic, usually on an appointment basis, and in the homes of those older people who are unable to attend a clinic. A chiropodist will also be able to advise on suitable footwear.

Private health plans

These arrangements need to be studied very carefully. They offer private health insurance which will save you from having to wait for treatment and for operations. However, the costs need to be looked at very carefully to see whether the expense of the insurance premiums really will provide sufficient cover in the event of long or serious illness. We provide details of just three schemes as well as of an organisation which can recommend a medical insurer which meets your needs. However, we are not necessarily recommending them.

▸ *The Private Health Partnership*
265a Otley Road, West Park, Leeds LS16 5LN (Tel: 0532-788855).

PHP says it can provide independent advice on all aspects of private medical insurance. It deals with all the various medical insurers (now over 30) and consequently has specialised facilities and rates not normally available to the public. In order to advise specifically, and because it is legally responsible for the advice it gives, it prefers its clients to complete a questionnaire detailing their personal circumstances. It charges a fee of £5.00 for providing individual advice and recommendations.

= ▶ *Private Patients Plan*
Has devised a *Retirement Health Plan* for those aged 60 and over. Details from Private Patients Plan, PPP House, Upperton Road, Eastbourne, East Sussex BN21 1LH (Tel: 0323-410505).

= ▶ *Budget BUPA*
Is another scheme which is aimed at protecting your health in retirement. Application for membership is open to you and your spouse, provided you are both under 75. Details from: Budget BUPA Centre, 1st Floor, Spruce House, Pinetrees, Chertsey Lane, Staines, Middlesex TW18 4SL
(Tel: Enquiries – free 0800-010383).

= ▶ *The Saga Private Healthcare Plan*
Saga Services Ltd, Freepost, PO Box 131, Folkestone, Kent CT20 1BR
(Tel: 0483-306171).

On enquiry, an information pack will be sent to you. There is no upper age limit. The minimum age is 60. You will have guaranteed acceptance without a medical examination or any health questions. Pre-existing conditions may be covered after two years free of treatment, advice, medication or consultation for those or related conditions.

Publications and resources

See also Section 15, 'Selected Further Reading'.

The Age Concerns of England, Wales, Scotland and Northern Ireland have a range of publications, a number of them concerned with health. Some of these have been mentioned in this Section. They will be glad to send you copies of their publications lists.

In particular, you may be interested in the *Age Well* newsletter produced in co-operation with Age Concern England. This is a very lively publication describing some of the many activities older people are undertaking and enjoying throughout the country. Copies may be obtained from: *Age Well*, Age Concern England, Astral House, 1268 London Road, London SW16 4ER (Tel: 081-679 8000).

= ▶ *Coping with Rheumatoid Arthritis*
By Heather Unsworth. (W and R Chambers Ltd, 43–5 Annandale Street, Edinburgh EH7 4AZ (Tel: 031-557 4571)), price: £3.95.

This is a practical guide to the day-to-day problems which have to be overcome by those diagnosed as having rheumatoid arthritis. It provides information on how the disease begins, likely symptoms and the longer-term prospects for individual people. Details of the various medical treatments and alternative therapies are given, together with self-help techniques which can be used.

Coping with Depression
By Ivy M. Blackburn. (W and R Chambers Ltd, 43–5 Annandale Street, Edinburgh EH7 4AZ (Tel: 031-557 4571)), price: £3.95.

This book is a guide to the stages and signs of depression and the techniques which may prevent it becoming a major problem. The author emphasises the importance of self-help and intends that the advice, information and sources of support will enable readers to lead a fuller, more enjoyable life.

Disabled Living Foundation
380–4 Harrow Road, London W9 2HU (Tel: 071-289 6111).

The DLF's publications list has a range of books. The Foundation also has papers and leaflets in specific areas in connection with a special service it offers. These include a Clothing Advisory Service and a Continence Advisory Service. It will be glad to send you its publications list or if you have a specific query, write to the particular advisory service or, if your query is more general, write to the enquiry service.

The Foot Care Book: An A–Z of fitter feet
By Judith Kemp. Available from Age Concern England, Astral House, 1268 London Road, London SW16 4ER, price: £2.95.

This is a detailed self-help guide giving advice on routine foot care written in a simple style and in enlarged type. It tells you what to do if there is a problem and where to go for advice. The book gives advice about choosing shoes and includes an A–Z of foot conditions covering a wide range of possible problems from athlete's foot and chilblains to ulcers, varicose veins and verrucas. As the book says: 'Though our feet may be the most downtrodden parts of our body, they are the basis for an active and independent lifestyle for everyone from the age of one upwards.'

Guide to Medicines and Drugs
Produced by the British Medical Association (Dorling Kindersley Limited, 9 Henrietta Street, London WC2E 8PS (Tel: 071-836 5411), second edition 1991), price £17.99 hardback; £9.99 paperback.

This 456-page book is accurately described as the essential family reference to prescription and over-the-counter medications including vitamins and minerals. It explains how drugs work, discusses possible side-effects and other potential problems, and gives profiles of the most widely used prescription and over-the-counter drugs. It is an invaluable guide for laypeople, helping each of us to understand our treatment.

The book is written in non-technical terms and helps the layperson, without medical training, to understand how a drug works and how useful it is for a particular condition.

It has been compiled by doctors and pharmacists familiar with the sorts of questions people want answered. The information is, of course, not intended to supersede the information given by a patient's doctor.

The book is beautifully produced with copious illustrations. It is easy to follow and to find the particular information you may be looking for.

▶ *The Health Directory*
(Bedford Square Press, 26 Bedford Square, London WC1B 3HU (Tel: 071-636 4066)), price £6.95.

The Health Directory lists around a thousand organisations set up to help patients and their families with many common (and not so common) health problems. The organisations include well-known national bodies and advice services as well as informal self-help groups. The groups are listed alphabetically, covering a wide range of problems. Whether you want the British Migraine Association, Coronary Prevention Group, Depressives Associated, National Back Pain Association, New Approaches to Cancer, Sickle Cell Society or Vegetarian Society, you can find them all here. Aimed particularly at the non-specialist, this book will also be a useful reference book for doctors, nurses and other professionals.

▶ *Health Education Authority publications*
Hamilton House, Mabledon Place, London WC1H 9TX (Tel: 071-631 0930).

The HEA has a very wide range of materials on every aspect of health including keeping fit, smoking and drinking. The titles include:

– *Action on Coronary Heart Disease in Asians* – this booklet describes a video, but nevertheless also stands on its own. Asian communities in the United Kingdom have higher mortality rates for coronary heart disease than the rest of the United Kingdom. The main risk factors are described, as well as how to avoid these. Price: £2.95.

– *AIDS and You* – an illustrated guide to HIV and AIDS, describing how you get HIV, safe behaviour, unsafe behaviour, what you can do about it, signs of AIDS, the tests – where to go, what to do. Price: £2.25.

– *Cancer: A guide to reducing your risks* – this booklet clearly describes what is cancer, the causes of cancer, and what you can do if you are at risk through smoking, drinking, sunbathing, eating too much of certain foods, viruses.

– *The Cervical Smear Test* – a leaflet describing why the test is necessary and how it is carried out.

– *Do You Take Sugar?* – a leaflet showing how sugar affects your teeth, and how to cut down on sugar.

– *Enjoy Healthy Eating* – a very well illustrated booklet showing the variety of foods we need to eat to keep us healthy and those we should cut down on. In addition, there are some very tasty recipes. Available free.

– *Exercise. Why Bother?: A simple guide to getting fitter for adults of all ages*. The booklet describes the advantages of fitness, the precautions you need to take before

you start any form of exercise, and the different types of exercise you can do from walking, swimming and cycling to bowling, exercise classes and yoga.
- *Making a New Start: A simple guide to keeping your heart young and enjoying it.* This leaflet describes how to cut down on eating fat and gives a table of the fat content of various foods. The headings are encouraging and include: 'Ten tasty things you can eat more of' and 'You don't have to give up your tipple'.
- *Passive Smoking: Questions and answers.* This leaflet describes passive smoking and how it can be harmful, and suggests how to avoid passive smoking.
- *That's the Limit: A guide to sensible drinking.* This leaflet describes those who are at risk, and provides a table showing the alcohol content in different drinks. It helps you to add up how much you drink and provides space for you to do this. It also describes sensible limits for men and women.

Health Education Board for Scotland publications
Woodburn House, Canaan Lane, Edinburgh EH10 4SG (Tel: 031-447 8044).

A wide range of publications includes *What Do You Expect at Your Age?*, written mainly for doctors; *Depression* and *Dementia*; and there is a well-illustrated book in the series *Eat To Your Heart's Content*, with mouth watering recipes.

Health and Healthy Living: A guide for older people
Available free from: Health Publications Unit, No. 2 Site, Heywood Stores, Manchester Road, Heywood,Lancashire OL10 2PZ.

This well-set-out booklet describes ways of living a healthy life-style, including the benefits of exercise for the body as well as keeping mentally active. It discusses looking after eyes, ears and teeth and describes common health concerns.

Health Wise: An intelligent guide for the over 60s
By James Le Fanu. (Papermac, Cavaye Place, London SW10 9PG (Tel: 071-373 6070)), price £10.99.

Written by a doctor, the books sets out to show how it is possible to increase the chances of a long life by having regular check-ups and taking anti-ageing drugs like Hormone Replacement Therapy. The author explains how to distinguish those symptoms which might be potentially serious and so require urgent medical attention. He also gives hints on how to get the best out of general practitioners and hospital consultants and how to bypass long waiting lists, and provides the essential information anyone will need in deciding which treatments are best.

How To ... books
Available from: How To Books Ltd, Plymbridge House, Estover Road, Plymouth PL6 7PZ (Tel: 0752-705251).

1. *How To Take Care of Your Heart*
By Mark Payne. With its clear layout, checklists and self-assessment charts, this

no-nonsense book demystifies the whole subject of heart disorders and explains step by step how to cut your risk of an attack and how to increase your chances of survival if one should happen. Fully illustrated with line diagrams, charts and tables and complete with glossary, useful addresses, further reading and index. Price: £5.95.

2. *How To Lose Weight and Keep Fit*
By Aine McCarthy, who says: 'People who exercise regularly and eat well look, feel and perform better than those who don't.' This user-friendly guide to fitness and weight controls provides a step-by-step approach tailored to the fitness needs of the individual. Price: £6.95.

The In Touch Handbook
Available from: Broadcasting Support Services, PO Box 7, London W3 6XJ. Braille and tape editions are also available. Price: £12.50.

This handbook has been produced by the team that produces the weekly Radio 4 programme. It has a wealth of information describing how to get help from the local authority, voluntary organisations and so on. It also describes very fully the financial benefits and allowances you may be entitled to and how to go about claiming them. There is a chapter on everyday living, and other chapters cover: housing; in the kitchen; getting around; reading and writing; leisure; computers for home, office, and handbag; travel and holidays; and tape newspapers and books. Aids and equipment are described, as well as details of services. In addition, up-to-date information on low vision aids is complemented by a chart with which people unable to contact an optometrist can be helped to choose a suitable magnifier.

The In Touch Bulletin
For details write to: In Touch, Room 6114, Broadcasting House,
London W1A 4WW.

A quarterly summary of all the broadcast information available free in print, braille and Moon script and on tape.

In Touch at Home
By Margaret Ford. Available from ISIS Large Print, 55 St Thomas' Street, Oxford OX1 1JG (Tel: 0865-250333). Price: £5.95 including postage.

In this book Margaret Ford has compiled hundreds of tips and ideas using the helpful suggestions of handicapped people. From safe cooking to moving furniture, this book provides helpful hints enabling people with visual handicap to run their homes efficiently and safely. It details potential hazards in each and decribes how to avoid them.

The Magic of Movement: A tonic for older people.
By Laura Mitchell. Available from Age Concern, Astral House, 1268 London Road, London SW16 4ER. Price: £3.95.

Laura Mitchell believes that regular exercise enhances the condition of both body and mind and in this book she presents a series of gentle exercises suitable for those with limited mobility. The exercises range from deep breathing to hand stretching. She also writes about eating and drinking and how important it is not only to eat and drink healthily but also to enjoy your meals. A great deal of Laura Mitchell's advice is about enjoyment in whatever you are doing. She also mentions clothing, massage, managing incontinence, and care of your feet. This is both a practical and enjoyable book.

Preventing Heart Disease
Produced by the Coronary Prevention Group. Available from: Consumers' Association, Castlemead, Gascoyne Way, Hertford X, SG14 1LH.

This book explains how your heart works and what can go wrong, and shows how smoking, being overweight, and having high blood pressure or high blood cholesterol levels can contribute to heart disease. It gives practical advice on eating healthily, taking exercise, stopping smoking and learning to tackle stress. For people who have angina or have already had a heart attack or heart surgery the pros and cons of drugs and surgery are explained, and there is information and advice on getting back to normal. Government, industry and health professionals also have a role to play in helping people to look after their hearts; the book outlines what you have a right to expect.

Saga Holidays Ltd
FREEPOST, Folkestone, Kent CT20 1BR.

Saga has a number of publications covering subjects of interest to older people. We give brief details of two in this Section:

1. *Saga Food Guide* by Carol Leverkus.
Price: £3.50. This book provides advice on basic nutrition which considers the foods which are valuable for preventing nutritional deficiency and ill health in later life. A chapter describes the best ways to cater for one or two people. Another chapter, 'A taste of health', is concerned with the most common diet-related illnesses. These may be due to an over-consumption of energy sources (calories), fat (especially saturated fat), sugar and salt, and to taking too few of the fibre-rich foods. Other chapters cover having fun with vegetables, feeding the grandchildren, and entertaining.

2. *Saga Health Guide* by Dr Muir Gray.
Price: £3.50. The subjects covered in this book include: body changes; exercises for fitness; aches and pains; looking after your heart; stress; sleeping well; common medical problems; and women's health. Although written by a doctor, the style is simple and uses layperson's language. It is a book you can easily dip into when you want to consult it on a particular subject or concern.

Scottish Council on Alcohol
137/145 Sauchiehall Street, Glasgow G2 3EW (Tel: 041-333 9677).

SCA produces a very interesting and lively publication four times a year: *Alcohol Update*. Subscription £8.50. It also has a range of publications, including two published in co-operation with Age Concern Scotland: *Why Spoil a Good Time?*, describing the effects of alcohol on people who are older and suggesting ways to enjoy drinking without drinking too much; and *Alcohol and Older People*, a leaflet prepared for those caring for older people.

Simple Relaxation
By Laura Mitchell. (John Murray Ltd, 50 Albemarle Street, London W1X 4BD (Tel: 071-493 4361)), price £4.95.

The author avoids complicated exercises or meditation and teaches you to recognise the pattern of stress all over your body. She equips you with precise orders to give yourself to change tension to ease. You do not have to stop whatever you are doing before carrying out the orders – they fit in with housework, office routine, meetings, driving, telephoning – in fact just those times and places when tension most often grips you and when you want to get free from it fast. Equally, you can use the method for resting or to help you get to sleep.

You and Your GP
(Bedford Square Press, 8 Regents Wharf, All Saints Street, London N1 9RL), price: £4.95.

Written from a consumer's point of view, this book is full of practical information on how to find and choose a GP who meets your needs, how to use your GP, and what his or her duties are medically and legally. It investigates the doctor–patient relationship and discusses problems which you may encounter in the delivery of care. There is information on your rights as a patient and on making complaints when things go wrong. The author also deals with arranging family care and care away from home. Finally, she covers other options including health insurance, private care and complementary medicine. In addition, an appendix gives a very useful glossary of common terms and procedures.

Your Health in Retirement
Available from Age Concern England, Astral House, 1268 London Road, London SW16 4ER (Tel: 081-679 8000). Price £4.50.

This book is a good source of information to help readers look after themselves and work towards better health. Produced in an easy-to-read A–Z style. Full details are given of people and useful organisations from which advice and assistance can be sought.

SECTION EIGHT

Planning for death and coping with bereavement

Advance planning for your death

The burden on others can be greatly relieved if, in various practical ways, you systematically prepare for your own death. You need realistically to face up to the inevitability of your own passing, and to make suitable prior arrangements.

Making your wishes known

It makes sense, and is sometimes vital, to commit your personal wishes to paper, offering clear guidance to those you leave behind.

Your last will and testament

First and foremost, if you have assets of any substance, it is of the utmost importance that you express your wishes as to their disposal by making a will. Should you die intestate (i.e. without having made a will), the rules which govern the distribution of your estate (*see* page 204) may not achieve what you would have wished and may not adequately provide for those you most care about. Section 2, 'More Money Matters', has basic advice about making a will.

Funeral arrangements

You may wish to make clear any feelings you have about the way your funeral is to be arranged or your body is to be dealt with (your personal representative will actually be entitled to the last word on this, but your wishes will normally be respected). One of the facts of death which has to be taken into account is that those who are bereaved are often in a confused psychological state – shock, despair, guilt, self-reproach or even disbelief. They may not have much idea of what to do, and are likely to feel that time itself is against them. Some may be too embarrassed to admit to a funeral director that what he is offering seems expensive. Some may be tempted, for a variety of reasons, to spend more lavishly than they can afford. Others may simply not take in what is said or realise what they have agreed to do. A great many of these problems can be anticipated and avoided by setting down and making known your own wishes. Death is a reality and though nobody wishes to be morbid in advance, there is great deal to be said, if death seems not too far away, in favour of calm discussion within the family. Openness in this, as in medical matters, is often more reassuring than the uncertainty of silence and fear of the unspoken. Those who will have the responsibility for meeting the requests of the deceased will also then have the opportunity to consider in advance what they will need to do.

Secular funerals

One of the questions you may wish to address (though it is somewhat for the bereaved as well) is whether you really want a religious service, which unless you are a regular churchgoer is likely to follow a routine formula and to be conducted by a stranger. If you hold no religious views or are antagonistic to religion, it may be more honest to make clear that you do not want a religious ceremony at your funeral. There is no obligation to have any funeral ceremony at all, but it is worth bearing in mind that there is a considerable psychological value for those bereaved to have some form of commemoration. In Holland, for example, it is common practice for people attending a funeral to stand and pay tribute to the deceased. The National Secular Society, 702 Holloway Road, London N19 3NL (Tel: 071-272 1266) or the British Humanist Association, 14 Lamb's Conduit Passage, London WC1R 4RH can give you information about alternative arrangements, and will, on request, usually be able to help by providing an officiant for a secular funeral ceremony. Alternatively (or as well), those you leave behind may be helped by a later secular memorial meeting, which they may find a more meaningful way in which to mark and honour the passing and the life of a loved one. This is something which can be arranged in a very personal way and shared by relatives and friends. Though it would obviously be something for the bereaved to order, you may wish to indicate in advance some readings and music which you particularly treasure.

Paying for your funeral in advance

More and more people are planning their funeral arrangements in advance and making sure that there will be adequate money to meet the costs involved. One way of making financial provision is by the traditional route of a life assurance scheme. Various kinds of policy and payment can be made either by the investment of a lump sum or by regular premiums for a set number of years or until death. A disadvantage is that such plans are usually for a fixed amount of cover, which because of rising prices may prove to be insufficient to meet the full cost of your funeral. Some plans, however, may provide for the amount to be received from the policy to be increased annually. If the person insured is very old, and hence not a good 'risk', it is likely to be difficult to obtain cover.

Age Concern recommends a scheme which is not insurance based. This is offered by Chosen Heritage Ltd, whom you can contact by writing to *Freepost*, Chosen Heritage, East Grinstead, West Sussex RH19 1EW or by telephoning free of charge on 0800-525555. There is a choice of differently priced plans, all of which allow the essential details of a funeral to be paid for in advance *at the prices relevant at the date of entering the plan*, either by a lump sum payment or by 60 monthly payments. These plans secure the chosen funeral irrespective of subsequent inflation; they meet the cost of not only the funeral director's services but some of the disbursements – crematorium fees (or an equivalent amount towards burial costs) and a payment for a minister of religion. There is no upper or lower age limit for applicants and discounts are available to those who apply through Age Concern (*see* page 324). The Age Concern fact sheet No. 27, *Arranging a Funeral*, mentions a number of alternative schemes.

The donation of your body or organs

If you want your body or any organs to be used for transplants or for medical research it is necessary to complete a donor card. These can be obtained either from the Department of Health (Leaflets, PO Box 21, Stanmore, Middlesex HA7 1AY) or from the British Organ Donor Society (BODY), Balsham, Cambridge CB1 6DL (Tel: 0800-444136), a voluntary organisation which can offer advice both to donors and the families of donors and recipients (*see* page 206). For medical reasons or simply because there are more whole body donors than are required for training purposes at a particular time, it is possible that when you die your body will not be needed. There is a much greater demand for organ donors, and BODY recommends that a multi-organ donor card should be used; there is room on this card to add 'Whole body donor'. There is no real age limitation for organ transplantation; eye corneas in particular are required for older recipients.

It is very important to let your family or a close friend know of your wishes regarding organ donation. The reason is that it will be your family or possibly a close friend who will be approached concerning your wishes. In practice, despite the need for organs, the circumstances under which they can be removed for use are very limited – usually if you die in an intensive care unit in hospital, where your heart can be kept beating after your brain death. Sometimes, however, if the prevailing conditions allow, certain organs can be removed after heart death: kidneys within one hour, corneas within 12 hours, skin within 24 hours, bone within 36 hours and heart valves within 72 hours. BODY has a fact sheet, *Organ Donation and Transportation*, which provides details.

If your whole body is to be donated, it is again very important that your family or a close friend is made aware of your wishes. It will be for them to take the immediate action required when you die. Ideally, they should contact their nearest medical school or, if in London, the London Anatomy Office, Rockefeller Building, University Street, London WC1E 6JJ (Tel: 071-387 7850). Consideration will be given to the place and cause of death and the condition of the body at the time of death. Acceptance is at the discretion of the Anatomy Department concerned.

Bodies may sometimes have to be refused for various reasons, for instance if there has been a post-mortem examination. If yours is accepted, the medical school concerned may keep it for up to two years before funeral arrangements can be made. This can then be a private occasion or a combined service for several donors. In the latter case all the arrangements and costs will be covered by the medical school. Again, BODY has a fact sheet, *Whole Body Donors*, with details.

Note that if the deceased had expressed an objection to the removal and use of any of his or her organs, the nearest relative cannot override that objection and agree to their donation. If the death is one that must be reported to a coroner, the coroner's consent is needed before organs or body can be donated.

Bereavement

Death is something from which most of us, other than in exceptional circumstances, are able to insulate ourselves. We know that it is inevitable, but we would rather not be reminded of it in advance. Society is now so ordered that other people's deaths seldom touch us in a personal or practical way: other people are employed to deal with it, and it is neatly sanitised away from our gaze. In such circumstances, the bereavement of others is likely to make us uncomfortable: we feel sympathy, certainly, but we would rather not get too close. We do not know what to say.

The result is that, more often than not, those who are bereaved find that they are denied expression of their sorrow. Precisely when emotions need to be communicated – to be let out – they have to be bottled up and kept private. While (up to a point) laughter at times of happiness is acceptable, tears in grief are not. We hope that the bereaved will not cry; we may even enjoin them to 'keep a stiff upper lip', essentially because, at least in the British culture, we are embarrassed by lamentation.

For the individual, therefore, the inevitable and often devastating pain and sense of loss experienced when a loved one dies often cannot be shared. Emotions are repressed: an unnatural avoidance of grief which hinders the process of recovery. When bereavement comes late in life, particularly if we lose a lifelong partner, the pain and distress are likely to be compounded by loneliness: people who enjoyed our company as a couple may not relate to us as individuals, and some of our old and best friends may also have died. There are fewer opportunities to strike out in a new direction, and it can be more difficult to rebuild our lives.

It helps if we can learn to understand our feelings, and to accept that it is all right, indeed natural, to mourn – to be unhappy and to express that unhappiness. Grief is not something to resist, but rather something that we have to work our way through.

Even with help and support, bereavement can last a long time. Most of us initially experience a sense of unreality and come to terms with the truth only gradually. We are gripped by a sense of dispossession, which may lead to despair and a feeling that life is no longer worth living. Or we may feel guilty about the past and opportunities missed: we could have done so much more for, been so much more to, the person who has died. There is a danger that we will make impulsive decisions at a time when we are not thinking rationally.

Many of us like to feel that we are self-sufficient. In bereavement, this can be a mistake. Inner strength may have its merits, but it is isolating. We need to turn outwards rather than inwards, however difficult this may be. We need not turn our backs on the past or try to shut out fond memories, but our attachment must turn away from what has passed and from those who are gone, and towards new experiences and new people. There is often a particular difficulty in this. Those who have lost a partner often find it hard to make new relationships without feeling a sense of guilt and disloyalty. There is a passage in Robert Butler and Myrna Lewis's *Love and Sex After Sixty* (Harper & Row Ltd, 1988) which seems to us to capture exactly the essential balance between past and future:

Once the period of mourning is over and the initial shock and grief have abated, you owe it to yourself to become realistic about your need to have a new life of your own. This means the appropriate preservation of your memories without excessive dwelling in the past. The usual cure for enshrinement is to take an active role in getting life moving again. This is an act of will and determination. It can happen only if the individual decides to make it happen. Removing from sight the personal possessions of the deceased will help. It may also be necessary to put away obvious marriage symbols, such as the wedding ring. It is not a betrayal of a past marriage to accept the present and build a future.

Practical arrangements

The most immediate problem after a death is that there are a number of practical responsibilities thrust upon the bereaved, numb with grief though he or she may be, which just have to be dealt with. In the following pages, we offer basic guidance to help bereaved people to cope with the arrangements which must be made. A number of books and leaflets listed at the end of this section will provide further, more detailed advice. They deal with the priority action necessary (which will depend on whether the death is in hospital or elsewhere, and whether it is expected or unexpected), the usual procedures for the issue of a medical certificate, the exceptional steps which must be taken if your doctor decides that the death has to be reported to a coroner and if a post-mortem is necessary, and what to do to register the death. We recognise, of course, that those personally affected are unlikely to feel much like studying a guidebook at such a time, and most of us would think it morbid to do so in anticipation of a loved one's death. Fortunately, in practice, there are usually friends and relatives to help, and those professionally involved will be able to offer guidance through the essential procedures.

Funeral arrangements

Dealing with the exceptions first, there is no requirement in law for a coffin to be used for burial or cremation, and some ethnic groups in fact do not use them (in practice, this would rule out cremation, because no cremation authority would accept a body without a coffin, partly on public health grounds and partly because the combustion process would be more difficult without a coffin). Neither is it obligatory to use the services of a funeral director.

Most people, however, at a time of personal distress, prefer to rely on the professional services of a funeral director. The problem here is that if they have never thought about it before, they are liable, at a time when they can hardly think straight at all, to make the wrong choices and to finish up with a funeral which costs a great deal more than they wish to pay or than they can afford.

There are a considerable number of funeral directors in the United Kingdom. Most of them provide a twenty-four hour service. This includes the supply of a coffin or a casket (respectively tapered or rectangular), a conductor, bearers, a hearse, and following cars. They lay out the body (and may embalm it), keep it on their premises (normally providing a room where it may be viewed), and transport the body and mourners as required. Some funeral directors provide facilities for those whose religion requires them to wash and dress their own deceased. They also co-ordinate and arrange payment for services provided by others, such as cemeteries or crematoria, organists, florists, caterers, etc., and will place an obituary notice in newspapers if required. They cannot and do not register the death; nor can they apply for social security benefits on a client's behalf, though they should be able to offer help and advice about them.

Around 80 per cent of all funerals in the United Kingdom are arranged by members of the National Association of Funeral Directors. Members are expected to comply with a code of practice, perhaps the most significant features of which are that they will give clients full information about the services offered, including a price list, offer those clients who require it a basic simple funeral, and provide a firm estimate.

These seem to us essential requirements on which a customer should insist, and it is disturbing to read that many funeral directors, in practice, still fail to provide a price list. We think, moreover, that it is reasonable to expect that the estimate should be itemised to show the various elements of cost. Funeral services are business transactions, like any other, and customers are entitled to know what they are paying for, and to choose to reject particular services either on grounds of cost or because they consider them inappropriate. We think, in fact, that customers, for whom the service is being performed, rather than being presented with various package deals, should be allowed to decide exactly how the arrangements are to be made: we believe that many people would much prefer to dispense with some of the trappings, the conventional expressions of mourning, and religious offices. The problem is that a bereaved person hardly feels like haggling and may easily be tempted into giving their loved one 'a good send-off'. That is a legitimate choice, so long as it is a choice. With the average price of a funeral now approaching £1,000, an equally valid alternative is to buy what we want and only what we want.

Funerals for people who have donated their bodies for research are normally arranged by the donee medical schools, while local authorities are under a statutory duty (section 46, Public Health (Control of Disease) Act 1984) to arrange funerals for those who have 'died or been found dead in their area, in any case where it appears to the authority that no suitable arrangements for the disposal of the body have been or are being made otherwise than by the authority'. Some local authorities, although prevented by law from generally providing funerals directly, have negotiated special low cost 'packages' with local firms. If you want this, it may be worth asking your local authority if any such service is available.

Do-it-yourself funerals

Relatively few people, we think, will want to carry DIY this far. It is, however, a perfectly feasible alternative, and one which must surely be seen as an intensely personal and loving final service to someone who has been dear to us in life. Some writers have focused on the difficulty of procuring a coffin. Funeral directors, we think not surprisingly, are unwilling to provide coffins (on which they may add a big mark-up) other than as part of their normal services. A coffin is, however, very easy (and cheap) to make, say from veneered chipboard panels: if you are not good at simple carpentry, we have no doubt that a friend or local carpenter would oblige. Better still, the Swiss newspaper *Neue Zürchen Zeitung* reported early in 1992 the invention of a paper coffin, said to be especially good for cremations. An estate car or van can be used to transport the coffin, and you will need four or more friends to carry it. If you do not want a religious ceremony, you can nevertheless ask a relative or friend to speak about the deceased.

Age Concern England's fact sheet No. 27, *Arranging a Funeral*, provides more detailed information. Also helpful (and inspiring) are Jane Spottiswoode's *Undertaken with Love* and Dr Tony Walter's *Funerals: And how to improve them*. See pages 210 and 212 for details of these publications, and page 208 for information about the Natural Death Centre.

Burial at sea

There is no legal objection to burial at sea, subject to the coroner being informed (the body is regarded as being taken out of the country) and a licence being obtained. Application for a licence under Part II of the Food and Environment Protection Act 1985 should be made to:

Fisheries Marine Environmental Protection Division
Ministry of Agriculture, Fisheries and Food (MAFF)
Nobel House
17 Smith Square
London SW1P 3JR

The usual conditions in the licence are that:
1. The body must not be embalmed.
2. The body must be in a paper shroud inside a wooden or solid-type coffin.
3. There must be sufficent weights in the coffin to sink it.
4. It must be put into the sea quite a long way out from the shore (the distance will be specified).

Registering a death

Death must be certified by the doctor concerned (two doctors if the body is to be cremated). This certificate must be taken to the Registrar of Births and Deaths for the area in which the death occurred (for the address see the relevant telephone directory or ask the doctor, local authority, post office or police). This must be done within five days (eight days in Scotland) unless the death has been referred to a coroner. Check when the Registrar will be available, and take with you the medical certificate of cause of death, the deceased's medical card (if any), any war pension order book, and, if the coroner held a post-mortem which established that death was due to natural causes, Form 100 (the coroner may sometimes send this direct).

The Registrar will issue two certified copies of the entry in the death register. Further copies can be obtained for a small fee. You are likely to need certificates for probate purposes or to release money from insurance policies, pensions, bank deposits, etc.

Administering the estate (English law only)

If there has been a will, responsibility for administering the estate will fall upon the executors, who act as the deceased's personal representatives. Building societies, pension funds, insurance companies and the Department of National Savings will usually release limited amounts to an executor on production of a death certificate. Otherwise, it will normally be necessary to have the will 'proved' and to produce a grant of 'probate' before money can be released. Circumstances can vary a great deal and you may well need detailed guidance. The Personal Application Department of Principal Registry of the Family Division, Somerset House, Strand, London WC2R 1LP (Tel: 071-936 6983 or 071-936 7464) should be able to help, though it cannot, of course, give legal advice. Similar services are available in district probate registries. These, and probate sub-registries, are located in many major towns in England and Wales.

If no will was made, the deceased is said to have died 'intestate' and a personal representative, usually the nearest relative, must administer the estate. Again, as under a will, limited amounts in National Savings building societies, insurances or pension funds will usually be released on production of the death certificate. Otherwise, the personal representative will normally need to apply to a probate registry for a grant of 'letters of administration'. This will authorise the personal representative to administer the estate and can be produced to allow the release of money as with a grant of probate. However, whereas an executor has full legal authority to administer the estate by virtue of the will and needs probate only by way of confirmation, a personal representative in intestacy has no authority unless and until letters of administration are granted. And whereas the estate under a will is distributed in accordance with that will, an estate in intestacy must be distributed in accordance with legal rules, namely the following:

If there is a surviving spouse:
In the case of a marriage with children, the surviving spouse is entitled to the first £75,000 of the estate (plus any interest accruing since the date of death), personal possessions, and a life interest in half of the rest of the estate, the children sharing the other half.

In the case of a marriage without children, the surviving spouse is entitled to the whole estate unless any of the deceased's parents, brothers and sisters or their children are alive; in this event, the surviving spouse is entitled to the first £125,000 (plus any interest accruing since the date of death), personal possessions, and half the rest of the estate, the above relatives (or some of them) sharing the other half.

If there is no surviving partner:
The children (if any) are entitled to equal shares of the estate; if any child has already died, his/her share will go to his/her children.

If there are no surviving children, the whole estate goes to one of the following groups of people in the priority shown:

1. the grandchildren;
2. the father and mother of the deceased;
3. brothers and sisters of the whole blood and the issue of any deceased brother or sister of the whole blood who died before the deceased;
4. brothers and sisters of the half blood and the issue of any deceased brother or sister of the half blood who died before the deceased;
5. grandparents;
6. uncles and aunts of the whole blood and the issue of any deceased uncle or aunt of the whole blood who died before the deceased;
7. uncles and aunts of the half blood and the issue of any deceased uncle or aunt of the half blood who died before the deceased.

If there are no surviving relatives, the estate passes to the Crown.

Further information on probate

Wills and Probate
(Consumers' Association, Castlemead, Gascoyne Way, Hertford X, SG14 1LH), price £9.95.

⇒▶ *Probate: Dealing with someone's estate*
(Age Concern England, Astral House, 1268 London Road SW16 4ER (Tel: 081-679 8000).

Fact sheet No.14, free in response to a 9" × 6" s.a.e.

Helpful organisations

⇒▶ *British Organ Donor Society (BODY)*
Balsham, Cambridge CB1 6DL (Tel: 0223-893636).

BODY is a voluntary society with a membership of people interested or involved in organ transplantation as recipient or donor families, medical professionals and others. Its aims are to give support to donor, recipient and waiting recipient families and to promote the carrying of the multi-organ donor card (*see* page 199 for further details).

Donor, recipient and waiting recipient communication is on a personal basis. BODY can therefore give support to involved families based on their own experiences. For donor families, the support is the same as for any grieving family who have lost a loved one. A helpful leaflet, *Carry the Card for Life*, and further information are available on request.

⇒▶ *The Compassionate Friends*
6 Denmark Street, Bristol BS1 5DQ (Tel: 0272-292778).

This organisation was founded in Coventry in 1969. It is now a nationwide organisation of bereaved parents, who have themselves experienced heartbreak, loneliness and social isolation and who seek to help other bereaved parents. While religious or philosophical beliefs are helpful to some bereaved parents, CF has no religious affiliation.

Initial contact with bereaved parents is in the form of a leaflet giving a local contact address. If this link is taken up, the parents will be put in touch with others in similar circumstances, and contact will be made by visits, telephone calls, letters or small meetings. A quarterly newsletter is also distributed to all members, initially free of charge. CF has a wide range of literature and operates a postal library.

⇒▶ *The Cremation Society of Great Britain*
Brecon House, Albion Place, Maidstone, Kent ME14 5DZ (Tel: 0622-688292/3).

Founded in 1874, the Society is the pioneer of cremation in Great Britain. It aims to 'save the land for the living', and works to promote and establish the practice of cremation among all members of the community. It has assisted local authorities in the setting up of new crematoria and has pressed the government departments concerned for law reforms so that cremation may be practised with the least possible restriction.

The Society is also a founder member of the International Cremation Federation, established in 1937 to promote cremation throughout the world.

Among a number of publications on cremation, the Society publishes a quarterly journal, *Pharos International*. Particularly helpful to those in doubt about cremation is the Society's leaflet, *What You Should Know About Cremation*, presently available free of charge.

Cruse – Bereavement Care

Cruse House, 126 Sheen Road, Richmond, Surrey TW9 1UR (Tel: 081-940 4818; Fax: 081-940 7638; Cruse bereavement counselling hire: 081-332 7227).

Cruse began in 1959 as an organisation of and for widows. The name itself was taken from the familiar Old Testament story about the widow who shared the last of her food with a passing stranger, and found that thereafter her barrel of meal and cruse of oil were replenished 'according to her need'. The service has since been extended to help all bereaved people through its central office and more than 125 local branches.

Cruse national membership is offered to those who do not have a nearby local branch. Counsellors are available to answer letters and talk on the telephone. Help is also available on practical matters, either by personal advice or information or through guidance as to where further relevant help can be obtained. This is backed by a wide range of publications, including fact sheets, leaflets and a regular newsletter, *The Cruse Chronicle*. For national members who are widowed, there are two contact lists, one enabling widows to get in touch with other widows, the other for widowers to contact widowers.

Cruse branches offer help to all bereaved people who live in their area. Counsellors are available to visit, at home or elsewhere, and regular social meetings are arranged, providing the opportunity to meet others and make new friendships. Advice on practical matters is available from specialists, and Cruse literature is, of course, available through the branch. Details of your nearest branch can be obtained from the Richmond office.

Although its name comes from a Bible story, Cruse is not affiliated to any religious organisation and offers its help to bereaved people of all faiths or none. Similarly, Cruse has no political affiliation, but it is concerned about the statutory provision of pensions and benefits. It is represented in Parliament and has close links with government departments.

Cruse is also involved in training and education. It runs courses and conferences, at national and branch level, for those who care for or about bereaved people, and works to increase society's understanding of bereavement and the needs it can create. In particular, many health care professionals turn to Cruse for information and training.

A publications list is available from Cruse House. This includes a wide range of relevant books (some of which are mentioned on page 209); fact sheets on practical subjects; and helpful leaflets on living through loss, depression, loneliness, and on friendship, sex and remarriage. A journal, *Bereavement Care*, is available on subscription for counsellors and others who work in the field of bereavement as health care staff, social workers and other caring professions.

208 Planning for death and coping with bereavement

▶ *Elderly Accommodation Counsel*
(*see* page 102 for details)

EAC's database includes information on hospices for those who are terminally ill. A search fee of £5 is normally chargeable.

▶ *Gay Bereavement Project*
Vaughan M. Williams Centre, Colindale Hospital, London NW9 5HG (Tel. Helpline: 081-455 8894; Tel. Admin: 081-200 0511), or ring London Lesbian and Gay Switchboard, 071-837 7324, which keeps a list of the Project's members.

The Gay Bereavement Project offers help especially in the first difficult hours and days of bereavement, to lesbians and gay men whose partners have died; a trained volunteer is on duty every evening ready to talk and to listen.

The Project also works to raise awareness of the fact that the death of a homosexual partner is just as traumatic as the loss of a spouse and that the feelings and needs of the bereaved partner need to be accorded the same kind of respect; and to educate lesbians and gay men that death is inevitable and that provision needs to be made 'for the day when "we" becomes "I"', especially since the normal rules of an intestacy will not provide for a gay partner.

▶ *The Hospice Information Service*
St Christopher's Hospice, 51–9 Lawrie Park Road, London SE26 6DZ
(Tel: 081-778 9252, ext. 262/3).

A resource and link for members of the public and health care professionals seeking information on the work of the hospice movement. Publications include: *Directory of Hospice Services in the UK and Ireland*; *Overseas Hospice Services*; *The Hospice Bulletin* (a quarterly newsletter); and *Choices*, listing details of conferences and courses relating to terminal care and bereavement both within the United Kingdom and, to a limited extent, overseas; and a range of fact sheets on various aspects of hospice planning and organisation. A modest charge is requested for printed materials to cover photocopying and postage, but the *Directory of Hospice Services in the UK and Ireland* is available free of charge on receipt of a large s.a.e. with a 34 pence stamp.

▶ *The Natural Death Centre*
20 Heber Road, London NW2 6AA (Tel: 081-208 2853; Fax: 081-452 6434).

This Centre, a non-profit association, was launched in the Spring of 1991 with the overall aim of helping to improve the quality of dying. It works towards breaking the taboo about freely discussing death and dying. People are encouraged through workshops, courses and in other ways to prepare for dying well in advance. A network of people is being built up, in which people who have had near-death experiences are particularly welcome, to act, if desired, as informal counsellors to the dying person and the family.

The Natural Death Centre wants to help ordinary families to take back control of the process of dying from the big institutions. It seeks to generate more support for those dying at home, both from the authorities and the surrounding neighbourhood, so that most people can die in familiar surroundings rather than in hospital. It also encourages research into the alleviation of suffering for the dying, and into alternatives to euthanasia.

The Centre also acts as a consumer body, offering impartial information about, for example, who are the good healers, counsellors and undertakers throughout the United Kingdom, and recommending relevant literature and best buys. It campaigns to prevent funeral suppliers selling their coffins only to the funeral trade, and for legislation to require all funeral directors to give price breakdowns over the telephone and written price lists on application.

The Centre will help people to draw up a 'living will', stating how much hi-tech medical intervention they want in the event of their terminal illness. Such 'living wills', the Centre believes, should be recognised by law.

The *Natural Death Handbook*, a compendium of personal experiences, is planned for 1993.

Further information

The following references are only a small selection of the wide range of publications dealing with bereavement and related matters. Fuller lists are available from Cruse, 126 Sheen Road, Richmond, Surrey TW9 1UR.

▶ *After the Death of Someone Very Close*
By Caroline Morcom (Cruse, 126 Sheen Road, Richmond, Surrey TW9 1UR), price 80 pence plus 30 pence postage and packing.

A Cruse counsellor guides the reader through some of the feelings experienced during the grief of bereavement.

▶ *Arranging A Funeral*
(Age Concern, Astral House, 1268 London Road, London SW16 4ER, December 1990).

A short, but surprisingly detailed, fact sheet, which sets out the essential information clearly and succinctly. Free in response to a s.a.e.

▶ *Bereavement*
(Help the Aged, St James's Walk, London EC1R 0BE (Tel: 071-253 0253)).

A free leaflet about the emotional and practical aspects of dealing with bereavement.

▶ Bereavement Care

A journal published three times a year by Cruse, 126 Sheen Road, Richmond, Surrey TW9 1UR. It is written for Cruse workers and others who help bereaved people in their professional work. It is available on subscription, price £8.50 a year including postage to individuals (£6.50 to Cruse members; £16.00 to libraries and organisations).

▶ Beyond Grief: A guide for recovering from the death of a loved one

By Carol Staudacher (Souvenir Press, 1988, available from Bookpoint Ltd, 39 Milton Trading Estate, Abingdon, Oxfordshire OX14 4TD (Tel: 0235-835001)), price (paperback) £7.95 (hardback) £14.95.

A helpful book, based partly on earlier literature in this field, but also substantially on interviews with those who work with the grieving and with people themselves dealing with the death of a loved one, and on personal experience. Its approach is systematic, with the text broken up under subject headings which make it readily accessible. The author begins with the paradox that despite its universality, grief comes to individuals as a stranger. She examines the various ways in which grief may be experienced and suggests strategies for dealing with these many reactions, and goes on to describe the feelings and the healing processes which follow death in particular circumstances. Finally, there are sections on getting and giving help. The book is valuable for its penetrating insight into the emotions of and responses to grief, and its pervasive theme of hope.

▶ Coming Home, A Guide to Dying at Home with Dignity

By Deborah Duda (Aurora Press, New York, 1987), available from Airlift, 26 Eden Grove, London N7 (Tel: 071-607 5798), price £13.05.

Recommended by The Natural Death Centre (*see* page 208) as the best book on dying at home.

▶ Deathing, An Intelligent Alternative for the Final Moments of Life

By Anya Foos-Graber (Nicolays-Hays Inc., Maine, USA, 1989), available from Airlift, 26 Eden Grove, London N7 (Tel: 071-607 5798), price £13.50.

One of two books recommended by The Natural Death Centre (*see* page 208) as the best reading on spiritual preparations for dying (the other is *Who Dies?* mentioned below).

▶ Funerals

A survey in *Which?*, February 1992.

▶ Funerals: And how to improve them

By Dr Tony Walter (Hodder & Stoughton Ltd, Mill Road, Dunton Green, Sevenoaks, Kent TN13 2YA).

One of two books recommended by The Natural Death Centre (*see* page 208) as the best reading on DIY funerals (the other is *Undertaken with Love* mentioned below).

▶ *Funerals Without God*
(British Humanist Association, 14 Lamb's Conduit Passage, London WC1R 4RH), price £3.

▶ *Help When Someone Dies (Guide FB29)*
(Department of Social Security)

A free guide to relevant social security benefits.

▶ *How to Direct Your Own Funeral: A practical handbook*
By Mary Illingworth (Bookstall Publications, 79a Gloucester Road, Bristol BS7 8AS, 1992), price £10.

Includes information on planning your funeral in advance, keeping the cost down, DIY funerals, alternative and 'green' funerals, burial at sea or in private ground, and helpful organisations.

▶ *Secret Flowers: Mourning and the adaptation to loss*
By Mary Jones (The Women's Press Ltd, 34 Great Sutton Street, London EC1V 0DX, 1988), price £2.95.

Writing out of her personal experience, the author revives the different stages of her grief and loss towards a kind of consolation: 'Death has given me one priceless gift, that of knowing I did love; once; deeply and truly. So I am safe, now and for ever.' This is a warm and compassionate book which recognises at the end that death is an incident in a love story, not the end of that story.

▶ *Talking About Bereavement*
(Health Education Board for Scotland, Woodburn House, Canaan Lane, Edinburgh EH10 4SG (Tel: 031-447 8044)).

A free booklet which briefly examines the nature of bereavement, how bereaved people react, social attitudes, what friends can do to help, and the wider support which is available.

▶ *Through Grief: The bereavement journey*
By Elizabeth Collick (Darton, Longman & Todd in association with Cruse, 126 Sheen Road, Richmond, Surrey, TW9 1UR, 1986), price £3.95 plus 65 pence postage and packing.

The author, a bereavement counsellor with Cruse (*see* page 207) and herself a widow, sets out to explain to those in grief the feelings, problems and reactions which usually accompany this devastating experience. Her description of the normal phases of grief is accompanied by personal accounts of some of those whose distress she has shared.

Cruse has also produced a *Through Grief* cassette (price £5.50 plus 60 pence postage and packing) containing a series of personal talks to bereaved people by Elizabeth Collick, based on the general pattern of her book and complementary to it. It is arranged in nine sections: Looking at Grief, Loss, Anxiety, Anger, Guilt, Reminiscence, Depression, Loneliness and Healing. The talks are direct and intended to bring the emotions of bereavement into the open, and thus to help listeners to a point of reassurance and self-awareness.

▶ *Undertaken with Love*
By Jane Spottiswoode (Robert Hale, 45-7 Clerkenwell Green, London EC1R 0HT (Tel: 071-251 2661), 1991), price £12.95.

One of two books recommended by The Natural Death Centre (*see* page 208) as the best reading on DIY funerals (the other is *Funerals: And how to improve them* mentioned above).

▶ *What to Do After a Death*
(Department of Social Security).

▶ *What to Do After a Death in Scotland*
(Scottish Home and Health Department)

Free booklets giving basic guidance on what you must do and the help you can get.

▶ *What to Do When Someone Dies*
(Consumers' Association), price £9.95, available post and packing free, from Consumers' Association, Castlemead, Gascoyne Way, Hertford X, SG14 1LH. For credit card orders phone 0800-252100 quoting Dept DFOP (freephone service).

A regularly updated guide to the practical arrangements following a death, including registering the death, obtaining medical and death certificates, and arranging the burial or cremation and the funeral. Recommended by The Natural Death Centre (*see* page 208) as the best book on 'red tape surrounding death'.

▶ *Who Dies? An investigation of conscious living and conscious dying*
By Stephen Levine (Gateway Books, The Hollies, Wellow, Bath BA2 8QJ, 1988), price £7.95.

One of two books recommended by The Natural Death Centre (*see* page 208) as the best reading on spiritual preparations for dying (the other is *Deathing*, mentioned above).

=▶ *Wills and Probate*
(Consumers' Association), price £9.95, available post and packing free, from Consumers' Association, Castlemead, Gascoyne Way, Hertford X, SG14 1LH. For credit card orders phone 0800-252100 quoting Dept DFOP (freephone service).

In our view an indispensable guide to the subject. Regularly updated, it is written for the layperson and includes advice on making your own will, inheritance tax and the administration of an estate.

SECTION NINE

Opportunities for volunteering

One of the wonderful things about volunteering is that, unlike a job which you may not enjoy all that much but which you have to stick with, you can take on the kind of work which suits you best and give it however much time you choose. You may find that you become so committed, and enjoy what you are doing so much, that you find yourself busier than ever. The variety of work you can undertake as a volunteer is endless. You now have the opportunity to follow interests you previously had no time for. These may take you out and about, or if you need to be at home a great deal or have difficulty going out you can take on jobs that can be done from your home. You could type at home for an organisation or, if you have a telephone, you can act as a link between others who are more active, or you can do some book-keeping, or run a raffle from home. Organisations will usually pay expenses so you do not need to be out of pocket.

Volunteers are needed to work as volunteer literacy tutors, to work in youth clubs, in Citizens Advice Bureaux or with a local victim support scheme. (The National Association of Victims Support Schemes is described on page 223.) Helping out with the tea trolley at the local hospital can be both useful and pleasurable as you meet patients who are ready for a chat. You may be able to help a local talking newspaper with the recording or general administration. The needs are endless.

Other more vigorous voluntary work is needed by conservation organisations who are keen to look after the local environment (clearing ponds, taking care of wildlife); even in cities there are opportunities to preserve and develop habitats for a range of wildlife.

Then again, volunteers with particular skills are needed to work in developing countries. Mature people are welcomed by agencies like Voluntary Service Overseas (VSO), who accept volunteers up to the age of 70. For details see later in this section.

Most organisations need help with fund raising and you may be able to help in a variety of ways. Fund raising needs to be imaginative to catch the public's eye, and this can make it great fun to be involved with.

There are many organisations concerned with the welfare of particular groups of people, including children, people with a disability and others who may need help of one sort or another. Almost any of the organisations we list in Section 14, Helpful

Organisations, will be glad of any offers of voluntary help either nationally or at local level.

Campaigning is another area of voluntary activity. It can be very hard work but very satisfying. It is also a wonderful way to make friends as you join with others to achieve a particular objective. It may be to have a zebra crossing put in on a road where it is very difficult to cross and where perhaps there have been pedestrian accidents or where you fear there may be. Or you could be campaigning for pensioners' rights. You may be fighting to keep the local hospital open. Very many benefits we enjoy have arisen as a result of determined campaigning on the part of people who were not prepared to take 'no' for an answer.

Our section on leisure gives details of organisations which, as well as providing leisure opportunities, will also welcome the active and regular involvement of volunteers. Sports associations, for instance, need coaches, umpires and people to help with events. The Sports Council arranges courses for people who would like to take up these activities. You need no longer just sit on the sidelines: even if you cannot take part in the sport, you can still be very actively involved.

We describe below just a few organisations who seek volunteers who have particular skills and who are prepared to share their skills and to make a definite commitment of their time.

If you would like to find out about local volunteering opportunities but are unsure about what you would like to do, you would find it helpful to visit a Volunteer Bureau. These have been neatly described as 'job shops for voluntary work'. Staff in Volunteer Bureaux will be glad to recommend voluntary work to suit your experience and preferences. All bureaux hold a wide range of general information about voluntary work, as well as details of current opportunities available locally. Some have a 'jobs board' so volunteers can browse first to get a few ideas. You will be offered an initial chat or interview, perhaps on the spot, or by appointment. This will give you a chance to explore what kind of voluntary work you are interested in if you have not already made up your mind, and what you can undertake. It will also give you an opportunity to find out what kind of current openings exist.

Some Social Service Departments have work for volunteers. If you would like to volunteer for work in a hospital you could ask if there is a Voluntary Service Co-ordinator in the hospital. Your local library will have a list of all local voluntary organisations; you could then contact any organisation you would like to help direct.

If you are uncertain about what becoming a volunteer for a particular organisation would involve you might find it helpful to buy *So You Want to be a Volunteer*, a helpful publication described at the end of this section.

Voluntary work and Social Security benefits

Your rights to Social Security benefits will not necessarily be affected if you do voluntary work or take a part-time job, but in some circumstances they could be. The Volunteer Centre UK has a standard form, agreed with the DSS, to enable Income Support claimants to record their out-of-pocket expenses. Forms are available from: The Volunteer Centre UK, 29 Lower King's Road, Berkhamsted, Hertfordshire HP4 2AB (Tel: 0442-873311). If you start voluntary or part-time work, you must tell:

- your Unemployment Benefit office, if you are signing on there for Unemployment Benefit or Income Support;
- your Social Security office, if you are getting any Social Security benefits or pensions;
- the Inland Revenue. You must declare all your earnings when you complete your tax return (*see* also below, 'Motor Mileage Allowances and Tax'). For paid voluntary work, be sure to show how much of your payments was for work done, how much for necessary expenses, how much for travelling and meals, and so on;
- your local council, if you are getting Housing Benefit or Community Charge Benefit.

For further information get Social Security leaflet FB26, *Voluntary and part-time workers: Your benefits, pensions and National Insurance contributions* from post offices or Social Security offices, or by writing to: Leaflets Unit, PO Box 21, Stanmore, Middlesex HA7 1AY.

Motor mileage allowances and tax

Volunteers who drive for the hospital car service and for voluntary organisations are usually paid a mileage rate for using their cars. The Inland Revenue is concerned that drivers may make a taxable profit if the mileage allowances they receive exceed the costs of running and maintaining the car for the miles travelled for the voluntary service. The tax charge is to be phased in gradually over a number of years. Tax will not be payable on the full amount of the profit element until 1995/6. The 1992/3 tax-free rates are as follows:

	Cars up to 1,000cc	Cars 1,001 –1,500cc	Cars 1,501 –2,000cc	Cars over 2,000cc
Up to 4,000 miles	25p	30p	38p	51p
Over 4,000 miles	14p	17p	21p	27p

Organisations which welcome volunteers

We give below just a selection of organisations which welcome volunteers. This gives some idea of the wide range of activities you can engage in.

Action Resource Centre
1st Floor, 102 Park Village East, London NW1 3SP (Tel: 071-383 2200).

ARC's role is to assist local communities by involving business and professional people in the work of community organisations. ARC acts as a broker of secondments and business volunteering from companies to community projects.

Secondments and volunteer placements can allow those approaching retirement to use their business and professional skills to help the community or to explore opportunities for further employment or volunteering.

ARC is a national voluntary agency with a network of area offices, supported by a head office in London.

Age Concern England
Astral House, 1268 London Road, London SW16 4ER (Tel: 081-679 8000).

Local groups work through volunteers. Each group is independent and therefore they often have very different programmes of activity. If you would like to know more about services or opportunities for volunteers in your area contact your local Age Concern group whose address you will find in the telephone book under *Age Concern* or *Old People's Welfare*. It will certainly always welcome any offers of help.

Age Resource

Age Resource is based at Age Concern England. It exists to encourage the development of volunteering opportunities for 'active elders' as they are described. It seeks to foster the potential capacity of many older people – those aged from around 50 and upwards – to be actively involved, and find personal satisfaction, in a variety of activities which are both economically and socially valuable. Age Resource has a very interesting newsletter and will be glad to send you a copy – available free of charge. It will also be glad to send you its awards brochure. Each year, Age Resource presents awards to schemes and projects which involve the creative potential and participation of active elders at all levels of community need and in all types of endeavour. The Awards Brochure is very interesting to read and will give you an idea of the broad range of activities being undertaken in all parts of the country. You may like to join in a particular scheme or to start a similar idea.

The Beth Johnson Foundation
Parkfield House, 64 Princes Road, Hartshill, Stoke-on-Trent ST4 7JL
(Tel: 0782-44036).

The Foundation has developed a scheme of Peer Health Counsellors. They are retired people who have an interest in self-health and want to share their enthusiasm with their peer group in the form of satisfying volutary work. They must be willing to undertake training and to attend monthly support meetings in addition to a regular commitment to the work of peer counselling.

Black Volunteering
See Resource Unit to Promote Black Volunteering on page 226.

British Executive Service Overseas
164 Vauxhall Bridge Road, London SW1V 2RB (Tel: 071-630 0644).

BESO was conceived to assist economic development in the developing countries. BESO's volunteer advisers are sent on short-term assignments to help public and private sector organisations. It is an independent charity and BESO volunteer advisers are mainly retired men and women with professional, technical or managerial skills. The cost of travel and related expenses is met for volunteer and spouse, but no consultancy fee is made.

A register of 2,000 volunteers is maintained, and others have but to be asked when their particular discipline is in demand. Industry, commerce, trade and utilities avail themselves of the service, as do governments. No charge is made, but the recipients are asked to meet the cost of accommodation, transport and subsistence. Assigment objectives and work conditions are defined and executive and project matched carefully. Volunteers must be prepared to travel and not be daunted by possible difficulties or work in remote places.

British Red Cross
9 Grosvenor Crescent, London SW1X 7EJ (Tel: 071-235 5454).

If you are interested in offering your voluntary services to the Red Cross you should contact your local group or centre. If you are accepted as a volunteer, you will receive whatever training is necessary. There is an upper age level of 70, although there may be lower age limits for certain activities.

Christians Abroad
1 Stockwell Green, London SW9 9HP Tel: 071-737 7811.

This organisation provides a service to anyone who is seeking information and advice about work overseas and also for those who want to do more in Britain for a more just and compassionate world. They aim to help you discover opportunities which are related to your skills, age, aims and circumstances. They have a range of leaflets, *A Place For You Overseas?*, one of which is written for the over 50s. A quote from an African bishop in the leaflet sets the scene. He says: 'Why do you only send young people? Don't you respect us enough to send older ones?' The leaflet points out that opportunities do exist for older people to work abroad, often through mission and volunteer agencies looking for skilled people at the request of overseas churches and other organisations. Sometimes older people are preferred because of their experience and maturity and in many cultures age gives a natural authority and commands respect.

Other leaflets include *A Place For You in Britain?*, *Community Work* and *Working for world development*.

Church Missionary Society
Partnership House, 157 Waterloo Road, London SE1 8UU (Tel: 071-928 8681).

Volunteers must be committed Christians with a degree, professional qualification or practical skill. People up to 70 (including married couples) can be considered for short-term placements working in partnership with churches overseas.

From time to time opportunities exist for volunteers to assist at the Society's offices in Waterloo or with local activities outside London. Generally, volunteers are required to have clerical or particular skills.

The Civic Trust
17 Carlton House Terrace, London SW1Y 5AW (Tel: 071-930 0914).

The Civic Trust works with a nationwide network of 1,000 local amenity societies who are caring for the places where we live and work. Societies are always looking for volunteers for a variety of work. You may also be interested to see their *Environmental Directory*, which lists organisations concerned with amenity and the environment. Each entry gives the address, telephone number and details of the organisations's aims and activities. Symbols indicate facilities, such as whether they give grants, offer an advisory service, membership, etc. Price: £4 including postage.

Scottish Civic Trust
Box 111, Glasgow G1 4EW.

Promotes the conservation of Scotland's heritage of old buildings while encouraging high standards of building for the future. It is the umbrella body for some 140 civic societies.

Civic Trust for Wales
4th Floor, Empire House, Mount Stuart Square, Cardiff CF1 6DN.

Established in 1964, it now supports and advises a network of more than 70 civic and amenity societies in Welsh towns and communities.

See also details of organisations mentioned in Section 12 on Arts, Sport and Leisure under Conservation and under Heritage.

Community Service Volunteers
237 Pentonville Road, London N1 9NJ (Tel: 071-278 6601).

CSV's Retired and Senior Volunteer Programme (RSVP) is for anyone who is aged over 50 and who has time to spare and wants to become involved in the community. RSVP aims to: benefit all older people, frail as well as fit; give older people the chance to use their skills and follow their own interests; provide group activities and, in particular, group support for the older people taking part. Volunteers are not confined to caring for and helping others. A wide range of activities is enjoyed by RSVP volunteers – RSVP will be glad to send you a leaflet.

Friends of the Earth
26-8 Underwood Street, London N1 7JQ (Tel: 071-490 1555).

Friends of the Earth (FOE) is one of the leading environmental pressure groups in the United Kingdom. It blows the whistle on those who destroy the environment, and puts pressure on those who have the power to protect it. FOE has a network of around 300 groups across the country and more than 230,000 supporters. The local groups always welcome new members who can quickly become involved in their activities. Each group decides on its programme of action and area of work. Subscription to FOE is £12. As a member you will receive *Earth Matters*, FOE's magazine.

Greenpeace
Canonbury Villas, London N1 2PN (Tel: 071-354 5100/071-359 7396).

Greenpeace has a network of around 200 Local Support Groups who organise various fund-raising initiatives such as street collections and sponsored events. Occasionally they may help with campaigns by lobbying MPs, gathering signatories for petitions and generally publicising campaign issues. If you would like to become involved, contact the Local Fund Raising Unit at the above address. They will be able to put you in touch with your Local Support Group.

International Cooperation for Development (ICD)
Unit 3, Canonbury Yard, 190A New North Road, London N1 7BJ
(Tel: 071-354 0883).

ICD, a department of CIIR (Catholic Institute for International Relief), has been recruiting experienced people to share their skills with communities in developing countries since 1965. Today, ICD development workers join with local people in south and central America, Namibia, Yemen and Zimbabwe, to implement programmes that challenge poverty and promote development.

ICD recruits people in response to requests for assistance from their partners overseas. The partners are either community organisations (such as peasant federations, women's groups, co-operatives or local development associations) or government ministries.

ICD development workers are employed in various capacities: as advisers in agricultural co-operatives, as health workers in urban and rural health care programmes, as trainers in peasant-run education programmes or as teacher trainers and lecturers. These are all challenging and professionally demanding posts.

ICD development workers receive a minimum two-year contract, a salary based on local rates, a UK allowance, accommodation and essential household equipment, return flights, a pre-departure grant, comprehensive insurance cover, language training and extensive briefings.

The posts to be filled are always highly specialised and ICD does recruit older people – as they comment, 'their experience can prove invaluable, though they must, of course, be physically fit'. Some posts entail living and working in harsh conditions and also possibly travelling through rough terrain. Certain posts, namely those for Zimbabwe, have an age limit set by the government of 50 years.

International Voluntary Service
Old Hall, East Bergholt, Colchester CO7 6TQ.

International workcamps are a unique form of voluntary service. The project benefits through the volunteers' work and the volunteers benefit through the experience of living and working as part of an international group. There is no upper age limit for volunteers though most do tend to be young. However, older people do regularly take part and are welcome.

Camps last from one to four weeks and there is a wide variety of work projects. They all have one thing in common. The workcamp takes place because the project needs outside support, but the work is designed to help the project become independent of the need for such support. The volunteers become involved in discussions about the nature of the work they are doing and the reasons why it is needed. Indeed some camps have a formal element of study built into their programme to enable this to happen to a greater degree.

The volunteers form international teams of between six and eighteen people, often of very different backgrounds and experience. Living together and working as a team towards common objectives helps to break down barriers and results in a greater understanding of differences in culture and outlook. In this way, workcamps promote international understanding and are a positive and very practical step towards peace.

Volunteers may find themselves working with children, or working with people with disabilities and mental health problems, or working on environmental improvement schemes or recycling projects, or they may attend work/study camps.

Workcamps in Britain are held at all times of the year, but most occur either between early June and late September or at Easter. The majority of volunteers on each camp are likely to be from other countries, from Western Europe, Eastern Europe and sometimes from the Third World.

Camps abroad take place mainly in the summer but there are a few at Christmas and Easter. Volunteers wishing to attend workcamps abroad should have previous experience of a workcamp in Britain or other relevant voluntary work. Most are held in Western Europe, some in the USA and Canada.

Workcamp volunteers have to pay a small registration fee and become members of IVS. Although volunteers pay their own travel expenses to and from the workcamp, food and accommodation, usually very basic, are provided.

If you are interested in going on a workcamp either in Britain or abroad you will need to write enclosing a $6\frac{1}{2}'' \times 9\frac{1}{2}''$ s.a.e. asking for further details, and stating at which time of the year you are available. The summer workcamp booklet costs about £1 to print, so donations towards the cost are welcome.

LinkAge

LinkAge aims to develop and foster links between the alternate generations: between young and old. For details *see* Section 12.

Marriage Counselling Scotland
26 Frederick Street, Edinburgh EH2 2JR (Tel: 031-225 5006).

Marriage Counselling Scotland selects suitable volunteers to train as marriage counsellors. Counsellors are women and men from all walks of life. They are carefully selected and trained for what can be difficult but rewarding work. The MCS seeks mature people, with some experience of life, who have a tolerant outlook and can listen to others. Local Marriage Counselling Services sponsor interested people for selection by the National panel. Counsellors should be able to help and support anxious and unhappy people as they work through their difficulties, without themselves becoming discouraged.

Counsellors may be of any marital status and there are no rigid age limits. Candidates who are considered to have the right potential are asked to attend a Selection Conference. This is a detailed and challenging procedure, designed to select individuals most suitable for training as marriage counsellors. In recent years, about one half of the candidates have been selected.

Basic training includes six residential weekends held over a two year period. If selected and trained you will need to be available for at least 120 hours counselling each year. In addition, there are regular meetings for case discussions and tutorials.

NACRO
169 Clapham Road, London SW9 OPU (Tel: 071-582 6500).

The National Association for the Care and Resettlement of Offenders (NACRO) is a charity and has limited opportunities for volunteering. Projects run through the Opportunities for Volunteering-funded Youth Activities Unit use volunteers, and these usually relate to locally-run, community-level initiatives that aim to recruit volunteers from the local community to organise, for instance, crèches, youth clubs, etc. These Units are in: South Saltley (Birmingham), Henley Green (Coventry), Salford Precinct (Salford), Brextowe Estate (Nottingham), Pleck (Walsall), Ferrier Estate (Greenwich), Rectory Park (Ealing), Hammersmith and Fulham. NACRO also runs a Resettlement Information Service and Resettlement Centre for prisoners and ex-prisoners in Birmingham, and education centres in Manchester and London that use volunteers. For more information about any of these services, please contact NACRO Information Department on the telephone number above.

If you are particularly interested in voluntary work with offenders, you should contact your local probation service, which will often use volunteers for a variety of its support services.

National Association of Leagues of Hospital Friends
2nd Floor, Fairfax House, Causton Road, Colchester, Essex CO1 1RJ
(Tel: 0206-761227).

The National Association is an 'umbrella organisation' which acts as a support and advice centre to its 1,243 affiliated members, having some 350,000 individual voluntary helpers. Together they raise over £20,000,000 per year for patients and health establishments they support and give over 6,500,000 hours of voluntary service each year. The range of services provided varies from League to League and includes shops, canteens, libraries, flower arranging and organising outings, as well as befriending and visiting patients.

If you would like to join a League locally, write or telephone the Honorary Secretary of the League of Hospital Friends at the hospital you would like to serve. If you have any difficulty in making contact, write to the National Association as above.

National Association of Prison Visitors (NAPV)
46b Hartington Street, Bedford MK41 7RL (Tel: 0234-359763/211803).

Prison Visitors are men and women, appointed by the Home Office, who voluntarily give up part of their spare time to visit and befriend a number of prisoners, some of whom may have no other visitors. Most Prison Visitors make weekly or fortnightly visits, during the evening or at weekends. Their visits are unsupervised and may take place in the privacy of the prisoner's cell. A Prison Visitor is a friendly representative of the outside world, reminding the prisoner that he or she is not forgotten or rejected.

If you are interested in this voluntary work, confident of your ability to meet and relate to prisoners from all backgrounds, and you live within easy travelling distance of a prison, you should write to the Governor for further information. The NAPV publishes a newsletter and will be glad to supply you with information.

National Association of Victims Support Schemes
National Office, Cranmer House, 39 Brixton Road, London SW9 6DZ
(Tel: 071-735 9166).

Victim Support relies upon the hard work of over 7,000 people who volunteer time and energy to help victims of crime. They contribute a wide range of skills and experience and there are many ways you could help, depending on the time you have to give. Because of the rapid growth of the number of Victims Support Schemes and the services they offer, there is always a demand for more volunteers. In some areas volunteers are needed with specific skills, such as the ability to speak or write another language. All Schemes appreciate volunteers who are good listeners and who are able to give practical advice and help.

If you offered your services you would receive comprehensive training and continuing support and have the opportunity to meet with other volunteers on a regular basis.

As well as the need for volunteers to visit victims of crime other volunteers are needed who do not provide direct support to victims but who use their skills in other ways. Some volunteers take on tasks such as fitting new locks in the victims' homes, or helping with the Scheme's office administration. The training of new volunteers relies upon the participation of those who have specialist knowledge, for example in insurance or in legal or medical fields. All Schemes have to raise additional money and the organisation of fund raising events requires ideas, energy and enthusiasm.

Schemes are listed in the telephone book and can also be contacted through the police. The National Office above can also put you in touch with your local scheme.

See also reference to Victims Support Schemes for those who are victims themselves in Section 6.

▶ *National Association of Volunteer Bureaux*
St. Peter's College, College Road, Saltley, Birmingham B8 3TE
(Tel: 021-327 0265).

The National Association of Volunteer Bureaux supports a network of around 300 volunteer bureaux throughout England, Wales and Northern Ireland. Volunteer bureaux recruit volunteers and place them with a wide variety of local voluntary activities and projects. They also recruit volunteers for projects and activities offered by other voluntary organisations and for statutory health and social services. Some volunteer bureaux also recruit volunteers for their own activities and projects. The volunteering opportunities offered by volunteer bureaux might include community driving, befriending and providing direct one-to-one services for elderly and vulnerable people, environmental project work, advice-giving and counselling, participation in community activities such as self-help groups, and so on.

Volunteer bureaux are listed in the local telephone directory under 'V'. Alternatively, the NAVB can provide potential volunteers with details of their nearest bureaux.

▶ *New Horizons Trust*
Paramount House, 290-2 Brighton Road, South Croydon, Surrey CR2 6AG
(Tel: 081-666 0201).

The Trust offers cash grants to community projects carried out by older people. The grants may be made available to any group coming forward with a useful and imaginative project, provided there are at least ten people in the group, at least half of them are over age 60, and the project is a new one that makes use of the knowledge and expertise of group members to benefit the community.

▶ *Oxfam*
274 Banbury Road, Oxford OX2 7DZ (Tel: 0865-56777).

There are approximately 27,000 volunteers serving in more than 870 shops, and others working in Oxfam offices, as well as all those who send donations. As a retired person you may be able to offer time and skills which Oxfam would be glad to have. Possible jobs are: typing and secretarial; general administration/finance; helping to organise fund-raising events; helping with emergency appeals – being at the end of a phone, available at short notice, duplicating letters, stuffing envelopes, sending out information sheets, thank-you letters and suchlike. Shop helpers are also needed.

If you do not know where your local office is, contact the address above. You could also ask Oxfam to send you a copy of its booklet *Volunteer for a Fairer World*.

Relate: National Marriage Guidance
Herbert Gray College, Little Church Street, Rugby CV21 3AP (Tel: 0788-73241).

People interested in becoming counsellors begin with informal conversations with members of their local marriage guidance council. These are followed by a formal interview to decide whether the council will 'sponsor' the candidate to be put forward for final selection. Sponsored candidates then attend a final selection conference where they work together on various tasks related to counselling and are individually interviewed by National Marriage Guidance Council tutors and external selectors.

On the basis of these tests and interviews, about half the selected candidates are accepted for counsellor training, which lasts for two years. The basic programme consists of six residential sessions, each lasting 48 hours. Training is free, but counsellors work without pay for a minimum of 120 hours a year. Most counsellors are women, although the Council is actively encouraging the recruitment of more men. Counsellors usually retire at 65, but this can be extended at the counsellors' request, provided they are able to maintain effective standards of counselling.

Religious Society of Friends
Friends House, Euston House, Euston Road, London NW1 2BJ (Tel: 071-387 3601).

Quaker International Social Projects (QISP) bring together volunteers of many different nationalities, cultures and backgrounds who give two to three weeks of their time to live and work on a project committed to improving quality of life. Working with local organisations they develop: play schemes; social work; environmental and manual work; women-only schemes; social activities in hospitals; study; or a combination of these, for example a playscheme with an environmental theme in Hackney, a joint Soviet/British project studying East/West issues, refurbishing tools to send to Nicaragua or taking long stay hospital residents to the Edinburgh Festival.

QISP also have partner agencies throughout Europe, Turkey and North Africa, so if you have some volunteer project experience, work-abroad experience or community work experience they may be able to offer you a placement abroad. British volunteers are sent abroad to do projects in over 20 countries, including in East and West Europe, Morocco and Turkey.

QISP projects are good fun and offer a chance to get away and meet others and learn new skills, as well as being of benefit to a local community. Anyone can be involved. Applications are welcome from individuals with a disability. Food and accommodation is free on a project and, if you are unwaged, it may be possible to help you with your travel costs. QISP particularly welcome older volunteers on their projects. Many volunteers/co-ordinators are retired and there is usually a wide age range on each project.

REACH – *Retired Executives Action Clearing-House*
89 Southwark Street, London SE1 OHD (Tel: 071-928 0452).

REACH was set up over ten years ago to place retired men and women with business or other professional skills in voluntary organisations throughout Great Britain. It finds only part-time, voluntary jobs, but with out-of-pocket expenses paid. REACH is itself a registered charity funded mainly by donations from companies and trusts. It makes no charge to either the volunteer or to the voluntary organisation. At the time of writing there are over 1,000 jobs waiting to be filled, so there is a good chance of finding something to make proper use of a particular expertise, not too far from home.

Resource Unit to Promote Black Volunteering – RUBV
Unit 117–19 Brixton Enterprise Centre, 444 Brixton Road, London SW9 8EJ (Tel: 071-738 3462).

RUBV is a new organisation launched in 1991. Its major aim is to promote Black Voluntary activities and Black Volunteering. RUBV works with individuals, volunteer organisers, and different organisations within the voluntary and statutory sectors at both local and national level. It aims to bring together people of different cultures, colour, race and religion to work together. For further details and for a copy of the quarterly newsletter *Black Echo* contact as above.

Retired and Senior Volunteer Programme
237 Pentonville Road, London N1 9NJ (Tel: 071-278 6601).

RSVP is part of Community Service Volunteers and is for anyone aged over 50 with time and energy to spare who wants to become involved in their community. There are 1,000 volunteers spead around the country who are undertaking over 100,000 hours of voluntary work each year.

RSVP volunteers do what they want to do and choose when they want to do it. Opportunities are as diverse as the volunteers themselves. Some volunteers are assisting in schools by listening to children read, helping by demonstrating skills and working in the school library cataloguing books, while others are helping to organise and run tenant groups and other associations, advice and counselling groups, lunch clubs and visiting services to older people who cannot go out and who live alone. If you join RSVP you will not work on your own – it is a cardinal principle that all volunteers work in groups. A group may consist of two or three people or many more. If you are interested send for an application form – enrolment meetings are held regularly.

The Samaritans

The Samaritans seek volunteers from those about to retire and from the recently retired to help maintain a 24-hour listening and befriending service at their 183 branches throughout the United Kingdom and Ireland.

Preparation classes for this work are held at frequent intervals. If you would like more details about the selection process, contact the local branch of the Samaritans – see your local phone book.

Save the Children Fund UK
Mary Datchelor House, 17 Grove Lane, Camberwell, London SE5 8RD
(Tel: 071-703 5400).

Save the Children (SCF) is the United Kingdom's largest international voluntary agency concerned with child health and welfare.

Organisations such as SCF appreciate the contribution made by volunteers to their work. SCF has over 800 branches of voluntary fundraisers in the United Kingdom, supported by a network of regional fund-raising staff. The combined efforts of volunteers in shops and branches raise approximately one-fifth of SCF's income. Branches always welcome new members and there are many ways in which individuals can contribute. Branch activities vary, ranging from coffee mornings to large prestigious events such as concerts and other similar social gatherings. Some volunteers may take on special responsibilities with the branch, such as becoming a press officer, school speaker or trading secretary.

SCF has a network of around 150 shops. Volunteers can become involved in various activities, including serving in the shop, pricing, sorting, ironing and accounting. As well as raising money, shops provide a focal point for SCF in the community.

The fund-raising department at Save the Children headquarters is always delighted to put potential volunteers in touch with their nearest branch or shop. Whatever their age, experience or time available, most people have something to offer.

Scottish Conservation Projects
Balallan House, 24 Allan Park, Stirling FK8 2QG (Tel: 0786-79697).

The Scottish Conservation Projects Trust (SCP) is Scotland's leading charity involving people in improving the quality of the environment through practical conservation work.

SCP offers a wide variety of 7–14-day residential Action Breaks throughout Scotland where volunteers can participate in practical conservation projects. The type of project includes deer fencing, building a drystone dyke (stone wall), planting native trees, restoring a small traditional building, constructing a pond for wildlife – and lots more.

Volunteers are of all ages – from 16 to 71 – and SCP encourages the older person. Both men and women enjoy working on the projects and they come from all walks of life: engineers, office workers, builders, students, housewives/househusbands, retired people and those who are unemployed.

Each volunteer pays £4 per day. Food and accommodation are provided. No work skill or experience is required. All skills are taught by the fully trained leader. There is one day off each week and participants enjoy getting to know each other, seeing the wonderful scenery and wildlife of Scotland – while achieving something different.

SCP also runs weekend training courses in environmental skills. Many of the skills used on Action Breaks are taught during these courses. In Falkirk, Edinburgh, Glasgow and Inverness SCP offers midweek opportunities to participate in practical conservation projects on the urban fringe. No experience is required. Full training is given.

Membership of SCP costs £12 p.a. (£6 retired). Members receive a members' newsletter twice a year; an Action Breaks programme twice a year; an Environmental Skills Training Programme twice a year; and a full colour Annual Review.

Skillshare Africa
3 Belvoir Street, Leicester LE1 6SL (Tel: 0533-541862).

Skillshare Africa sends skilled and experienced co-operantes to work in southern Africa, where there is a real need for outside help. The skills and experience of the co-operantes are matched with aims and needs of the local people. Between 60 and 80 Skillshare Africa co-operantes are working in southern Africa at any one time, and their abilities cover almost every skilled and professional field from civil engineering to social work, from boat building to environmental education, from welding to small business advising, from handicrafts to plumbing.

If you have the right qualifications and a number of years' experience, and are able to pass the medical, you are welcome to apply whatever your age. As well as the qualifications and length of experience specified in the Vacancy List/Job Description other qualities are also valued such as flexibility, maturity, sensitivity to local values and a sense of humour. All contracts are for two years to enable you to make the best, most lasting contribution you can.

Skillshare Africa would be glad to send you details and a copy of the Possible Future Vacancies List.

Society of Voluntary Associates – SOVA
Brixton Hill Place, London SW2 1HJ (Tel: 081-671 7833).

SOVA specialises in training local volunteers and involving them in work with offenders and their families. The volunteers who work with the Probation Service are known as Voluntary Associates (VAs). They are people from a wide variety of backgrounds who bring different skills and experience – what they have in common is a genuine interest in helping offenders and their families in their own communities. Qualifications and experience are not necessary.

Some of the examples of the kinds of work in whichs VAs are involved include: befriending people on probation; supporting the partners and families of people in prison; teaching literacy or numeracy skills; visiting or writing to people in prison; helping to find work or accommodation; group work in a variety of settings; providing support to individuals or families in court.

VSO (Voluntary Service Overseas)
317 Putney Bridge Road, London SW15 2PN (Tel: 081-780 2266).

VSO is a registered charity dedicated to assisting developing countries. Each year, in response to requests from 45 countries, VSO sends more than 700 volunteers to share their skills and their lives with people in Third World communities. Volunteers come from all walks of life and are aged between 20 and 70. There are doctors, bricklayers, midwives, diesel mechanics, agriculturalists, business advisers, nurses, social and community workers, small business advisers, financial managers, electricians, teachers, librarians, and many, many other skills in demand each year. Volunteers must be prepared for a two year commitment. VSO pays return fares, equipment grants, a mid-tour grant after one year in post, resettlement grant on return to the United Kingdom, National Insurance payments, and also payments to a specially arranged endowment plan. Language training and some skills-adaptation courses are provided by VSO. Accommodation overseas is provided by the employer and payment is made from the employer based on local rates. VSO will be pleased to send you further details.

The Volunteer Centre UK
29 Lower King's Road, Berkhamsted, Hertfordshire HP4 2AB (Tel: 0442-873311).

The Volunteer Centre UK can provide information if you want to volunteer for the first time or if you are already involved and want to know more. The Centre also runs events and training courses for those whose work, paid or unpaid, involves organising volunteers, and also co-ordinates UK Volunteers Week, which takes place annually from 1 to 7 June. For full information and a free catalogue of services, send a s.a.e. to the above address.

If you are particularly interested in voluntary work concerned with the environment, The Volunteer Centre can provide you with a list of organisations in your area that work with the help of volunteers. Contact: Jonathan Pinkney-Baird, Training and Development Officer (Environment).

Volunteer Reading Help
National Office, Unit 111, 156 Blackfriars Road, London SE1 8EN
(Tel: 071-721 7156).

Volunteer Reading Help is a national charity which links volunteers from the local community with children aged 6 to 11 who teachers feel would benefit from one-to-one help. Volunteers give their time to each child in a way no teacher can ever hope or be expected to do. They include people aged 18 to 80 from all cultures and backgrounds. Each volunteer works with the same three children individually, for half an hour each, twice a week in a local primary school. They talk, read, play games and help build each child's confidence and interests in books. Before being accepted for training, volunteers are interviewed and a medical reference is taken. Training takes place over three sessions of $1\frac{1}{2}$ hours each. Training courses are held once a term. Fares to and from school are paid. Volunteer Reading Help has branches in inner London, Bolton, Bristol, Liverpool, Nottingham, Oxford, Reading, Surrey, West Dorset, West Oxfordshire and West Kent. There are plans to start others.

Volunteer Stroke Service – VSS
Manor Farm House, Appleton, Abingdon, Oxfordshire OX13 5JR (Tel: 0865-862954).

VSS helps people who suffer from speech and associated problems as the result of a stroke. It also aims to help their families. Each patient is offered a small team of volunteers who visit him or her singly for about an hour at a time on a regular weekly rota basis. There are also weekly groups where patients meet, and where the need arises, smaller groups of patients and volunteers are formed. Outings and entertainments are arranged for the groups from time to time.

Volunteers need no special qualifications and will be offered relevant training sessions. They are briefed about individual patients. Volunteers establish a relaxed neighbourly relationship with the stroke patient and use common interests, games, puzzles, and other simple methods to stimulate and help overcome the difficulty of speech, memory, handling money, numbers, telling the time, etc.

Each scheme is run within a Health District by a part-time organiser who is given an instructive seminar and in-service training.

The VSS is managed by The Stroke Association, of which it is a part, on behalf of Health Authorities which provide the funding.

Women's Royal Voluntary Service
234-44 Stockwell Road, Brixton, London SW9 9SP (Tel: 071-416 0146).

The WRVS has over 160,000 members regularly serving in various capacities, with several more thousand able to be deployed in an emergency. The range of activities varies in every locality and includes organised meals, hospital services, clothing stores, emergency services, family welfare including children and family holidays, old people's welfare, and the welfare of offenders and their families.

WRVS members work independently and with the Health and Local Authorities to provide welfare services, not otherwise available, for young, old, ill, lonely, disabled and troubled people.

For many jobs, volunteers need not commit themselves to more than two or three hours a fortnight. Evening and weekend jobs are available. WRVS offers much scope for the ideas and talents of retired people, women at home, and others with the time and will for further involvement. No one needs to feel bored or underused, and members may work in teams or on their own as they prefer. The work is rewarding and companionable. Reliability and kindness are more important than special skills.

WRVS is non-political and non-sectarian, and does not raise funds. There is no subscription. Wearing uniform is optional. Men volunteers are welcomed.

A range of leaflets is available to tell you more about volunteering with the WRVS. Either contact the address above or contact any WRVS office (*see* under *Women's Royal Voluntary Service* in the telephone book.)

=▶ *Youth Clubs UK*
Keswick House, 30 Peacock Lane, Leicester LE1 5NY (Tel: 0533-629514).

There is a local association office in each county, and all of these welcome volunteers. Each youth club has a wide range of activities, including artistic, sporting, health development, etc. Each club also arranges a number of events each year. Volunteers are welcome to help with activities. Contact Youth Clubs UK to find out about local youth clubs.

Publications

=▶ *Voluntary Agencies Directory*
Published semi-annually by the National Council for Voluntary Organisations, 8 Regents Wharf, All Saints Street, London N1 9RL. Price: £10.95. Or by post from Plymbridge Distributors Ltd, Plymbridge House, Estover, Plymouth PL6 7PZ (Tel: 0752-695745). Price: £12.30 including postage and packing.

The directory includes some 1,800 national voluntary agencies, ranging from household names to specialist self-help groups. Names and addresses are listed alphabetically with summaries of aims and activities. Symbols indicate charitable status, local branches, use of volunteers, number of paid staff, size of organisation, trading companies and library/information room.

A list of useful addresses following the directory section includes professional and public advisory bodies which are relevant to the work of voluntary organisations. There is an extensive classified subject index, plus a list of abbreviations and acronyms.

=▶ *Directory of National Voluntary Organisations for Scotland*
Editor: Anne Boyle. Published by the Scottish Council for Voluntary Organisations, 18–19 Claremont Crescent, Edinburgh EH7 4QD (Tel: 031-556 3882). Price: £7.50 including postage (SCVO members £6).

With 496 entries ranging from the Aberlour Child Care Trust to Youth with a Mission (Scotland) Ltd, the eighth edition of the Directory (1990) reflects the growth and diversity of the voluntary sector in Scotland. Entries include a statement of aims and activities as well as contact and publications details for each organisation. Alphabetical and classified indexes are included, along with a list of professional and advisory bodies.

=▶ *Volunteer Bureaux Directory*
Available from: National Association of Volunteer Bureaux, St Peter's College, College Road, Saltley, Birmingham B8 3TE (Tel: 021-327 0265).
Price: £3 to members; £6.50 to non-members including postage and packing.

The Directory lists contact names and addresses of volunteer bureaux who are members of NAVB in England, Wales and Northern Ireland. The Directory gives the address, telephone number, hours of opening and name of the volunteer bureau organiser of each volunteer bureau. It also gives details of other useful contacts. While there is not yet a bureau in every town, where they do exist they will most probably be listed under 'V' in the phone book.

So You Want to be a Volunteer
Available from: The Volunteer Centre UK, 29 Lower King's Road, Berkhamsted, Hertfordshire HP4 2AB (Tel: 0442-873311). Price: £3.

This publication provides guidance for those wishing to consider becoming a volunteer and provides a checklist of questions to ask the organisation requiring volunteers. It also provides details of questions likely to be asked by the organisation. A reading list, information sheets, and leaflets on insurance and expenses are included.

Volunteer Work
Available from: Central Bureau for Educational Visits and Exchanges, Seymour Mews, London W1H 9PE (Tel: 071-486 5101). Price: £3 in good bookshops; £4 by post from the Bureau.

A wide range of opportunities exist in developed and developing countries, especially for those with skills or experience, and this directory provides valuable guidance and information. Some one hundred organisations are listed, recruiting volunteers for medium- and long-term projects in Britain and 153 countries worldwide. Each agency's orientation, philosophy, countries of operation and projects are detailed, together with the qualities and skills required as well as terms of service.

SECTION TEN

Carry on learning

Many of us miss out on further education or training when we are young, for one reason or another, and would now like to catch up. Or we may have developed different interests as we have matured and now have a wish to learn more about these. In either event, retirement may provide us with the opportunity to study those subjects which really interest us. They may not necessarily lead to qualifications but the studying, in itself, can be profoundly satisfying. Others will choose to take courses leading to qualifications and achieving these will prove to be immensely encouraging after a lifetime when perhaps we felt that our scholastic achievements were not all they could have been had we had different opportunities.

If you have never had the opportunity to study or it is a long time since you sat down to study seriously, you may feel too daunted at the prospect of your ever achieving anything worthwhile. We would recommend those who are interested but nervous to give it a try. It is quite remarkable how older people, with very little educational background, have nevertheless been able to enjoy studying, once they have mustered enough determination to go ahead. In order to follow a course of study you need two things: the desire to learn, and the self-discipline to allocate several hours a week to your studies. Probably the hardest part is starting; once you have embarked on a subject you have chosen because of its interest to you, you will be carried on by the sheer enthusiasm of finding out new things.

Adult education can provide people with a 'second chance to learn' – often a first real chance to those whose schooling, for whatever reason, was inadequate for their needs. Adult education is provided by a number of different sources, and varies from area to area. Further education colleges, adult education institutes, university extra-mural departments, home study courses (e.g. the Open University and Open College) are all potential providers in the field, offering a wide range of subjects for study or recreation. For further information contact your local education authority (LEA) adult education service. The Education Department will be listed in the telephone book under the name of the council.

We describe below a range of opportunities to give you some idea what is available but, of course, we cannot give details of local adult education provision.

Open learning

It is the coming of open learning which has changed the way in which courses for adults are set out and which provides an altogether more congenial way of studying. You can work at home, at your workplace, at a college or learning centre, even on a journey.

There is no universally agreed definition of open learning. The essential idea, however, is that of opening up new opportunities for people to learn. Different open learning schemes may do this in different ways – for example by dropping all entry requirements; by enabling learners to study what they like, when and where they find most convenient, using whatever teaching media best suits them, and at their own individual pace; by providing special tutorial help; by allowing learners to decide their own learning objectives and how (if at all) they are to be assessed. With open learning you can work at your own pace with no pressure to move on before you have fully understood the section you are working on, and you can work when it suits you.

Most open learning programmes involve the use of specially prepared self-instructional materials (packages). These packages may be separate units or modules, each of which may occupy only a few hours or days of study time. Or several may be put together to form a complete 'course' which may take a learner weeks or months to work through. Learners will usually (but not necessarily) work through the packages on their own – but they may meet together with other learners from time to time, and they may have occasional, but none the less crucial, contact with a tutor and perhaps a counsellor.

Local classes

It can be relatively easy to join in a local evening class (some day classes may also be available) where there are many subjects on offer. These may range from the academic or vocational to the practical – pottery, carpentry and so on. Classes are open to anyone and some local authorities offer concessionary rates for retired people. Enrolment usually takes place in mid-September and many local papers carry details of the courses on offer in advance – local libraries also have information. The most popular get booked up quickly, so you would need to be there early on the day of registration.

Local authorities are always looking for tutors who can take evening classes. If you have a particular interest or hobby you may be able to offer yourself as a tutor and you may be surprised how satisfying it can be to draw your information together and to structure it so that you can share your knowledge and pass on your enthusiasm to others. Never mind if your subject has not been taught locally before – all the more important that a class be started. A word of warning, however. Some evening class subjects do not immediately appeal to enough people to warrant keeping the class going. This happened to us. Somewhat nervously, but with great enthusiasm, we set off to lead an evening class on the subject of the history of recorded sound – unfortunately no one came! However, don't be put off. Our hobby remains intact and no doubt you will have better luck.

Universities and colleges

These frequently accept older students and some will accept you on your past experience, not just exams taken. They have adult or community or extra-mural departments which provide a range of interesting short courses. If you apply for a degree course and have never had a student grant before, you are eligible for one whatever your age.

Television

A number of the television companies transmit regular educational programmes and also provide back-up materials. The BBC publishes a magazine *Resources for Adult Learning and Training* which, as well as having interesting articles, also gives details of the various programmes which have been scheduled. Only recently, the BBC had a campaign aimed at encouraging viewers to take up second chance education or training. It is well worth sending for this guide just to see the wide range of programmes and resources that are on offer in your own sitting-room. To get a copy, write to: BBC Education, BBC White City, 201 Wood Lane, London W12 7TS (Tel: 081-752 5650).

The Independent Television Commission publishes information on educational programmes for adults on ITV and Channel 4. All those television companies granted licences from 1 January 1993 are committed to providing some local education/social action programming which is written into their licences. Many of the successful applicants are also interested in providing series of programmes for adult education which can be networked.

For details of educational programmes for adults on ITV and Channel 4 contact the Independent Television Commission, 70 Brompton Road, London SW3 1EY (Tel: 071-584 7011).

Home study courses

▶ *National Extension College*
18 Brooklands Avenue, Cambridge CB2 2HN (Tel: 0223-316644).

This is an educational charity founded to provide adults with high-quality home study courses. It provides distance learning courses for Open University preparatory and GCSE and A levels, as well as special interest courses. It also provides a distance learning tuition service for London University external degrees and diplomas and for certain professional examinations. You do not need to have any qualifications to start an NEC course. NEC has students aged 16 to 80 +, nearly half of whom left school aged 16 or less. One-fifth left school with no qualifications at all. NEC's Fresh Start courses may be of particular interest to you if you feel rusty about studying.

Its *Guide to Courses* contains full details of over 100 courses in which you might be interested.

In its Distance Learning courses for individuals, NEC enrols about 7,000 students annually on over 80 courses in subjects as diverse as mathematics, English literature, economics and psychology. The NEC Learning Support Department advises by telephone or letter 13,000 students and potential students annually and co-ordinates the work of 500 home-based tutors. NEC takes care to make the course material interesting and puts an emphasis on learning activities. It places great emphasis on the number of activities in its texts. These activities can be exercises, experiments, observational activities or tape activities. One student wrote: 'In spite of not having studied formally for thirty years I had no difficulty in coping with the study units.' In study guidance you will be given plenty of help in mastering skills essential to successful study, for example how to take notes and set out the results of experiments.

NEC took care to point out to us that their distance learning courses 'are particularly suitable for elderly people because they provide an opportunity for studying at home and many of our students are retired'.

In addition to their courses, NEC provides a range of learning resources for students to use as they choose, as distinct from the tutor-supported course materials. The 'Catalogue' makes interesting reading in its own right. NEC would be glad to send you a copy.

Open College of the Arts

Houndhill, Worsbrough, Barnsley, South Yorkshire S70 6TU (Tel: 0226-730495).

The Open College of the Arts, an educational trust, caters for those who would like to develop their artistic abilities but who prefer or need to work mainly from home.

OCA uses methods broadly similar to those of the Open University. Specially written course manuals guide students through a programme of activities lasting up to nine months, and students get regular help from OCA's network of 300 tutors who are practising artists or writers, or teachers in universities, polytechnics and colleges. Many courses can progress into a second and even a third year, and a range of day- and summer-schools are available to students.

Anyone can join. There are no entry requirements or age limits; among the ten thousand students who have already taken an OCA course are people of all ages from the late teens to 89 and in every conceivable occupation. Courses can be taken by complete beginners and by those who already have some experience but are looking for a more disciplined and wide-ranging approach.

Courses with tutorial support begin in the autumn. Courses include: Art and Design; Painting; Textiles; Sculpture; Garden Design; Music; The Art of Photography; Starting to Write; History of Art.

Many students do not seek formal assessment of their work, but others need or want to know the level of their achievement. The OCA Award can be applied for at the end of your course.

The Open University

Open University courses are specifically designed for home-based study. Age is no barrier. The youngest students are in their teens, and the oldest graduate (so far) was 93 when he received his degree.

More than 250 courses are available, ranging from self-contained study packs on everyday topics to degree-level subjects. Courses vary in length from those that involve a few hours of work for a few weeks to those that take nine months at the rate of 12 to 14 hours each week. You do not need previous qualifications to take any OU course. Nor do you have to take any test or face any interview to enrol on these courses.

There are courses covering the arts, computing, personal and community interests, environmental education, management, educational studies, science, social sciences, mathematics, and technology. No entry qualifications are required and the University is open to all over the age of 18 who are resident in the European Community. Entry is on a 'first come, first served' basis; hence early application is advisable.

The main element of study is the specially written course material. In addition, courses may utilise television and radio, audio and video cassettes, slides and home kits. Though study at home is the basis of Open University study there are opportunities for tuition and group discussions at local study centres. Tuition and counselling are also carried out by telephone or letter. Many courses run week-long residential summer schools at conventional university campuses. If anyone with a disability requires special help, he or she may take a personal assistant, or the residential schools office will find such a helper. This will incur no extra cost for the student. In certain circumstances, students may be excused residential school attendance.

To give local assistance to students the University has 13 Regional Centres and more than 260 study centres nationwide. Students are allocated to tutors who are responsible for commenting on and marking their work as well as holding occasional face-to-face tutorials. The University encourages the formation of self-help groups among students. It provides services such as telephone tutorials for those who live in the more remote areas.

The Open University provides certain advice and services specifically to meet the needs of disabled students. These include: assistance at residential schools; cassette tapes of course material for those unable to deal with written text; transcripts of broadcasts; study weekends for persons with particular handicaps; advice on the accessibility of courses to those with specific disabilities; and advice on study techniques. These services come from different areas within the University, and there is an Adviser on Education for students with disabilities to advise and to liaise with the different departments and with outside bodies.

If you would like further information, write to the Central Enquiry Service, The Open University, PO Box 200, Milton Keynes MK7 6AG. You can contact The Open University Adviser to Disabled Students at: the Open University, Walton Hall, Milton Keynes MK7 6YZ.

You can also contact the Enquiry and Admissions Service at your nearest Open University Regional Centre. It is usually best to telephone or write initially so that an appointment can be made with the appropriate member of staff. This service is free and puts you under no obligation. The Regional Centres are as follows:

- London
  Parsifal College, 527 Finchley Road, London NW3 7BG (Tel: 071-433 6161).
- South
  Foxcombe Hall, Boars Hill, Oxford OX1 5HR (Tel: 0865-328038).
- South West
  4–5 Portwall Lane, Bristol BS1 6NB (Tel: 0272-299641).
- South East
  St James's House, 150 London Road, East Grinstead, West Sussex RH19 1ES (Tel: 0342-410545).
- West Midlands
  66–8 High Street, Harborne, Birmingham B17 9NB (Tel: 021-428 1550).
- East Midlands
  The Octagon, 143 Derby Road, Nottingham NG7 1PH (Tel: 0602-240121).
- East Anglia
  Cintra House, 12 Hills Road, Cambridge CB2 1PF (Tel: 0223-61650).
- Yorkshire
  Fairfax House, Merrion Street, Leeds LS2 8JU (Tel: 0532-451466).
- North West
  Chorlton House, 70 Manchester Road, Chorlton-cum-Hardy, Manchester M21 1PQ (Tel: 061-861 9823).
- North
  Eldon House, Regent Street, Gosforth, Newcastle upon Tyne NE3 3PW (Tel: 091-284 1611).
- Wales
  24 Cathedral Road, Cardiff CF1 9SA (Tel: 0222-665636).
- Scotland
  60 Melville Street, Edinburgh EH3 7HF (Tel: 031-226 3851) and at 2 Park Gardens, Glasgow G3 7YE (Tel: 041-332 4364).
- Northern Ireland
  40 University Street, Belfast BT7 1SU (Tel: 0232-245025).

Costs of courses and financial help – grants and awards

Costs range from about £10 for a simple study pack on a modern novelist to £240 for a course in the BA degree programme and £975 for a course in the MBA programme.

So how do you go about seeking help with the costs? In the first instance, local authorities' social services departments or local education authorities should be approached for financial assistance relating to: preparatory studies; tuition fees; kit deposits; set books; summer school attendance; summer school assistant's travelling expenses; or travel to tutorials. The Open University also has its own limited funds to help those on low incomes.

The Open College
Freepost, Warrington WA2 7BR.

The Open College represents a new national approach to skills training, with the emphasis on learning rather than teaching. It increases opportunities for vocational education and training by making open learning readily available to anyone, whatever their age, education or occupation. You can take a course leading to a qualification which will prove your skill to others, or you can choose a course which will give you personal satisfaction. All Open College courses are designed to be practical, to teach you things you could not do before.

Courses can include videos, audio tapes, workbooks and other learning materials with advice and tutorial support available, if required, through a network of local centres. The training aims to be responsive and flexible, designed to meet the needs of employers and individuals.

More detailed information about how the College operates is contained in its prospectus. As well as describing the courses available it offers guidance on where help can be obtained and which qualifications or credits courses lead to. There is also a Centres list which will tell you where to go for the Tutorial Support to help you make the most of your course and give you help on any qualifications.

Learning together

University of the Third Age
1 Stockwell Green, London SW9 9JF (Tel: 071-737 2541).

'After the First Age of childhood, and the Second Age of work, family and social responsibility, comes the Third Age.'

U3A provides opportunities for all kinds of constructive activities and involves older adults in the creation and organisation of their own programmes, of a broadly eduational kind. It consists of 20,000 members in over 160 local groups run by and for older people. No qualifications are needed and none is given: U3A is dedicated to learning for pleasure. Each group decides its own study plan and organises its own activities using the skills, knowledge and experience of its members – so you may find yourself a learner one week and a leader the next.

Local U3As are completely free to decide their own programmes. They must raise whatever funds are needed by subscriptions or donations. U3As vary in size from 10 to 1,000 people and the range of activities and study groups is enormous but always depends on the wishes of the membership. Resources and help are available to anyone interested in starting a new U3A. Libraries, local media and word of mouth are used to bring interested people together.

As more members join, the variety of activities increases. Social, cultural, sporting and travel activities begin to develop. U3A believe that once one's Second Age is over, there can begin a time of creativity and fulfilment.

The Third Age is a national newspaper, published three times a year. It is available from local U3As. A national individual membership is available for £5.

A list of names and addresses of all local U3As is available from the address above on receipt of a 4" × 10" s.a.e.

Study holidays and courses

A wide range of educational short courses are available – the subjects include: painting, music, crafts, yoga, cookery, crafts, wine tasting, china restoration, sociology, realising self-esteem, caring for antiques, modern languages, pottery, arts, history, social science, flower arranging, music appreciation, archaeology, literature, education, gardening, architecture, photography, nature studies, writing, lace making and film making. Courses may be for a weekend or longer.

Details of these courses are published every January and August in *Time to Learn* (£3.95), produced by the National Institute of Adult Continuing Education, 19B De Montfort Street, Leicester LE1 7GE (Tel: 0533-551451).

Saga Study Holidays

Described as 'education for enjoyment', these holidays are not just for the academically-minded – they include something for everyone, from appreciation of Shakespeare to pottery for beginners. Saga's Study Holidays consist of seven nights full or half board accommodation at university and college centres with lectures, film and slide shows and a number of course-related excursions to places of interest or extra tuition sessions on practical courses. In each group, numbers are limited to ensure a friendly atmosphere and to give you the opportunity to talk directly to your lecturer.

Courses include: 'Theatre Appreciation', involving a full day with the National Theatre and a visit backstage at Sadlers Wells; 'Orchestral Music Appreciation', including a full day seminar with the London Symphony Orchestra; 'Welsh Music and Song', including a full day excursion to Llangollen and a visit to the European Centre of Folk Studies; 'Scottish Art and Architecture', including visits to classical buildings; 'British Painting from 1600 to 1914'; 'The History of English Pottery'; 'Architectural Styles in London', including visits to buildings of interest; 'Scottish Life and Letters'; 'The Life and Times of William Shakespeare'; 'Painting and Photography'; 'Pottery for Beginners'; 'How to Trace Your Family Tree'; 'Creative Writing'; 'Gardening'; 'Bridge Courses'; 'Computing for Beginners'; 'Transport Heritage'; 'Scottish Heritage'; 'Welsh Heritage'; 'Scotland before History'; 'Prehistoric Wessex'; 'Field Study of the Highlands'; 'Scottish Wildlife'. Prices from £161.

For further information on Saga Study Holidays ring 0800-300 500 and talk to a Holiday Adviser free of charge. Saga also offers a wide range of other holidays. For details see Section 13. *See also* details of Special Interest Holidays and Courses in Section 13.

Retirement courses

You may find that your local education authority arranges pre-retirement or post-retirement courses; it would be worth enquiring. We describe below the work of a college which specialises in retirement courses, but mostly not on a residential basis.

Retirement Education Centre
Bedford College of Higher Education, 6 Rothsay Gardens, Bedford MK40 3QB (Tel: 0234-360304).

The Centre offers a wide range of mostly non-residential 'Preparation for Retirement Courses' for men and women nearing retirement as well as over 40 study courses each week for those who have already retired. Courses range from practical subjects such as doll's house making and cookery to more academic subjects such as languages, literature, natural sciences, etc. Sporting activities are also arranged using the facilities of the town in off-peak periods. There is a full range of educational visits and excursions organised; these include residential visits both at home and abroad.

Preparation for retirement courses include: financial planning; taxation; state pension; benefits; concessions; budgeting; savings; investments; wills; health; diet; exercise; caring for others; leisure activities; home improvement; energy saving; to move or not; voluntary and/or paid work possibilities; personal relationships; case studies; videos; role play; coping with age and bereavement.

There are also study courses on a wide range of subjects including: Art; Italian; British Geology and Scenery; Bridge; Cookery; German; Environmental Studies; Lip Reading; Music and Movement; Gardening; International Politics; Yoga; Swimming; How We Lived Then; Batik; Small Scale Woodwork; Guitar; and Choir.

Fees: all courses comply with fees laid down by the Local Education Authority. Post-retirement students pay 30 per cent of the adult course – that is £16 for the year of 34 weeks. In addition, students are required to become subscribing members of the Centre for £10 a year.

Travelling Fellowships

The Winston Churchill Memorial Trust offers Churchill Travelling Fellowships for people to make studies overseas related to their trade, profession or interests, in order that they might bring back knowledge and experience for the benefit of the community. Each year applications are sought from UK citizens, with no age limits and no special qualifications required. Awards are offered in different categories each year. Those for a particular year are described in the annually updated leaflet. If awarded a Fellowship, you will receive a grant which will cover all your Fellowship expenses: return air fare, daily living, travel within the countries being visited, essential equipment and, in certain cases, home expenses. Grants usually cover a stay overseas of about eight weeks.

For further information apply to: The Winston Churchill Memorial Trust, 15 Queen's Gate Terrace, London SW7 5PR (Tel: 071-581 0410).

Helpful organisations

=▶ *Age Concern England*
Astral House, 1268 London Road, London SW16 4ER (Tel: 081-679 8000).

Age Concern England has a fact sheet, *Leisure Education*. It aims to supply basic and general information about all aspects of leisure education for older people. It covers national resources; the media and talking books; interest holidays; how and where to find out what's available locally; and suggestions for further reading. The fact sheet is available free from the Education and Leisure Officer on receipt of a large s.a.e. Locally, a number of local Age Concern groups have education programmes.

=▶ *Council for the Accreditation of Correspondence Colleges*
27 Marylebone Road, London NW1 5JS (Tel: 071-935 5391).

The Council is the only organisation in the United Kingdom officially recognised as responsible for the award of accreditation to correspondence colleges. Its principal objects are as follows:

(a) to promote education by setting standards for all aspects of tuition, education or training conducted wholly or in part by post, to investigate the manner in which such activities are carried out and to grant, where appropriate, the award of accreditation stating that the activities of the college conform to such standards; and
(b) to protect the educational interests and progress of students and to ensure that a satisfactory and responsible service is provided by accredited correspondence colleges.

An information leaflet listing accredited correspondence colleges and the courses offered is available free of charge from the Council's offices.

=▶ *National Adult School Organisation*
MASU Centre, Gaywood Croft, Cregoe Street, Birmingham B15 2ED
(Tel: 021-622 6400).

Adult schools are described as 'groups which seek to deepen understanding, and to enrich life, through friendship, study, social service and concern for religious and ethical values'. Groups meet in their own premises, halls or members' homes.

A Study Handbook containing 40 topics for discussion is produced each year and forms the basis for over 100 Adult School groups situated in various parts of the country. All are welcome to attend any of these groups which are informal, self-help, friendly discussion groups. The work of the groups is co-ordinated by the National Adult School organisation, through a number of County Unions. In addition to the Study Handbook,

NASO publishes a monthly magazine, *One and All*, and organises Summer Schools, lecture schools, international visits and other educational opportunities.

National Association of Women's Clubs
5 Vernon Rise, King's Cross Road, London WC1X 9EP (Tel: 071-837 1434).

A Women's Club is a non-political, non-sectarian group open to all women, whatever their age and interests. A wide range of activities caters for all tastes, but as NAWC is an educational charity, the emphasis is on self-development. Many activities are carried on within the clubs, from the practice of various crafts to taking part in choirs and in drama and keep fit groups, and listening to speakers on a wide range of subjects. Outings are also arranged to theatres, exhibitions and local industries. Members have the opportunity to attend Weekend Schools or One Day Workshops held in various parts of the country.

Skill: National Bureau for Students with Disabilities
336 Brixton Road, London SW9 7AA (Tel: 071-274 0565).

The Bureau is a national voluntary organisation developing opportunities in further, higher and adult education, training, and employment throughout the United Kingdom. It is concerned with the special educational needs of students of any age who have physical and sensory disabilities, learning disabilities or emotional problems.

A network of 14 regional groups support members in all areas of the United Kingdom through meetings, newsletters and other locally directed activities.

Membership to the Bureau is open to: local authorities; education and training bodies; student unions; professional and voluntary bodies; and individuals who have an interest in the work of the Bureau.

The Bureau publishes a journal, *Educare*, which aims to cover any subject which facilitates and enhances the teaching, learning and work experience of students with disabilities and learning difficulties.

Workers' Educational Association
17 Victoria Park Square, London E2 9PB (Tel: 081-983 1515).

The WEA is a voluntary movement operating throughout England, Scotland, Wales and Northern Ireland through 800 Branches in 19 Districts. WEA offers you the opportunity to continue learning throughout your life. You may wish to develop new skills or to extend what you learned earlier. Whatever your past educational experience the WEA has a course for you.

The WEA is a democratic organisation – members determine the choice, content and location of courses; they administer the WEA's classes; and they determine the level of fees that students should pay.

Courses may be as short as one day or may be a term or more of evening classes. They may be in the form of a conference, seminar, residential course or study tour. They are held in a variety of locations such as local schools, colleges and community centres.

Courses include: history and science, education for the unemployed, courses to help you improve your skills at work or return to education after a break, creative arts such as writing, video, and crafts, education for school governors, parents, and trade unionists, education for women, pre- and post-retirement education, health education. Costs: some courses are free; costs of other courses are kept to a minimum.

The WEA also publishes a range of resources for learners, tutors and policy-makers. For further information and details of your local WEA District, contact the national office as above.

Books and publications

▶ *Open Learning Map of Scotland.*

Produced by the Scottish Council for Educational Technology for the Training Agency, the Map shows the location of 65 centres providing open learning. The information for each centre includes the name of the person to contact for further details and details of the subjects offered. Many of the centres produce brochures on their open learning service and will supply copies on request.

Copies of the Map are available free of charge from: Information Resource Centre, Scottish Council for Educational Technology, Dowanhill, 74 Victoria Crescent Road, Glasgow G12 9JN (Tel: 041-334 9314).

▶ *Study Holidays*

A complete holiday guide to language courses in Europe. Actually staying in another country, learning formally and informally, can be an ideal way to become confident and fluent in another language. This guide provides detailed information on courses throughout Europe where you can receive expert tuition, put language skills into practice and enjoy a range of social, cultural or sporting activities. There is also practical information on travel and entry regulations, sources for bursaries, grants and scholarships, and useful publications.

Available from the Central Bureau for Educational Visits and Exchanges, Seymour Mews, London W1H 9PE (Tel: 071-486 5101). Price: £7.95 from good bookshops or £8.95 by post from the address above.

SECTION ELEVEN

Getting around and about

Most older people continue to remain mobile and active, even though it may sometimes be a struggle. This section looks at help that is available to make it easier to travel.

Travel concessions

Bus travel

Local authorities have powers to operate a concessionary fares scheme for travel on buses – free or at reduced rates for residents over pension age (60 for women, 65 for men). The nature and extent of such concessions vary from area to area depending on local authority policies. To find out about concessions and bus passes to which you may be entitled, ask at your town hall, local Age Concern group or Citizens Advice Bureau.

Coach travel

A number of coach travel firms offer concessions – sometimes as much as a third off standard fares. It would be worth enquiring what various companies are offering before booking your journey. You can either contact a coach firm directly, or alternatively your local travel agent would be able to give you details.

National Express, in particular, has a Discount Coach Card, costing £6 a year, which entitles anyone over the age of 60 to concessionary coach fares.

Rail travel

Senior Railcard

The Senior Railcard is available to anyone over 60 and offers a wide range of ticket discounts for a whole year. A Railcard can be bought from most British Rail stations or rail appointed travel agents for £16. To obtain your Senior Railcard you need to give proof of your age – your pension book, passport, NHS medical card or your birth certificate will suffice. Your Railcard gives you one-third off the following tickets:

- Saver Returns – Friday off-peak travel
- Cheap Day Returns – off-peak travel
- Standard Day Returns – travel any time (but see note below)
- Standard Singles – travel any time (but see note below)
- Standard Open Returns – travel any time
- Rail Rovers (except Network SouthEast Rail Rovers) – see special leaflet for more details
- First Class Singles and Returns – travel any time
- All-zone One-day Travelcards – travel on London Underground

There is no discount on many trains into London on peak morning services.

If you have particular queries about the Railcard you can contact your railway station or The Railcard Manager, Room 433, Euston House, 24 Eversholt Street, London NW1 1DZ (Tel: 071-928 5151, ext. 40157 or 24083).

Rail Europ Senior Card

Once you hold a Senior Railcard, for only £7.50 extra you can also buy a Rail Europ Senior card which will provide you with discounts on travel to Europe. You can make savings on travel to 19 countries, including many in Eastern Europe.

Shipping services discounts

Through rail/ship journeys on the Red Funnel Group Services to and from the Isle of Wight discounts are available to Senior Railcard holders. British Channel Island Ferries also offer reductions on their services to Guernsey and Jersey. From time to time other shipping companies offer reduced prices to Senior Railcard holders.

Disabled Person's Railcard

A leaflet describing the concessions available to disabled people is available from local rail stations or main post offices.

The Disabled Person's Railcard costs £14 a year and offers the following discounts:

- one-third off Savers and Supersavers
- one-third off Network AwayBreaks
- half-price Cheap Day Returns (one-third from 3 January 1993)
- one-third off Open Returns
- one-third off Standard Singles
- half-price First Class and Standard Day Returns (one-third from 3 January 1993)
- reduced rate London Underground tickets (until 2 January 1993)
- reduced price One Day Travel cards, subject to a minimum price
- reductions for cardholders and accompanying passengers on some MotorRail services

To qualify for a Disabled Person's Railcard you will need to be a person:
(a) in receipt of Attendance Allowance, Disability Living Allowance, Severe Disablement Allowance, or Industrial Disablement Benefit; or
(b) in the Motability scheme; or
(c) with at least 80 per cent disability and receiving War and Severe Disablement Pension; or
(d) with epilepsy with a continuing liability to seizures in spite of treatment by drugs.

Air travel

Several airlines offer concessionary fares to elderly people on domestic flights.

Assistance with travel

Travelling by rail

If you have a disability or have difficulty walking or managing on your own, then British Rail will help you if you give them notice of your journey in advance. They will provide help at your departure, interchange or arrival station. They can also help you plan your journey by advising you on the stations and trains best suited to your needs, and where stations are unstaffed or lightly staffed. British Rail prefer a couple of days' notice but will do their best to help even if you can give only a few hours. There is no charge for the service.

If you need assistance or special arrangements, contact your local Area Manager by letter or telephone giving the following details:
— date of travel and departure time of train;
— destination station and any intermediate stations where a change of train is necessary;
— the nature of your disability or difficulty;
— means of transport to and from stations (taxi, private car, etc.) and whether you are being met at your destination;
— whether you are travelling alone or with a companion;
— whether a wheelchair will be required at stations.

A useful leaflet sets out the arrangements. It is called *British Rail and Disabled Travellers* and is available from stations.

Carelink is a special bus service which provides a link between the main British Rail London terminal stations and the Airbus services to Heathrow from Victoria and Euston. Each bus has a lift and, like Airbus, can take people in wheelchairs. Buses run every hour, every day of the week, on a clockwise circular route: Euston, St Pancras, King's Cross, Liverpool Street, Waterloo, Victoria, Paddington, Euston. Further details, including fares and times, from LRT Unit for Disabled Passengers, 55 Broadway, London SW1H 0BD (Tel: 071-222 5600).

Travelling by air

Airlines are usually very helpful to travellers who have a disability or who cannot walk very far without help. If you are going to need assistance it is necessary to contact the airline well in advance of your journey. Depending on the severity of any disability, the airline may require a 'medical certificate of fitness for air travel' to be completed by the traveller's doctor. Not all airlines want this, and it is important to check at the time of booking.

It is worth noting that folding wheelchairs are carried on aeroplanes free of weight restrictions.

Helpful organisation

▶ *Tripscope*
63 Esmond Road, London W4 1JE (Tel: 081-994 9294).

Tripscope provides a free nationwide travel and transport information service for disabled and elderly people, 'WHEREVER you live, WHATEVER your journey'. It can offer help with information about any travel problem which a disabled or elderly person may have in getting from place to place. It can also point the way to assistance with all those other matters which may be a bother – from accessible loos to wheelchair hire. It should be noted, however, that Tripscope is neither a travel agency nor a booking agency.

Low speed scooters and buggies

A range of these vehicles is now available. They can be a great boon for those who lead active lives but who find walking any distance difficult. They are broadly divided into Class 2 vehicles, which are limited to a maximum speed of four miles per hour, and Class 3 vehicles, with a maximum speed of eight miles per hour. Among other legal requirements, Class 3 vehicles must be fitted with a speed indicator and a device which the user can operate to limit the speed to four miles per hour. Such vehicles, when driven by a person with a physical disability, are not treated as motor vehicles for the purposes of the Road Traffic Acts and can be driven on pavements at speeds of up to four miles per hour. A driving licence is not required, nor need you pay vehicle excise duty or take a test, although training is strongly recommended.

A considerable number of different models are available, all of which are stylishly designed. Most are battery-powered and some, where space permits, can be used indoors as well as outdoors. Most of the buggies have optional hoods. Accessories include walking stick clips, shopping baskets, waterproof capes, leg aprons, lights, and mirrors. Most can be modified to suit a user's special needs and some can be dismantled for storage or to go in a car boot.

It is important, when choosing your vehicle from the glossy brochures, to ensure it suits your needs and is precisely what you want, and that you have compared it with other makes and with other models. You need to know, in particular, the range of the battery if the vehicle is driven by a person of your weight and in your own locality (which may be hilly!). It is wise to insist on a demonstration, and this should always be carried out in your home area, where you are going to drive. It is also important to bear in mind that maintenance costs may be substantial – replacement tyres, batteries, other parts, and labour charges. Some firms make a high charge just for a call-out.

Before buying your scooter or buggy it would be a good idea to contact one of the Disabled Living Centres (for details see Section 4), who would be glad to advise you on the types most suitable for your needs. More detailed information is given in our guide, *Motoring and Mobility for Disabled People*, 1991, price £4.50 plus postage and packing, available from RADAR, 25 Mortimer Street, London W1N 8AB (Tel: 071-637 5400).

Driving

Being able to continue to drive a car is obviously a great advantage in getting out and about. Except in special circumstances (i.e. in the case of certain prescribed disabilities), driving licences are valid until we reach the age of 70, and even then they can be renewed (see below). Older people, on the whole, have a good reputation on the road. They tend to have a better understanding of their own limitations and are generally prepared to take more care and to drive within their limitations. A few insurance companies have recognised this and offer concessions to retired drivers.

You need to make certain that your sight is up to standard by wearing glasses, if necessary, and making sure that they have been prescribed recently enough to have accommodated any deterioration in your vision. The legal requirement is that you should be able to read in good daylight (with the aid of glasses if worn) a registration mark fixed to a motor vehicle at a distance of 20.5 metres where the letters and figures are 79.4 mm high.

Anyone who uses a hearing aid should ensure that it is regularly tested and that the batteries are kept up to standard.

Always make sure that, if you are taking medicines or tablets, it is safe to drive – your doctor will advise you.

It is wise to give yourself plenty of time for your journey and to take regular breaks during the journey so that you are not driving when you are tired.

Motor insurance

It is always wise to shop around for insurance. If you use a broker, she or he should be serving your best interests by looking around for the company best able to suit your requirements. We mention below some companies that provide policies targeted towards older people, but it is always desirable to look at various options and not to settle on a company until you have compared benefits and costs.

▶ *Age Concern Insurance Services*
Garrod House, Chaldon Road, Caterham, Surrey CR3 5YZ (Tel: 0883-346964).

ACIS offers a motor insurance policy said to have been specially designed to provide motorists aged 60 and over with wide-ranging cover at extremely competitive premiums.

▶ *Norwich Union Fire Insurance Society Limited*
PO Box No. 6, Surrey Street, Norwich NR1 3NS (Tel: 0603-622200), or contact your local insurance adviser.

Norwich Union's Motoring Gold insurance is said to be competitively priced and to provide valuable additional benefits for motorists aged 55-75 who are fully retired and in good health, and have at least four years no-claim discount and no serious motoring offences.

▶ *Saga Services Ltd*
Freepost, PO Box 131, Folkestone, Kent CT20 1BR.

Saga says that it specialises in arranging car insurance with low premiums for more mature and experienced drivers, and that in many cases the costs will be found to be lower than other reputable insurers in the United Kingdom.

Driving licences

Driving licences are administered and issued by the Driver and Vehicle Licensing Agency (DVLA), Swansea SA6 7JL.

Term of licence

Licences are normally issued until the age of 70. They may then be renewed, but will run for only three years or less, depending on the circumstances, with the possibility of further renewals. A fee of £6 is payable for such renewals. In the event of a licence being refused or revoked, the applicant/licence holder has a right of appeal to a Magistrates' Court (or Sheriff's Court in Scotland) against the decision and the Licensing Centre will notify the individual of this right where appropriate.

Fitness to drive

The question of fitness to drive is an all-important one for older people. Your licence may be revoked if you have one of a number of prescribed disabilities (*see* our guide, *Motoring and Mobility for Disabled People*, described on page 256, for details).

Essentially, you should mention any disability likely to cause the driving of a vehicle to be a source of danger to the public or one which may in time become such a danger. Applicants for licences are under a legal obligation to declare any such disability, while licence holders are similarly required to inform the DVLA 'forthwith' if during the currency of a licence they become aware that they are suffering from a prescribed disability not previously disclosed, or if a previously notified disability has become worse. (Temporary disabilities – those reasonably expected to last less than three months – which the licence holder has not previously suffered are outside this obligation.) If you need to declare a disability which may affect your driving, write to: Drivers Medical Branch, DVLA, Swansea SA1 1TU.

When such facts are disclosed, a medical-in-confidence form will normally be issued. This asks the person concerned to describe his or her medical condition in greater detail and give permission for all his or her doctors and specialists to make reports to the Medical Adviser at the DVLA. Medical reports are made on a doctor-to-doctor basis from the applicant's GP and, if appropriate, consultant. If consent is withheld, the law provides for the revocation or refusal of a driving licence if the licensing authority has reasonable grounds for thinking that a person may have a disability.

In the ordinary way, the medical reports are considered by the Medical Adviser who will then normally make a recommendation about the issue of a licence. If, however, there is still some doubt about the effect that an applicant's or licensee's condition might have on his or her ability to drive safely, she or he may be asked to attend an examination by an independent doctor in the local area.

Restricted licences

The fact that a driver is disabled does not necessarily mean that his or her licence will be restricted in any way. We have been assured by the Department of Transport that where a licence can be granted or continued, the aim of the DVLA is to give the maximum entitlement possible, bearing in mind the safety of the driver and others. If, as a result of medical enquiries or following a driving test, the Medical Adviser at the DVLA considers that a disabled driver might need to have any or all vehicles which he or she is entitled to drive suitably adapted, the licence will be restricted. Such restrictions are typically worded: 'Entitled to drive ... with controls adapted to suit disability'.

Further information

Motoring and Mobility for Disabled People (*see* page 256).

The Orange Badge scheme

This scheme of parking concessions for disabled people operates under Regulations made in accordance with the Chronically Sick and Disabled Persons Act 1970. The issue of badges is controlled by local authorities who must be satisfied that strict eligibility rules are met. They have power to refuse renewal or require the return of badges if they are persistently misused. Able-bodied people not entitled to the concessions who misuse the Orange Badge to park where they would otherwise not be permitted to do so commit an offence under section 117 of the Road Traffic Regulation Act 1984, punishable by a fine on top of that which may be imposed for any ordinary traffic offence involved.

Eligibility

The badge, which may be used on any motor vehicle (including a taxi or hired car), or a Class 3 'invalid carriage' driven by or carrying a badgeholder, is available if:

(a) you receive Mobility Allowance, War Pensioners' Mobility Supplement, or the higher rate of the mobility component of the Disability Living Allowance (DLA); or
(b) you are registered blind; or
(c) you use a vehicle supplied by a government department, or receive a grant towards your own vehicle; or
(d) you have a permanent and substantial disability which means you are unable to walk or have very considerable difficulty in walking. (Your doctor may be asked a series of questions to help the local authority to determine whether you are eligible for a badge. People with a psychological disorder will not normally qualify unless their handicap causes very considerable difficulty in walking.)
(e) you have a severe disability in both upper limbs, regularly drive a motor vehicle, but cannot turn the steering wheel by hand even if the wheel is fitted with a turning knob.

Category (d) is open to interpretation. Our understanding is that, in order to qualify, the applicant's degree of impairment must either be of the standard required for the higher rate of the mobility component of the DLA (*see* page 5) or almost of that standard, so that he or she would be physically incapable of visiting shops, public buildings and other places unless allowed to park close by. In all cases, entitlement depends on ability to walk, and considerations such as difficulty in carrying parcels are not taken into account. The applicant's inability to walk or very considerable difficulty in walking must be permanent and not just spasmodic.

However, whereas the mobility component of DLA is not normally available to applicants over 65, there is no upper age restriction in the Orange Badge Scheme.

Issue

Badges are issued by local authorities (normally the Social Services Department) for a period of three years from the date of issue. They remain the property of the authority.

The badge

To limit misuse, the Orange Badge has been redesigned in the form of a personal passport-type document with a space for a photograph of the holder to be displayed. Two passport-size photographs should accompany your application. The badge should be displayed only when you are using the parking concessions, when it must be displayed on the dashboard or facia panel of the vehicle with the front facing forward so that the relevant details can be seen from outside the vehicle.

In England and Wales you also need a special parking disc which can be used to show your time of arrival. This is for use in places where parking is subject to a time limit.

Parking concessions

If and when you are issued with an Orange Badge, you will be provided with guidance on the scope of the concessions and the places (e.g. parts of central London) where the scheme does not apply. It is important to appreciate that the Orange Badge is not a licence to park anywhere.

Exemption of Orange Badge holders from wheelclamping

Section 105 of the Road Traffic Regulation Act 1984 exempts the cars of Orange Badge holders from wheelclamping, but police can remove a car if it is parked dangerously or is causing an obstruction.

Further information

Department of Transport leaflet, *The Orange Badge Scheme*. (Be sure to get the version with a blue flash 'EFFECTIVE FROM MARCH 1992' – at that time significant changes were made in the scheme.)

Community transport schemes

Dial-a-Ride schemes

Dial-a-Ride services are by now a familiar part of transport services in many parts of Great Britain. They are usually run by voluntary organisations, but with funding from transport authorities or some other public source. Their great merits are that they provide transport which is accessible to people with physical disabilities on a door-to-door basis at low cost. The snags are that the services are invariably limited (there may be waiting lists before you can even be considered as a user), notice usually has to be given and and there are normally restrictions on the number and length of journeys you can make. The concept is imaginative, appropriate and needed, and deserves to be funded more generously and more systematically so that such services can be integrated into public transport provision throughout the country on a scale which realistically meets demand. (We would stress, however, that improvement of Dial-a-Ride services should not be seen as a substitute for making conventional public transport services accessible to all passengers.)

Because the services are locally based, and have emerged as the result of local initiative, the scope and type of services and indeed the vehicles used vary from place to place. Some schemes take only wheelchair users, while others accommodate other mobility impaired people. Some schemes operate very narrowly within their own districts, while others will travel further afield. Sadly, funders may impose restrictions on how the services are operated, so that parsimonious grants can be spread as widely (and thinly) as possible. Typically, difficulties are experienced in having to book a long time in advance, and even then finding that the trip you want cannot be arranged at the time you want it, and in not being able to get to where you want to go if it lies outside the boundaries of the scheme.

Clients are usually asked to make a contribution to costs, but this will not normally exceed that charged on ordinary public transport over a comparable distance.

One thing Dial-a-Rides all have in common is the belief that citizens with disabilities have a right to transport services appropriate to their needs in common with the whole population. They have a right to travel for business or pleasure, at no greater expense than their fellow citizens, at times when they choose.

Other community transport

As well as local Dial-a-Rides, there are various local, non-commercial community transport services designed to meet the needs of people who are without private transport and who cannot use, or who feel uneasy about using, public transport. Such projects aim to provide affordable, accessible vehicles, available to anyone who wants to use them.

Some community transport projects use donated vehicles and/or raise funds to buy or lease vehicles to build up a fleet. Other projects focus on vehicle pooling, which is a system of organised vehicle sharing, managed and co-ordinated by the project team, which is responsible for maintaining and administering the vehicle. This is an extremely cost-effective concept for vehicles which would otherwise be underused. It allows a cheaper, more efficient and reliable service for groups who use their vehicles only occasionally. Community transport projects attempt to maximise the use of such vehicles (thereby reducing their operating costs) while ensuring that the owners can use them whenever they need to. Such schemes usually operate on a self-drive basis, much like a commercial company but a great deal cheaper.

Some schemes are based on volunteer drivers using their own cars, and a number of organisations specifically provide escorted transport services. We know of the following, operating on a national basis:

British Red Cross Society
9 Grosvenor Crescent, London SW1X 7EJ (Tel: 071-235 5454).

Red Cross Transport and Escort Service provides volunteers to drive cars and ambulances, and, if needed, qualified escorts, to enable housebound and other handicapped people to make journeys that would otherwise be impossible for them. Red Cross drivers and/or escorts will undertake long or short journeys to assist people with hospital appointments, family visits, and difficulties with a route or with luggage, or just to give support.

Charges for this service, which cover the expenses of the volunteers, are kept as low as possible.

Enquiries about this service, or any of the other wide range of services offered by the British Red Cross, should be made to your local Branch, whose address and telephone number will be listed in the telephone directory under 'B' or 'R'.

St John Ambulance
1 Grosvenor Crescent, London SW1X 7EF (Tel: 071-235 5231).

Many divisions run road ambulances, using volunteer drivers and nurses and charging only mileage costs and expenses. Contact your local division for help (address in local telephone directory). Nursing facilities and loans of equipment are often possible.

Women's Royal Voluntary Service
234–44 Stockwell Road, London SW9 9SP (Tel: 071-416 0146).

Some local branches of the WRVS will arrange, on an occasional basis and with reasonable advance notice, to meet disabled people at interchange stations and escort them to their connecting coach or train, usually by public transport or taxi. Escorts will assist generally but cannot offer nursing or medical care.

Information about commercial ambulance services can be obtained from the Disabled Living Foundation, 380–4 Harrow Road, London W9 2HU (Tel: 071-289 6111).

Further information

Voluntary and Community Transport Schemes Directory

The Department of Transport has produced a directory giving details of over 700 voluntary and community transport schemes throughout the country. The information is held on a computerised database, broken down into sections such as county, type of service and facilities offered. The data will be kept up to date, and print-outs as required can be obtained free of charge from: The Disability Unit, Room S10/21, Department of Transport, 2 Marsham Street, London SW1P 3EB (Tel: 071-275 5257).

Care with a chair

In shops, banks and post offices there are now far fewer seats than there used to be. This makes for considerable problems for those of us who can manage reasonably well provided we can sit down occasionally. Some shops have been willing to put chairs out if they have the problem pointed out to them. To help this process along, Margot Knowles, who had to give up work early because of back problems, began the We Care with a Chair campaign to persuade shopkeepers and others to have chairs ready for people who need them and to put a sticker up to say so. Margot told them that knowing that a chair is available on their premises would make all the difference to people who would otherwise give up – or never set out.

Age Concern groups in Scotland, Wales, Northern Ireland and England are helping to spread the idea throughout the United Kingdom and many other organisations have helped to promote the idea.

As well as welcoming the scheme yourself you might feel you could help to spread this useful and simple idea. Age Concern England would be glad to send you, free of charge, some stickers and leaflets to give to shopkeepers, banks, post offices, etc. Please send a large s.a.e. to Age Concern England, Astral House, 1268 London Road, London SW16 4ER.

Books and publications

▶ *Getting About Safely*
(Broadcasting Support Services, PO Box 7, London W3 6XJ), price £1.75.
Also available on audio cassette from RNIB (PO Box 173, Peterborough PE2 0WS).

A survey by RNIB in 1991 showed that only about five per cent of Britain's estimated one million blind people have received any mobility training. Elderly blind people are even less likely than people of working age to have had such training. This booklet in the series of In Touch Care Guides explains how people who are visually handicapped can learn to move safely indoors and outdoors. It describes the types of mobility training that are now available and some of the initiatives that are now being undertaken to make the outdoor environment safer for people with very poor sight.

▶ *Motoring and Mobility for Disabled People*
By Ann Darnbrough and Derek Kinrade (RADAR, 25 Mortimer Street, London W1N 8AB (Tel: 071-637 5400), 1991), price £4.50 plus postage and packing.

This book covers every aspect of motoring for drivers and passengers with a disability. This fifth edition has a new chapter on facilities for getting about without a car. It is particularly helpful in clarifying the factors to consider in buying a car or low speed vehicle.

=▶ *Mobility*
(Help the Aged, St James's Walk, London EC1R 0BE (Tel: 071-253 0253)), free in response to a 6" × 9" s.a.e.

This advice booklet discusses fitness, health and exercise, as well as briefly describing walking aids, wheelchairs, stairlifts, personal vehicles and community transport schemes, with guidance as to their availability and sources of further information.

SECTION TWELVE

Arts, Sport and Leisure

In this section of the Directory we give just a taste of the many activities open to people of all ages, but with an emphasis on those with some facilities or consideration for older people. Some of us will have had a range of interests all our lives, and retirement gives us the opportunity to develop these and to enjoy them to a greater extent than was previously possible. Others of us will not have had much opportunity to take up hobbies or arts or sports activities and now there is a chance to develop ideas we may have had at the back of our minds for years. The Dark Horse Venture, an exciting initiative, has been set up to encourage older people discover their hidden abilities and talents – for details *see* page 297.

You may have always enjoyed sports, either taking part or as a spectator. If you still want to be involved in sport, we are assured there are many local sports clubs who would warmly welcome help with administration, coaching, serving on committees, helping with events and activities and just generally being encouraging.

Most retired people have to manage on a limited income and often this does not allow much extra cash to follow new interests. However, we have tried to cover both those activities which cost very little – rambling, scrabble playing – and those which can be expensive – collecting antiques and visiting the theatre. Because some older people have disabilities, we have also given some information on special facilities available. Further information can be given by the Disabled Living Foundation and other Disabled Living Centres on special aids and on equipment which is available to help you follow your particular interest. They will also give you details of special organisations who will be glad to help.

Keeping fit

There is a great emphasis on keeping fit nowadays. This involves taking as much exercise as you can. Many sports activities, even those undertaken very gently, provide just the right exercise we need. A very useful little booklet, *Exercise. Why Bother?*, is a simple guide to getting fitter for adults of all ages. As well as giving advice on strength and stamina it describes sensible precautions you should take before you start taking exercise. In addition, it lists a range of activities from jogging and running to bowling and weight training. Each activity is assessed for its exercise value and practical points are made. The booklet is available free from the Health Education Authority, Hamilton House, Mabledon Place, London WC1H 9TX.

Activity holidays

Whether it is learning a new sport or leisure interest or carrying on with a long enjoyed interest, it can be great fun to take part in an activity holiday. For details of these *see* Section 13. In particular, *see* details of the *RAC Activity Holiday Guide Great Britain and Ireland*. Saga, the specialist holiday organisation for older people, arranges a wide choice of activity holidays.

Local authority services

Local authorities throughout the United Kingdom arrange leisure and sporting activities for local people of all ages. It would be worth enquiring to find out if there is a local Leisure Centre or its equivalent and what facilities there are for older people in the area. They may be able to assist you by making facilities, equipment or finance available. They will also have contact with local sports clubs, coaches, instructors, etc.

Your local library provides, as well as books, periodicals, tapes, records and local history material, information about what is available and happening in your area – whether it is provided by the local authority or a local interest group.

Antiques

Saga arranges 'Antique Appreciation' holidays. For details of Saga holidays *see* Section 13.

▶ *The British Antique Dealers' Association*
20 Rutland Gate, London SW7 1BD (Tel: 071-589 4128).

The BADA is the trade association for approximately 400 leading antique dealers in Britain. BADA will supply anybody who requires it with a free list of its members. The Association says: 'The antiques buying or selling public is assured of a highly professional service wherever the BADA logo is displayed.' BADA has its own code of practice whereby the authenticity of all items sold by a BADA member is guaranteed. BADA is obliged to make a full refund of the purchase price, at any time after the sale, in the event that there has been a mistake in the description of an item.

BADA also has an Antiques Consumer Information Service providing guidelines on buying and selling; a Guarantee and Arbitration Service; advice on experts; lists of antiques fairs; information on restorers; Antique Societies to join; information on looking after antiques.

Archaeology

▶ *The Council for British Archaeology*
112 Kennington Road, London SE11 6RE (Tel: 071-582 0494).

The Council says 'Many elderly people enjoy working on excavations. It seems to be a hobby that has lain dormant for many years, and retirement offers the perfect opportunity to get involved. Many amateur archaeologists are retired, and do a great deal of work on the conservation/cataloguing side. The only problem seems to be our backs which can object to too much bending especially if one wants to trowel!'

Other aspects of archaeology may be better suited to older enthusiasts: field walking, landscape studies, and the investigation of buildings are particularly rewarding.

Subscription is £10.50 (1992) and includes receipt of *British Archaeological News*, which gives details of digs.

Archery

▶ *The Grand National Archery Society*
7th Street, National Agricultural Society, Stoneleigh, Kenilworth, Warwickshire CV8 2LG (Tel: 0203-696631).
Liaison Officer for Disabled People: Mrs N. Douglas, c/o Webb, Bush Farm, Clunton, Craven Arms, Shropshire SY7 OHU (Tel: 0588-7330).

Quite a lot of elderly archers can carry on, as it is a sport that can be enjoyed at one's own pace and does not entail dashing about. There are about 1,200 clubs stretching from the Shetlands to Cornwall, and the Society will be glad to put you in touch with the nearest one. There is a coaching scheme for all levels: Club, County, Region, National, and International. Beginners are advised not to buy equipment before having a practice session at a club where they will be given advice on the suitability of equipment. It is possible to adapt equipment to overcome any particular disability or weakness. Most clubs will normally give six lessons for a small fee before the beginner has to join (or leave).

Arts

Saga organises painting holidays. For details of Saga holidays *see* Section 13. *See also* Music, page 281.

Many arts activities are carried on throughout the country and, often, there is far more taking place locally than many of us are aware of. Retirement could provide just the opportunity to take part in a range of arts activities and to pursue an interest for which there has never been time before.

Arts Councils – national

The national Arts Councils aim to foster the arts and to fund arts activities within their own countries. They will be glad to send you a report of their activities, and a publications list.

- *Arts Council (England)*
  14 Great Peter Street, London SW1P 3NQ (Tel: 071-333 0100).

- *Arts Council of Northern Ireland*
  181a Stranmillis Road, Belfast BT9 5DU (Tel: 0232-381591).

- *Scottish Arts Council*
  19 Charlotte Square, Edinburgh EH2 4DF (Tel: 031-226 6051).

- *Welsh Arts Council – Cyngor y Celfyddydau*
  9 Museum Place, Cardiff CF1 3NX (Tel: 0222-394711).

Regional Arts Boards

Regional Arts Boards in England have specific responsibility for funding and promoting the arts in their regions. They will also have names and addresses of local arts activities. They can be contacted as follows:

- *Eastern Arts Board*
  Cherry Hinton Hall, Cherry Hinton Road, Cambridge CB1 4DW
  (Tel: 0223-215355).

  Area covered: Bedfordshire, Cambridgeshire, Essex, Hertfordshire, Lincolnshire, Norfolk and Suffolk.

  See also Artlink East listed in the Shape Network on page 264.

- *East Midlands Arts Board*
  Mountfields House, Forest Road, Loughborough, Leicestershire LE11 3HU
  (Tel: 0509-218292).

  Area covered: Derbyshire (excluding High Peak District), Leicestershire, Northamptonshire, Nottinghamshire.

- *London Arts Board*
  20 Gainsford Street, Butlers Wharf, London SE1 2NE (Tel: 071-403 9072).

  Area covered: the area of the 32 London Boroughs and the City of London.

- *Northern Arts Board*
  9–10 Osborne Terrace, Jesmond, Newcastle upon Tyne NE2 1NZ
  (Tel: 091-281 6334).

  Area covered: Cleveland, Cumbria, Durham, Northumberland, Metropolitan Districts of Newcastle, Gateshead, North Tyneside, Sunderland and South Tyneside.

- *North West Arts Board*
  12 Harter Street, Manchester M1 6HY (Tel: 061-228 3062).

  Area covered: Lancashire, Cheshire, Merseyside, Greater Manchester and High Peak District of Derbyshire.

- *Southern Arts Board*
  13 St Clement Street, Winchester SO23 9DQ (Tel: 0962-855099).

  Area covered: Berkshire, Buckinghamshire, Hampshire, Isle of Wight, Oxfordshire, Wiltshire and East Dorset.

- *South East Arts Board*
  10 Mount Ephraim, Tunbridge Wells, Kent TN4 8AS (Tel: 0892-515210).

  Area covered: Kent, Surrey, East Sussex, West Sussex.

- *South West Arts Board*
  Bradninch Place, Gandy Street, Exeter EX4 3LS (Tel: 0392-218188).

  Area covered: Avon, Cornwall, Devon, Dorset (except districts of Bournemouth, Christchurch and Poole), Gloucestershire and Somerset.

- *West Midlands Arts Board*
  82 Granville Street, Birmingham B1 2LH (Tel: 021-631 3121).

  Area covered: County of Hereford and Worcester, Shropshire, Staffordshire, Warwickshire, Metropolitan Districts of Birmingham, Coventry, Dudley, Sandwell, Solihull, Walsall and Wolverhampton.

- *Yorkshire and Humberside Arts Board*
  21 Bond Street, Dewsbury, West Yorkshire WF13 1AX (Tel: 0924-455555).

  Area covered: Metropolitan Districts of Barnsley, Bradford, Calderdale, Doncaster, Kirklees, Leeds, Rotherham, Sheffield, Wakefield; Counties of Humberside, North Yorkshire.

The National Association of Decorative and Fine Arts Societies (NADFAS)
8A Lower Grosvenor Place, London SW1W OEN (Tel: 071-233 5433).

NADFAS consists of member societies throughout the United Kingdom, mainland Europe, Australia and South Africa. Each autonomous society organises a programme of illustrated monthly lectures, study days and visits to art galleries, museums, cathedrals, and country houses which are related to the decorative and fine arts. NADFAS also assembles small groups of volunteers country-wide who have become involved in a wide variety of projects, such as book refurbishing, cataloguing and archival listing, textile preservation, making furniture case covers, costume covers and replica costumes, cleaning of armour, ceramics, metals and statuary, house and garden guiding and stewarding.

NADFAS also arranges tours for its members in the United Kingdom and abroad. All tours have a high artistic, cultural or educational ingredient. They are led by an organiser and accompanied by a lecturer. A colour brochure is produced every year and is available to each member.

NADFAS News is published by the Association twice a year and distributed to all members. National events, tours, study courses and information for volunteer groups are featured, together with notice of exhibitions and articles relating to the decorative and fine arts. Membership is through local societies – details from the office above.

National Art Collections Fund
20 John Islip Street, London SW1P 4JX (Tel: 071-821 0404).

The Fund helps museums and galleries across the country to buy works of art to enrich their collections. There are over 33,000 members. Membership costs £15 per year, and members receive free entry into all art museums and galleries in Britain, as well as the magazine *The Art Quarterly* four times a year, the well illustrated *Review*, and lectures, concerts and private views all over the country.

The Shape Network

The Shape Network is a federation of some eighteen independently-constituted local services. The services vary in size and style of approach, but all broadly work to improve and increase access and involvement of disabled, elderly and other underrepresented groups in all aspects of the arts.

For further information about the Network, contact your nearest Shape service, or write to the Chair, Shape Network, c/o East Midlands Shape, 27a Belvoir Street, Leicester LE1 6FL. The following list gives the main contact addresses only. Many services have district offices – contact the nearest service to you for details:

Shape London
1 Thorpe Close, London W10 5XL (Tel: 081-960 9245 voice; 081-960 9248 minicom).

Shape London is an organisation which develops the arts with, by and for people with physical, mental or sensory disabilities, elderly people and people recovering from mental illness, through participation in arts activities and events. Shape organises workshops in varied locations such as day centres, hospitals, hostels and community centres. Shape also organises training courses for artists and staff, and tours performances and exhibitions. In addition, it provides information and advice to a wide range of individuals and organisations, and liaises with other arts and disability bodies to establish joint projects and initiatives.

- *Artlink East*
  c/o Eastern Arts, Cherry Hinton Hall, Cherry Hinton Road, Cambridge CB1 4DW (Tel: 0223-215355).

- *Artability South East*
  St James Centre, Quarry Road, Tunbridge Wells, Kent TN1 2EY (Tel: 0892-515478).

- *East Midlands Shape*
  27a Belvoir Street, Leicester LE1 6FL (Tel: 0533-552933).

- *Artlink Lincolnshire and Humberside*
  Central Library, Albion Street, Hull HU1 3TF (Tel: 0482-224040).

- *Shape Bucks*
  Room H, Old Child Assessment Unit, Royal Bucks Hospital, Aylesbury, Buckinghamshire HP19 3AB (Tel: 0296-395035).

- *Southern Artlink*
  St John Fisher School, Sandy Lane West, Oxford OX4 5LD (Tel: 0865-714652).

- *Artlink West Midlands*
  Garage Arts and Media Centre, 1 Hatherton Street, Walsall WS1 1YB (Tel: 0922-616566).

- *Artshare South West*
  Bradninch Place, Gandy Street, Exeter EX4 3LS (Tel: 0392-218923).

- *Artshare Avon*
  6-8 Sommerville Road, St Andrews, Bristol BS7 9AA (Tel: 0272-420721).

- *Artshare in Gloucs.*
  Guildhall Arts Centre, 23 Eastgate Street, Gloucester GL1 1NS (Tel: 0452-307684).

=▶ *Equal Arts*
Whinney House, Durham Road, Low Fell, Gateshead, Tyne and Wear NE9 5AR (Tel: 091-487 8892).

=▶ *North West Shape*
Back of Shawgrove School, Cavendish Road, West Didsbury, Manchester M20 8JR (Tel: 061-434 8666).

=▶ *Shape Up North*
191 Bellevue Road, Leeds LS3 1HG (Tel: 0532-431005).

Affiliated to the network:

=▶ *Artlink Edinburgh and Lothians*
4 Forth Street, Edinburgh EH1 3LD (Tel: 031-556 6350).

=▶ *ProjectAbility*
18 Albion Street, Glasgow G1 1LH (Tel: 041-552 2822).

=▶ *Disability Scotland*
5 Shandwick Place, Edinburgh EH2 4RG (Tel: 031-229 8632).

=▶ *Arts for Disabled People in Wales*
Channel View Centre, Jim Driscoll Way, The Marl, Grangetown, Cardiff CF1 7NF (Tel: 0222-377885).

=▶ *Merseyside Disability Arts Forum*
Crawford Arts Centre, Mill Lane, Liverpool L15 8LY (Tel: 051-722 0805).

Basket-making

=▶ *The Basket-makers' Association*
Secretary: Vivienne Jones, The Vineyard, Bury Green, Little Hadham, Ware, Hertfordshire SG11 2ES (Tel: 0279-651525).

The aims of the Association are to promote better standards of design and technique in the practice and teaching of basket-making, chair seating, and allied crafts, and to ensure the continuity of these skills by encouraging the production of tools and materials.

The Association arranges day schools, residential courses and demonstrations. In addition, an up-to-date index of experienced and expert craftspeople is maintained for commercial and conservation purposes. Members, who pay a subscription of £10 p.a., receive a quarterly newsletter.

Birdwatching

See the Royal Society for the Protection of Birds, and the National Extension College on 'Birds and Birdwatching' under the heading 'Environment' later in this section.

Bowls

Saga provides holidays for bowls enthusiasts. For details *see* Section 13.

Most areas have facilities for bowling, and your local leisure centre or the leisure department of your local authority will be glad to give you information. Locally there may be facilities for both indoor and outdoor bowling. Outdoor there may be Crown Green bowling or Flat Green bowling. Indoor bowling may include Short Mat (6' x 40') bowls. The different types require separate skills.

▸ *English Bowling Association*
Lyndhurst Road, Worthing, West Sussex BN11 2AZ (Tel: 0903-820222).

The members of the EBA include: International Bowling Board, British Isles Bowling Council, English Bowls Council, English Women's Bowling Association, English Indoor Bowling Federation, British Crown Green Bowling Association. For further information on any of these organisations contact EBA. The Official Year Book contains details of local clubs, and of the various matches and championships. The EBA also has a list of events.

Brass rubbing

▸ *Monumental Brass Society*
c/o Society of Antiquaries of London, Burlington House, Piccadilly, London W1V 0HS.

A member, paying a subscription of £12, will receive invitations to three General Meetings with lectures, discussions and an opportunity to meet other members as well as an invitation to apply for the annual excursion to churches of special interest. There is also an opportunity to attend an annual conference during a weekend in September. Members receive, each year, a copy of the illustrated Transactions containing original articles on brasses and incised slabs; and, three times a year, a Bulletin containing information about current activities, exhibitions and new literature.

Chess

▸ *British Chess Federation*
9a Grand Parade, St Leonards-on-Sea, East Sussex TN38 0DD (Tel: 0424-442500).

The British Chess Federation is an 'umbrella' organisation to which are affiliated a multitude of local chess clubs and specialist societies. The Federation carries information on correspondence chess. It will be glad to send you information about local chess clubs and tournaments, and a publications list.

▶ *British Postal Chess Federation*
Secretary: Malcolm Peltz, 14 Linden End, Aylesbury, Buckinghamshire HP21 7NA.

Membership of the British Postal Chess Federation is open to British groups which organise correspondence chess and to individuals as Vice-Presidents. Associations, clubs, etc. pay an annual fee based on their active correspondence chess playing membership. The official journal of the Federation, *Information Circular*, is sent to all members. This publication contains details of all games played by British players in the CC Olympiads, European CC Team Championship, North Atlantic Team Tournament and international friendly matches as well as many of the games played in the British championships.

The annual subscription for a BPCF Vice-President is £6. This includes the *BPCF Information Circular*. This is also available to non-members at £4 for a year's subscription of four issues. Sample copies are available on request.

A booklet, *Correspondence Chess*, is available describing the Federation's activities.

▶ *British Correspondence Chess Society*
David Wilkinson, 17 Speedwell Road, Birmingham B5 7PS (Tel: 021-440 3072).

The Society, affiliated to the British Postal Chess Federation, organises tournaments, matches and competitions for players of all strengths including beginners. A continuous tournament runs non-stop with as many free entries as wanted, whenever wanted. The BCCS provides entry to national and international correspondence chess events. Membership includes the free bi-monthly magazine *Chess Post*, which includes articles and news and has information on games and results. Annual subscription £9.

▶ *British Correspondence Chess Association*
86 Mortimer Road, London N1 4LH (Tel: 071-254 7912).

Postal chess, played against as many or as few opponents as you choose and with a move every two days, enables you to analyse every position as it arises and so improve your knowledge of the game. The BCCA Championship starts in the autumn and offers five opponents and a total of ten games. The Association has a quarterly magazine, *Correspondence Chess*, containing many interesting (annotated) games, chess news, and articles, plus a regular Results Bulletin and an annual Grading List.

Country dancing

▶ *The Royal Scottish Country Dance Society*
12 Coates Cresent, Edinburgh EH3 7AF (Tel: 031-225 3854).

The Society encourages older people to keep on dancing and to keep fit. It says it need not be over-energetic, and it can be very enjoyable. There are groups throughout the United Kingdom and the world involving over 27,000 members. The *Bulletin* gives details of groups and lots of information about all the activities. A Summer School is run each year, roughly from mid-July to mid-August, and courses of one week or two weeks are available.

Croquet

▶ *The Croquet Association*
Hurlingham Club, Ranelagh Gardens, London SW6 3PR (Tel: 071-736 3148).

Croquet is gaining in popularity and new clubs are regularly formed. It requires delicate skill rather than strength and tactical ability rather than quick reflexes.

You can join the Association for £13 as a Subscriber (i.e. non-Tournament) Member and for this you receive six issues of the *Croquet* magazine, with a lot of information about local clubs' activities, tournaments, equipment and coaching. As a member you will also have the opportunity to purchase mallets at reduced prices, to improve your own play by attending Croquet Association coaching courses, or to qualify to become a referee, handicapper or tournament manager. In addition, members can attend the two major tournaments, 'Open Championship' and 'President's Cup', free of charge. These are held at Hurlingham in July and September.

Embroidery

▶ *Embroiderers' Guild*
Apartment 41, Hampton Court Palace, East Molesey, Surrey KT8 9AU
(Tel: 081-943 1229).

The Guild is an educational charity, having over 150 affiliated branches. It arranges workshops, lectures and exhibitions and publishes the *Embroidery* magazine, in which all aspects of the craft are regularly covered – patchwork, design, collage, canvas work, quilting, ecclesiastical embroidery and metal thread. Full member subscriptions for those over 60 are £12.50; others £20. The Guild will be glad to inform you of the details of the nearest branch.

Environment

There are many organisations now concerned with environmental matters which welcome members to help them with the very pressing problems facing our environment. Working locally, members can have a significant impact on local policies and can join in campaigning activities, practical ways of dealing with local needs, from protecting wildlife (even in towns) to planting trees to encouraging recycling and controlling pollution.

It is only relatively recently that environmental matters have come to be discussed so widely, and if we are to understand this debate we have a lot to learn – and this can seem rather daunting. However, evening and day classes are often held on this subject. Your library would know about classes held locally. Some open learning colleges also provide courses (for details about open learning see Section 10). One of these colleges, the National Extension College, provides a course 'Birds and Birdwatching'. For details see below.

There is also a political party, the Green Party, which is particularly concerned with the environment as well as with other issues. Its address is: 10 Station Parade, Balham High Road, London SW12 9AZ (Tel: 081-673 0045). There will be a local Party near to you.

The Council for the Protection of Rural England (CPRE)
Warwick House, 25 Buckingham Palace Road, London SW1W OPP
Tel: 071-976 6433).

CPRE states that it is the only independent environmental group working for the whole countryside. CPRE has a strong impact wherever decisions shaping the countryside are made – from town hall, Parliament and Whitehall to Brussels – using the expertise of the Westminster office and local branches, which cover the whole countryside.

In its work, CPRE uses careful research, constructive ideas, reasoned argument and a knowledge of how to get things done.

CPRE has a membership of 45,000. CPRE's county branches and district committees are run largely by volunteers.

If you are interested in campaigning for the countryside together with others, the national office above will be glad to put you in touch with your local branch.

English Vineyards Association
38 West Park, London SE9 4RH (Tel: 081-857 0452).

The EVA represents the interests of English vine growers and wine makers. It has over 550 full members and associates. Full members have vines in excess of half an acre. Anyone else, with or without vines, may apply to be an associate. Members receive the magazine *The Grape Press*. If you are interested in visiting a vineyard send for the free leaflet *English Vineyards Open to Visitors*, but please enclose a s.a.e.

Forestry Commission
231 Corstorphine Road, Edinburgh EH12 7AT (Tel: 031-334 0303).

The Forestry Commission has a wonderful range of literature about the many forest areas it controls and the facilities it provides. The booklets include *Forests for Birds*, *Forests for Wildlife*, *Why Grow Trees?* and many more. Contact the forest area you plan to visit for local information. The Forestry Commission has a list of forest areas in a booklet *Forest Visitor Information*. For details of forest holidays see Section 13.

Friends of the Earth (FOE)
26–8 Underwood Street, London N1 7JQ (Tel: 071-490 1555).

FOE is one of the leading environmental pressure groups in the United Kingdom. Local groups welcome new members to help in the wide variety of activities they undertake in helping to care for the environment.

Greenpeace
Canonbury Villas, London N1 2PN (Tel: 071-354 5100/071-359 7396).

Greenpeace has a network of around 200 local support groups which organise fundraising initiatives. Occasionally they may help with campaigns. Greenpeace, while concerned with the environment generally, has a particular concern for the sea and all the life within the waters.

National Extension College
18 Brooklands Avenue, Cambridge CB2 2HN (Tel: 0223-316644).

The NEC course 'Birds and Birdwatching' is intended for anyone who enjoys birdwatching and who wants to know more about the subject. It covers a wide range of topics, including how to recognise birds, the skills needed for birdwatching, the various habitats of birds, their life history and breeding methods, how birds fly, their social behaviour and evolution, and ecology and conservation. Not only is the course full of fascinating information, it also includes practical activities to keep you firmly in touch with the everyday life of birds, for example setting up a place to study birds in their natural habitat, or listening to bird-song. The course has been prepared and revised with the co-operation of the Royal Society for the Protection of Birds. Price: £115 with tutor support.

Royal Society for the Protection of Birds (RSPB)
The Lodge, Sandy, Bedfordshire SG19 2BR (Tel: 0767-680551).

The RSPB exists to conserve wild birds and the environment in which they live. They do this by buying land to create new reserves, improving land for wildlife, campaigning by opposing developments that threaten the environment, advising landowners and planners, and researching the needs of birds, so that they can base all their actions on facts, education and the fostering of a concern for wildlife, protecting our rarest breeding birds through wardening schemes, and co-operating with conservation organisations.

By joining the RSPB you will join in the Action for Birds Campaign. You will receive the beautifully illustrated *Birds* magazine four times a year, and you will enjoy free entry to over 100 RSPB reserves. As a member you will also be able to join in activities in your region and attend exhibitions, talks and film shows. Single membership: £18; joint membership £22.

▶ *The Wildfowl and Wetlands Trust*
Slimbridge, Gloucester GL2 7BT (Tel: 0453-890333).

From a very small beginning, the Trust has grown to manage 3,600 acres of wetland at eight sites and is the world's foremost authority on wildfowl and wetland conservation. It has 53,000 members, including Bird Adopters. The Trust offers five different types of bird for adoption: wild ducks, geese and swans, and, from their captive collections, flamingos and Hawaiian Geese. All bear uniquely numbered leg rings, which helps the Trust to identify your individual bird. Wild ducks travel far and wide during their lifetimes and many Duck Adopters have enjoyed hearing of their bird turning up somewhere in Europe, Scandinavia or even the countries of the former Soviet Union.

Wildfowl and Wetlands Centres are at: Slimbridge, Arundel, Caerlaverock, Castle Espie, Llanelli, Martin Mere, Washington and Welney. The Trust will be glad to send you details. The leaflets about the various centres are outstandingly illustrated. There is also a magazine, *Wildfowl and Wetlands*, price £1. For details of membership contact as above.

Family history and genealogy

▶ *The Federation of Family History Societies*
5 Mornington Close, Copthorne, Shrewsbury, Shropshire SY3 8XN (Tel: 0743-65505).

This society was formed as a result of the growing interest in the study of family history. It now has a membership of 150 societies throughout the world, including national, regional and one-name groups. Its principal aims are to co-ordinate and assist the work of societies or other bodies interested in family history, genealogy and heraldry and to foster mutual co-operation and regional projects in these subjects. Membership is open to any society or body specialising in family history or an associated discipline.

The Federation will be glad to send you a list of family history societies. It also has a leaflet, *Tracing your Ancestors*.

▶ *Society of Genealogists*
14 Charterhouse Buildings, Goswell Road, London EC1M 7BA (Tel: 071-251 8799).

The Society is a charity and promotes and encourages the study of genealogy and heraldry. Members have access to the library with its collection of parish registers, printed and typescript family histories, and its vast indexes. The quarterly magazine is sent to members. Members pay an entrance fee when first joining of £7.50. The annual subscription for those living within 25 miles of Trafalgar Square is £25; for others £16. Non-members may use the library on payment of fees: £2.55 an hour, £6.15 for $3\frac{1}{2}$ hours, £8.15 for the day.

Films and film making

▶ *British Federation of Film Societies*
Film Society Unit, 21 Stephen Street, London W1P 1PL (Tel: 071-255 1444).

The BFFS is served and financially assisted by the British Film Institute. The BFFS publishes a monthly journal, *Film*, which is distributed to all film societies. The Federation will be glad to send you details of local film societies.

▶ *Institute of Amateur Cinematographers Ltd*
24c West Street, Epsom, Surrey KT18 7RJ (Tel: 0372-739672).

IAC promotes the amateur film movement and protects the interests of amateur film makers. It will provide advice on scripting, shooting, editing, sound, lighting, animation, presentation, and technical matters. There is also a special music advisory service to help amateurs who have difficulty in choosing the right music for their soundtracks. Members are kept in touch through *Amateur Film Maker* the IAC's own bi-monthly journal. There is a reduced subscription for older people.

Flower arranging

▶ *National Association of Flower Arrangement Societies of Great Britain*
21 Denbigh Street, London SW1V 2HF (Tel: 071-828 5145).

The Association will be glad to put interested flower arrangers in touch with local groups.

Gardening

▶ *Gardening*
Published by and available from: The Disability Information Trust, Mary Marlborough Lodge, Nuffield Orthopaedic Centre, Headington, Oxford OX3 7LD (Tel: 0865-64811 ext. 372). Price: £11 post free.

This is one in the series Equipment for Disabled People. The book provides information on aids and equipment to make gardening easier if you find any of the tasks physically difficult.

The book discusses: garden design; garden tools: forks, spades, hoes, rakes, tool handles, pruners, secateurs, flower gatherers, lawn mowers, lawn shears and edgers; plants in the garden; plant supports; weed problems; stools; wheelbarrows; patio gardens; hanging baskets; wildlife; greenhouses and accessories; plant propagation; indoor gardening; hand tools; safety; gardening for profit; gardening for food; gardening for blind people; buying wisely; clubs for disabled gardeners; lists sources of information; and has a select bibliography.

Gardening for Disabled Trust
Hayes Farmhouse, Hayes Lane, Peasmarsh, East Sussex TN31 6EX.

The Trust can provide grants to disabled people throughout the United Kingdom. Help may be given to: adapt private gardens to meet special needs; make grants towards tools, raised beds, paving and greenhouses; provide information on garden aids and techniques.

Through its Garden Club the Trust gives advice on garden design, answers horticultural questions, operates a service for exchanging plants and seeds, and shares experiences that may help with difficulties and problems. The Garden Club also publishes a quarterly newsletter with articles of special interest to disabled gardeners.

Gardening in Retirement
By Isobel Pays, with an Introduction by Percy Thrower (Age Concern England, Astral House, 1268 London Road, London SW16 4ER). Price: £1.95 including postage and packing.

This is a practical guide for beginners and experts alike. The introductory chapter for beginners is particularly useful as it explains the basics of planning what you want from your garden or window box, and details a range of tools which make gardening easier for older people. The book covers planning indoor ornamental gardens and growing fruits and vegetables, and explains how to grow plants from seeds and cuttings. It has helpful illustrations and colour photographs.

Gardens of England and Wales
Published by The National Gardens Scheme Charitable Trust, Hatchlands Park, East Clandon, Guildford, Surrey GU4 7RT (Tel: 0483-211535). Price: £2 from bookshops or £2.75 including postage and packing, from this address.

There are over 2,800 gardens opening in aid of the scheme, which are mostly private and not normally open to the public. The guide states admission prices (in some cases there are reductions for pensioners), whether or not teas are served, whether plants are sold, and directions to the garden. The wheelchair symbol is included to show those gardens accessible for visitors in wheelchairs.

The Hardy Plant Society
Tricia King (Administrator) Bank Cottage, Great Comberton, Pershore, Worcestershire WR10 3DP (Tel: 0386-710317).

The Society has some 8,000 members with whom it shares information about the less well-known, as well as the more familiar, hardy plants, how and where they may be obtained and how best cultivated. There are close links with the National Council for the Conservation of Plants and Gardens. There are 23 county-based local groups. Visits and tours are arranged. Some are to gardens closed to the public and some to gardens abroad. Members can obtain seed from the Seed Exchange scheme, which offers more than 2,500 varieties, many unavailable commercially. A newsletter is issued three times a year with information on local groups, current events and other items of interest. Many local groups produce newsletters too.

There is also a HPS Correspondence Group – the subscription is £2 in addition to the HPS subscription of £8.50 for a single person and £10 for two members living at the same address. The address for the HPS Correspondence Group is: Jane Lucas, 37 Horndean Avenue, Wigston Fields, Leicester LE8 1DP.

▸ *Horticultural Therapy*
Goulds Ground, Vallis Way, Frome, Somerset BA11 3DW (Tel: 0373-464782).

Horticultural Therapy promotes the view that gardening is for everyone and aims to help people overcome any obstacles to their enjoyment of gardening. To do this HT offers practical help, through its services, to anyone needing help and, in particular, to anyone who has a disability. It publishes a most imaginative magazine, *Growth Point*, with pull-out pages which can be kept for their particular information. It includes articles and information of interest to the small-scale gardener and the professional horticulturist. The layout of interestingly organised print, spiced with cartoons and other graphics, makes it a joy to read. The Information Service provides a wide range of information on designing a garden for easier working and on tools which can take the main strain out of gardening.

Membership subscription to HT is £15 p.a. (£12.50 for registered disabled people), or £10 if you would just like to receive *Growth Point*.

Available from Horticultural Therapy are two very useful books:

▸ *Gardening is for Everyone: A Week-by-Week Guide for People with Handicaps.*
By Audrey Cloet and Chris Underhill (Souvenir Press). Price: £4.95.

In this imaginative and detailed guide keen would-be gardeners will find a host of ideas for every week of the year which are within the scope of those whose mobility may be restricted. Designed with beginners in mind, it explains every technique with text and clear drawings, showing how to grow potatoes in containers, how to create a garden indoors, how and when to sow and plant, and how to make decorative pictures from pressed flowers, seedheads and grasses.

▸ *Able to Garden: A Practical guide for disabled and elderly gardeners*
(Batsford Books).

This book is a compendium of many of Horticultural Therapy's most practical leaflets. It has been edited by Peter Please, a garden designer and former training officer for HT. It includes line drawings by HT's magazine *Growth Point* editor Val George, plus photographs. The first half of the book, *Down to Basics*, covers just that – the structure of the garden and how to create it: surfaces, lawns, beds, containers, the shed, the greenhouse, tools (including useful addresses), hardwood cuttings and sowing. The second section, *Handy Ideas*, covers more specific areas, with a host of ideas, from small labour- and money-saving hints to a complete range of winter gardening activities. Price: £12.95 hardback; £7.95 paperback. Available in bookshops or by post (add £2.50 or 70 pence post and packaging respectively) from Horticultural Therapy as above.

The National Society of Allotment and Leisure Gardeners
Hunter's Road, Corby NN17 1JE (Tel: 0536-66576).

Free advice is available to members in connection with all horticultural and gardening matters. A variety of leaflets are produced. There is also a seed and insurance scheme whereby you are supplied with seeds at approximately half the price you would pay in the High Street stores. If you are not a member of an Association that is affilated to the Society, you can become a member of the Society by taking up one 10p share on joining, also making an annual contribution of not less than £5 for the support of the Society.

The Royal Horticultural Society
80 Vincent Square, London SW1P 2PE (Tel: 071-834 4333).

RHS membership gives you unlimited privileged visits to some of the finest gardens and flower shows, a monthly magazine, free practical advice and access to a wide range of lectures and demonstrations all over the United Kingdom. As an RHS member, you get free entry to Wisley and Rosemoor, plus six other fine gardens – at Harlow Carr near Harrogate, Ness in the Wirral, Bodnant in North Wales, Hidcote Manor in Gloucestershire, and Nymans and Sheffield Park in Sussex. Members receive the magazine *The Garden* – a mix of gardening history, new insights into plants and techniques, and insiders' views of gardens the world over. Membership also gives you news of the programme of over 250 lectures and demonstrations run nationwide. The RHS also publishes a Programme of Events and a very full publications list.

Individual membership: £21 (plus £5 enrolment fee); Family membership: £36 (plus £5 enrolment fee).

Scotland's Gardens
(Scotland's Gardens Scheme, 31 Castle Terrace, Edinburgh EH1 2EL (Tel: 031-229 1870). Price: £2 plus 50p postage and packing.

Saga arranges practical gardening holidays as well as a Gardens of Britain holiday. For details see Section 13.

Visually impaired gardeners

RNIB's booklet *Gardening without sight*, by Kathleen Fleet, for visually impaired gardeners who enjoy growing flowers or vegetables in their garden, allotment or indoors. Price: £2.50. Available in print, braille or on tape. Contact the Leisure Department, Royal National Institute for the Blind, 224 Great Portland Street, London W1N 6AA for details.

Come Gardening magazine and the Cassette Library for Blind Gardeners. An annual subscription of £2 covers receipt of the *Come Gardening* magazine each quarter (in braille or on tape) and use, at any time, of the Cassette Library for Blind Gardeners. Cheques and postal orders, made payable to Horticultural Therapy, should be sent to: Tim Spurgeon, Horticultural Therapy, Goulds Ground, Vallis Way, Frome, Somerset BA11 3DW (Tel: 0373-464782). When writing you are asked to supply your name and address in block capitals and not to send cassettes as you will be given full particulars about these in reply to your enquiry.

Golf

Golf is not just a sport for those who live in the country and play on 18-hole courses. Some clubs have long waiting lists and are expensive, but there are now many municipally owned 9- and 18-hole courses and smaller pitch and put courses. Driving ranges are also popular where you can hit a bucket full of balls and you don't even have to collect them! If walking distances is a problem then a golf buggie might be a help. Your district council recreation department or the leisure department of your local authority will be glad to tell you of any such facilities locally. Your local library would also have this information. Residential golfing holidays are run both in the United Kingdom and also overseas by several commercial holiday operators.

The Golf Club – Great Britain
302 Ewell Road, Surbiton, Surrey KT6 7AQ (Tel: 081-390 3113).

The Club has over 4,000 members. It seeks to educate members about the rules and etiquette of golf including the correct completion of score cards. This allows for handicaps to be controlled centrally, thus enabling the achievement of uniformity throughout the country. Having a handicap certificate enables members to match their skills against others in tournaments and competition. Up until now, many golfers who were not affiliated members of The Council of National Golf Unions, and thus within those particular handicapping rules, were excluded from entering competitions because they could not produce a handicap certificate. Each month there is a prize for the best net score in the various handicap categories and an annual prize for the most improved golfer.

Society for One-Armed Golfers
Contact Don Reid, 11 Coldwell Lane, Felling, Tyne and Wear NE10 9EX (Tel: 091-469 4742).

The Society holds regular meetings. Apart from a week-long annual championship, weekend and one-day events are organised by regional convenors in England, Scotland and Ireland. Members pay an annual subscription of £3.

Heritage and history

United Kingdom

=▶ *British Association of Friends of Museums*
548 Wilbraham Road, Manchester M21 1LB (Tel: 061-881 8640 (home), 061-236 8585 (office)).

The Association aims to give the many Societies of Friends of Museums in the British Isles a means of exchanging ideas and uniting to present these ideas to government, the public and the press. The word 'Museum' includes any institution preserving our cultural heritage. The Association will be glad to give you details of any local Friends groups where these are known. Annual subscription is £7.50 p.a. for individuals, who receive copies of the Broadsheet which is published three times a year. There is also a very interesting annual publication, *The Museum Visitor*.

=▶ *Civic Trust*
17 Carlton House Terrace, London SW1Y 5AW (Tel: 071-930 0914).

The Civic Trust is concerned with improving and regenerating the environment in the places where people live and work rather than the world of showpiece houses and landscape. It has no membership scheme but it is the national organisation covering the whole of the United Kingdom and is closely involved with local amenity groups. It will be glad to give you the name of your nearest group.

The Civic Trust has published an *Environmental Directory* which lists over 300 organisations concerned with amenity and the environment. Each entry gives the address and telephone number of the organisation, and details of its aims and activities. Symbols indicate facilities, such as whether an organisation gives grants, offers an advisory service, membership, etc. Price: £4 post paid. A publications list is available.

=▶ *Historic Houses Association*
Friends Membership Department, PO Box 21, Letchworth, Hertfordshire SG6 2JF (Tel: 0462-675848).

HHA represents over 1,000 owners of historic houses, parks and gardens in private ownership in the United Kingdom. Friends of HHA enjoy visiting country houses. They can visit 270 HHA members' properties free of charge and can become involved in the HHA's work at a regional level. Individual membership subscription is £20.

=▶ *The Historical Association*
59a Kennington Park Road, London SE11 4JH (Tel: 071-735 3901).

You do not have to be a famous historian to join the Historical Association – all you need is curiosity in the past and a belief in the value of history. *The Historian*, the Association's quarterly illustrated members' magazine, is sent free to all members. A wide range of 'Out and About' days are organised which are publicised regularly in the magazine, and members are given preference when booking and a reduction on the cost of the day. Individual membership subscription is £20.

England

British Association for Local History
Shopwyke Hall, Chichester, West Sussex PO20 6BQ (Tel: 0243-787639).

The Association is the national 'umbrella' organisation exclusively for the service of local history. Members have the opportunity to take part in seminars and courses, to visit places not normally accessible to the general public and to receive *The Local Historian* at a favourable subscription, as well as BALH's other regular publication *Local History News* which is free. Subscription is £15 p.a.

The Georgian Group
37 Spital Square, London E1 6DY (Tel: 071-377 1722).

Membership entitles you not only to take part in activities and to receive free copies of the newsletter and illustrated Journal, but also to make a practical contribution to the 'continuing battle of our heritage' as the leaflet describes it. Annual subscription £20.

Historic Houses, Castles and Gardens
Published by British Leisure Publications, Windsor Court, East Grinstead House, East Grinstead, West Sussesx RH19 1XA (Tel: 0342-326972). Price: £6.90.

This guide, in full colour throughout, includes over 1,300 properties giving details of opening times, admission charges, locations, collections and catering facilities.

History Today
83-4 Berwick Street, London W1V 3PJ (Tel: 071-439 8315).

If you are only half interested in history, this well-illustrated magazine will whet your appetite for the subject. It has a wide range of well-researched articles written in an easy style which bring alive different periods of history. The subscription for this monthly magazine is £25.

London Appreciation Society
17 Manson Mews, South Kensington, London SW7 5AF.

The main events take place on Saturday afternoons but weekday and evening outings are also planned. The Society specialises in the 'unusual' and one of its aims is to take its members to places not normally open to the public. The Society exists to enjoy and appreciate London as it is. Each year the Society prints its *Blue Book*, which is a list of events. Details will be sent to anyone interested on receipt of a s.a.e. (28p stamp on an envelope $6\frac{1}{2}'' \times 9\frac{1}{2}''$). Subscription £5.

=▶ *The National Trust (England, Wales, Northern Ireland)*
36 Queen Anne's Gate, London SW1H 9AS (Tel: 071-222 5097).

The Trust not only looks after 250 historic buildings but also preserves, for us all, and for all time, gardens and landscaped parks, countryside, including woods and downland, lakes, mountains and half of our finest remaining coastline, prehistoric Roman sites, relics of our industrial past, more than a thousand farms, 59 traditional villages and hamlets, nearly 200 shops, and nature reserves. It also has holiday cottages and organises summer festivals. Members have free entry to National Trust properties where the public has to pay. The Trust also publishes a booklet *Facilities for Disabled and Visually Handicapped Visitors* which is free, and there is a *Guide to National Trust Events*. Individual subscription is £21 p.a.

Scotland

=▶ *The Architectural Heritage Society of Scotland*
The Glasite Meeting House, 33 Barony Street, Edinburgh EH3 6NX
(Tel: 031-557 0019).

Formerly the Scottish Georgian Society, the AHSS exists to protect the architectural heritage of Scotland and to promote the study and appreciation of the built heritage of all periods. There are regional groups throughout Scotland offering a wide range of activities for members, as well as Cases Panels which monitor and comment on planning applications affecting listed buildings and buildings in conservation areas. The Society publishes an annual Journal and twice-yearly newsletters. Current individual membership is £12 p.a.

=▶ *Friends of Historic Scotland*
PO Box 157, Edinburgh EH3 5RA (Tel: 031-244 3099).

Friends of Historic Scotland have free entry to over 300 historic sites and monuments. In your first year you will also have half-price entry to English Heritage and Welsh Cadw sites. After that they are free too. You will also receive a free *Sites Directory* and a free regular newsletter. Subscriptions: Adult £13, Family £21, Reduced (persons aged 60 and over/young people up to 21 years in full-time education) £9, Senior Citizen Couple (husband and wife aged 60 and over) £13.50.

=▶ *The Friends of the National Museums of Scotland*
Chambers Street, Edinburgh EH1 1JF (Tel: 031-225 7534).

As a member you will be entitled to attend private views of exhibitions and collections and lectures, as well as to take part in expeditions to places of interest. You will receive the publication *The Reporter*, which is published every two months. Subscription £10, Senior Citizens £5. A publications list is available; it includes *Robert Burns, Farmer, The Scenery of Scotland, Scotland's Industrial Past*, and many more.

National Trust for Scotland
5 Charlotte Square, Edinburgh EH2 4DU (Tel: 031-226 5922).

Membership entitles those who belong to free entry to over 100 Trust properties and they receive the quarterly publication *Heritage Scotland: The National Trust for Scotland guide to over 100 properties*. This guide is also available to non-members at a cost of £1 including postage and packing. Subscription for Senior Citizens (over 60) is £10 for individuals and £16.50 for couples. Also available is a free leaflet: *Information about Trust Properties for Disabled Visitors*. Send a 24p s.a.e. for a copy.

Saltire Society
9 Fountain Close, 22 High Street, Edinburgh EH1 1TF (Tel: 031-556 1836).

The Society and its local branches are interested in all things Scottish: Scotland's past, present and future. Its main concern, however, is with the present and the future. It seeks to preserve all that is best in Scottish tradition and to encourage every new development which can strengthen and enrich the country's cultural life. Membership subscription £10, senior citizens £5.

Scottish Language Society
Lynn Corrigan, Secretary, 5 Caledonian Crescent, Edinburgh EH11 2DB
Tel: 031-337 7599).

The Society is a charity and exists to promote the Scottish language in literature, drama, the media, education, and in everyday usage. It publishes the twice-yearly *Lallans*, the magazine for writing in Lowland Scots, as well as a newsletter in Scots. Membership subscription is £5 for individuals.

Wales

Heritage in Wales
Brunel House, 2 Fitzalan Road, Cardiff CF2 1UY (Tel: 0222-465511).
Ty Brunel, 2 Ffordd Fitzalan, Caerdydd CF2 1UY.

Heritage in Wales is the membership scheme of Cadw: Welsh Historic Monuments, having care of ancient monuments. Some of the sites cannot easily be visited by people with disabilities or difficulties in getting around, being isolated and accessible only on foot over ground that is sometimes quite steep. Anyone wanting detailed information about specific sites should contact Jenny Gittins at the telephone number above. Members enjoy free entrance to all historic sites in the care of Cadw and half-price admission to English and Scottish sites. As a member, you will receive a Cadw information pack with details of the sites under Cadw's care, and a newspaper published three times a year. You will also qualify for a 10 per cent discount off Cadw gifts and souvenirs. The membership subscription is £10 p.a. for senior citizens.

=▶ *National Trust*
See National Trust under heading England above.

Jigsaws

=▶ *The British Jigsaw Puzzle Library*
8 Heath Terrace, Leamington Spa, Warwickshire CV32 5LY (Tel: 0926-311874).

This is a lending library in which jigsaw puzzles are exchanged by post and personally. Members pay by subscription (annually £58, half-yearly £36, or quarterly £26). All puzzles are wooden, without picture guides. They vary considerably in size and difficulty. The Library caters both for the connoisseur and for the less practised.

Judo

=▶ *British Judo Association*
7A Rutland Street, Leicester LE1 1RB (Tel: 0533-559660).

The BJA organises a Veterans Championships every year. You do not have to belong to a local club to enter but you must have reached a certain grade. Most clubs offer self-defence judo for older people. All clubs accept members of all ages.

Meteorology

=▶ *Royal Meteorological Society*
104 Oxford Road, Reading, Berkshire RG1 7LJ (Tel: 0344-422957).

Anyone with a genuine interest in meteorology and related sciences such as oceanography and hydrology is welcome to join the Society. Members receive the monthly magazine *Weather* without charge and may receive the *Quarterly Journal* and the *Journal of Climatology* at a subtantial discount.
  Membership subscription is £29 for a Fellow.

Music

See also Section 13 for holiday music courses.
  Saga arranges holidays for music lovers. You can enjoy recitals in stately homes or study musical appreciation or enjoy opera, or you may like to join the Edinburgh Festival. For details of Saga holidays *see* Section 13.

Arts, sport and leisure

▸ *British Music Education Yearbook*
Published by Rhinegold Publishing Limited, 241 Shaftesbury Avenue, London WC2H 8EH (Tel: 071-240 5749). Price: £11.50 plus £2 postage and packing.

Although mainly directed at ways of studying music for younger age groups, the book does provide information about studying music at all levels and right across the age spectrum. There is a Recreational Courses list providing details of short musical courses, residential or not, organised throughout the year right across the country.

Rhinegold also publishes *Classical Music* magazine fortnightly, which has news, reviews and features covering classical music, opera and dance, and makes interesting reading for anyone interested in the field and wishing to keep up with what is going on. Price: £1.80 per issue, or £36 post-inclusive for an annual subscription.

▸ *The Galpin Society - for the study of musical instruments*
38 Eastfield Road, Western Park, Leicester LE3 6FE (Contact Pauline Holden).

This is an international learned society with a worldwide membership of individuals and institutions. It publishes a journal annually, containing original research into the history, development, use and manufacture of musical instruments. It organises meetings both in the United Kingdom and abroad, when members are able to see collections not normally open to the public. Annual subscription for individuals is £15.

▸ *National Federation of Music Societies*
Francis House, Francis Street, London SW1P 1DE (Tel: 071-828 7320).

There are over 1,300 choirs, orchestras and music societies affiliated to the NFMS. For information on local societies contact the NFMS.

▸ *National Music and Disability Information Service*
Dartington Hall, Totnes, Devon TQ9 6EJ (Tel: 0803-866701).

By serving as a central resource for a wide range of information, contacts and advice, the NMDIS strives to ensure that no one is prevented from enjoying or participating in music in any form or at any level merely because of disability. The NMDIS will answer queries by letter or telephone on any music-and-disability-related matter. In addition, the Service publishes a wide range of resource material: information papers, conference and seminar proceedings, and a small amount of piano music for one hand. The publication list is available on request.

A quarterly newsletter, *Music News*, is available on subscription. The newsletter includes articles about recent events, new publications and audio-visual materials, a diary section of forthcoming courses, conferences and events, and details of new initiatives. *Music News* is available in both print form and on tape.

▸ *The Society of Recorder Players*
Hon. Sec. Anne Blackman, 469 Merton Road, London SW18 5LD (Tel: 081-874 2237).

The Society has 46 regional branches which welcome players of all standards. However, not all branches provide tuition for beginners. For details of your nearest branch contact the Society as above. The Society publishes *The Recorder Magazine* (quarterly) and *A Teacher's Guide to the Recorder*, and has a videotape *The Recorder and its History*.

Netball

▶ *All England Netball Association Limited*
Netball House, 9 Paynes Park, Hitchin, Hertfordshire SG5 1EH (Tel: 0462-442344).

▶ *Scottish Netball Association*
Kelvin Hall Sports Complex, Argyle Street, Glasgow G3 8AA (Tel: 041-334 3650).

▶ *Welsh Netball Association*
82 Cathedral Road, Cardiff, South Glamorgan CF1 9LN (Tel: 0222-237048).

These Associations are most keen to welcome members over 50. Both women and men can join in activities but playing is primarily for women. They welcome older people, who can do so much by helping with events as well as administration, serving on committees, umpiring and coaching – courses are available to train you to become an umpire or coach. In particular help is needed with clubs for very young people. Helping in this way is neither expensive (expenses would usually be met) nor energetic. The Association has a list of local County Associations.

Numismatics

▶ *The British Association of Numismatic Societies*
c/o Bush Boake Allen Ltd, Blackhorse Lane, London E17 5QT.

BANS has 61 affiliated societies, including the Royal and British. The Association exists to help further the study of numismatics in this country by bringing societies together. It holds an Annual Numismatic Congress at different centres (usually in April). It also runs an annual weekend lecture course (usually in September), and one-day courses from time to time. BANS will be glad to put you in touch with a local group.

▶ *The British Numismatic Society*
c/o Royal Mint, Llantrisant, Pontyclun, Mid Glamorgan CF7 8YT
(Tel: 0443-222111) (Contact: G.P. Dyer).

The *British Numismatic Journal*, published annually by the Society and distributed to all paid-up members, provides the results of the most recent scholarly research into the history of the coinage, and records significant new numismatic discoveries. Books may be borrowed personally or by post from the extensive library. Subscription for ordinary membership is £24. An entrance fee of £1 is also charged on election.

Oral history/reminiscing

Age Exchange
The Reminiscence Centre, 11 Blackheath Village, Blackheath, London SE3 9LA (Tel: 081-318 9105).

Age Exchange is a charity and the Reminiscence Centre, set in an old-fashioned shop dating back to the 1920s, is a place for people to enjoy reminiscing with others, to look at a display of items from the past, to see exhibitions and shows based on memories, and join in a programme of events and activities which run throughout the year. Open 10 a.m. to 5.30 p.m., Monday to Saturday. There is a café and access for disabled people.

Those interested in writing and talking about their lives are able to meet others who have an interest in their stories and are invited to contribute to the memory bank.

The Centre also provides a resource and training base for those who work with older people. It stocks current literature on reminiscence, life history publications and visual resources, tapes and exhibitions. The growing collection of objects suitable for use in reminiscence work is available for hire.

The Oral History Society
Department of Sociology, University of Essex, Wivenhoe Park, Colchester CO4 3SQ (Tel: 0206-873333).

The Society is a charity and has 800 members in over 20 countries. Members keep in touch with the network of oral history in Britain and worldwide through the journal *Oral History* and through meetings which are held in London, Manchester, Bradford and Edinburgh – each on a special theme such as *Oral History* and Women's History, Black History, Labour History, the Middle Classes, Health Care and Community History. The Society runs workshops on Reminiscence Therapy and on Reminiscence Drama.

Oral History, is available twice-yearly. Subscription (including membership fee) is £12 for individuals.

Reminiscence
Help the Aged, St James's Walk, London EC1R OBE (Tel: 071-253 0253).

Reminiscence is a publication produced by Help the Aged which includes reports on reminiscence projects around the United Kingdom. It also includes information on courses and training.

Orienteering

British Orienteering Federation
Riversdale, Dale Road North, Darley Dale, Matlock, Derbyshire DE4 2HX (Tel: 0629-734 042).

The Federation will be glad to send you details of local contacts and general information, including a fixtures list and guidance on how to get started in this fascinating leisure activity.

Painting

See Arts page 260 and Courses and Special Interest Holidays and Saga Holidays Section 13.

Philately

National Philatelic Society
107 Charterhouse Street, London EC1M 6PT (Tel: 071-251 5040).

A regular magazine, *Stamp Lover*, is sent free to all members, including a checklist of articles which have recently appeared in the British philatelic press, plus news of newly published books. There is also a monthly stamp auction. An Exchange Packet is provided for those who want an easy and convenient way of buying and selling from home. Annual subscription: £12.50 p.a.

Photography

The Royal Photographic Society
The Octagon, Milsom Street, Bath BA1 1DN (Tel: 0225-462841).

The Society, a registered charity, was founded in 1853, only fourteen years after the public announcement of the discovery of photography. Membership is worldwide and is open to anyone who is interested in photography. Amateurs and professionals are equally welcome.

The RPS has established a National Centre of photography at Bath. This comprises exhibition galleries for both contemporary and historical photography; a library; a research area for both images and apparatus; a modern lecture theatre; a sales area (which also operates a mail order service); and a restaurant. The Society has chair lifts for disabled visitors, which enables them to visit all of its galleries. As a member you will receive *The Photographic Journal*, the Society's own monthly magazine, and the bi-monthly *Journal of Photographic Science*. You will also benefit from reduced entrance fees for Society conferences, field trips, weekend instructional workshops, etc.

You can take advantage of preferential accommodation rates in numerous hotels and guest houses in the United Kingdom and elsewhere. Annual membership subscription is £49 (£29 for over-65s).

Saga arranges photography holidays. For details of Saga holidays, see Section 13.

Radio

▶ *British Wireless for the Blind Fund*
Gabriel House, 34 New Road, Chatham, Kent ME4 4QR (Tel: 0634-832501).

The Fund exists in order to provide radios or radio cassette recorders on a free permanent loan basis to registered blind people resident in the United Kingdom, who are in need and who enjoy listening to the wireless. All sets are distributed through local agents, who also issue the free allocation of batteries provided by the Fund – four sets per year. Headphones are also provided if these are needed. The local agent also deals with any repair or maintenance of sets directly, with the Fund paying any costs.

Railways

▶ *The Railway Correspondence and Travel Society*
20 Leckhampton Place, Old Station Drive, Leckhampton Road, Cheltenham GL53 0DD.

The Society has 19 branches around the country where fortnightly or monthly meetings are held during the winter months. In the warmer months, trips out are organised to places of interest to a railway enthusiast. The Society has published a large number of definitive works on the histories of locomotives of the four British pre-nationalisation railway companies and their pre-grouping constituents, as well as books of a more general railway interest.

The Society has a large library based in Uxbridge, from which members can borrow books either by a personal visit or through the post. The magazine *The Railway Observer* is published monthly.

Rambling

▶ *The Ramblers Association*
1–5 Wandsworth Road, London SW8 2XX (Tel: 071-582 6878).

Many older people belong to the 330 local Ramblers' groups. There is a special reduced membership rate of £7 for individuals and £9 for couples. This entitles you to receive the bi-monthly magazine *Rambling Today* and the Year Book, which lists bed and breakfast accommodation. You are also entitled to use the map library and membership covers your local group. Most rambles are for half days or full days.

See also details of walking and rambling holidays with Saga holidays and with Countrywide holidays in Section 13.

Reading

If you are interested in reading and are not near a bookshop, or have mobility problems, then you will find it difficult to buy the books you really want. We describe below firms who will supply books of your choice.

Blunt Fin Ltd
PO Box 860, Bristol BS99 5JF (Tel: 0272-467599).

Blunt Fin describes its service as being 'particularly useful to those who are of limited mobility, living abroad, studying specialised subjects or just tired of the impersonal attitude of high street stores'. If a book is in print Blunt Fin will obtain it for you. All they need to know is your area of interest, by subject, title or author, and they will send you personalised listings of the books which are in print.

The Good Book Guide
Braithwaite & Taylor Limited, 91 Great Russell Street, London WC1B 3PS (Tel: 071-580 8466).

The imaginative and straightforward consumer advice offered by *The Good Book Guide* – through its colour illustrated publications – makes browsing at home possible. In each issue of the *Guide* (bi-monthly with a special Christmas issue) some 500 new hardback and paperback books are objectively and concisely reviewed by professional book reviewers in 20 different subject areas. All of these books are available through the 24-hour dispatch service. *Bookpost* is another service through which any book currently in print can be ordered via the *Guide*. A complimentary copy of the *Guide* and full information about its services can be obtained from the address above. The annual subscription, entitling you to receive a year's issues of the guide, is £17 and there are tokens with each guide. These, if used, offset the entire subscription.

Large print books

The Partially Sighted Society would be glad to let you know of publishers producing large print books. Their address is: Queens Road, Doncaster, South Yorkshire DN1 2NX (Tel: 0302-368998).

Large print publishers, who would be glad to send you catalogues, include:
– ISIS Large Print, 55 St Thomas' Street, Oxford OX1 1JG (Tel: 0865-250333).

- Chivers Press Publishers, Windsor Bridge Road, Bath, Avon BA2 3AX (Tel: 0225-335336).
- Ulverscroft Large Print Books Limited, The Green, Bradgate Road, Anstey, Leicester LE7 7FU (Tel: 0533-364325).

Books, newspapers and magazines on tape

▶ *National Library for the Blind*
Cromwell Road, Bredbury, Stockport, Cheshire SK6 2SG (Tel: 061-494 0217).

Although the majority of books are in braille, there are also large collections in Moon type and large print. As well as being a large lending library of reading material and also music, the NLB produces many hundreds of books in braille of all kinds every year – from best-sellers to books of reference and the classics.

▶ *The Talking Newspaper Association (TNAUK)*
90 High Street, Heathfield, East Sussex TN21 8JD (Tel: 0435-866102).

The Association has voluntary groups in over 500 areas in the United Kingdom which produce tape versions of local newspapers for distribution to visually and physially handicapped people in their areas. The Association itself produces tape versions of about 100 national newspapers and magazines.

TNAUK will send details of your nearest Talking Newspaper and a list of national papers and magazines on tape. The Association publishes the *TNAUK Guide to Tape Services for the Handicapped*, which is a very useful reference to material it would otherwise be difficult to find. Costing £5 including postage and packing, the Guide has:

- listings of local and national newspapers and magazines on tape
- health information tapes
- educational and professional information on tape
- tape libraries
- reading services
- sources of religious material on tape
- special interest tape sources
- tape magazines and clubs
- indexes of material on tape (by title, subject and county).

Rowing

▶ *Amateur Rowing Association*
6 Lower Mall, London W6 9DJ (Tel: 081-748 3632).

Rowing has a very well developed system to ensure competitive participation at all ages. The sport today is essentially a competitive activity, but this does not mean that it is exclusively for those who have rowed in their youth. The Veteran categories begin at 27 years of age with discrete categories following at 32, 38, 45, 52 and 60 years of age. The ARA says, 'while the Veteran categories are normally populated with those who have learnt to row in their youth there is absolutely no reason why novices to the sport should not enter in their 30s, 40s and possibly 50s. It would probably be ill-advised for anyone older than this, unless extremely fit, to take the sport up.'

There are some 550 clubs in England with others in Scotland, Wales and Ireland through which entry into the sport can be made. Normally these clubs provide all the boats required, from single-seater sculls to those for eight people. Training and coaching facilities are also generally available. The annual subscription for these clubs would be typically set at about £50. Beyond this there is a charge for being registered as a member of the Amateur Rowing Association and also a charge for entering each Regatta. There are specialised Regattas for Veteran oarsmen and -women.

Running

▶ *The Running Sixties*
Contact: Jim Bennett, Secretary, 120 Norfolk Avenue, Sanderstead, Surrey CR2 8BS (Tel: 081-657 7660).

The objects of this club include the promotion of running or jogging for people over 60 with the aim of improving fitness and a general sense of well-being, while at the same time creating opportunities for joint recreational ventures.

Some members run annually in the London Marathon, while some members run frequently in road races in the UK and abroad as well as in other events including relay races.

Runners and joggers of all abilities are welcome to join. Contact the Secretary for further details and please enclose a s.a.e.

Sailing

▶ *Royal Yachting Association*
RYA House, Romsey Road, Eastleigh, Hampshire SO5 4YA (Tel: 0703-629962).

The RYA is the governing body for the sport of sailing, windsurfing and powerboating. It can provide a range of back-up services to those who enjoy the excitement of racing and the pleasures of cruising under power or sail. It manages training schemes which cater for everyone, from beginners to the most experienced. As a member you will receive *RYA News*, the quarterly house magazine of the RYA. You can also make use of legal advice on yachting matters. In addition, you will also have entrance to the RYA lounge at the Boat Show. Subscription: £16 p.a.

British Federation of Sand and Land Yacht Clubs
Contact: Mike Hampton, 23 Piper Drive, Long Whatton, Loughborough, Leicestershire LE12 5DJ.

Landsailing is becoming a popular sport and the BFSLYC is able to provide the equipment and trained instructors to help newcomers. It is said that landsailing is remarkably easy to learn. With proper instruction the complete novice can be sailing solo in less than an hour. The Federation will be glad to send you details of local clubs which have permission to sail on beaches and airfields. For details send a large s.a.e. to Mike Hampton.

Skiing

Nordic cross country skiing is popular with all ages but has special attractions for older people. Unlike Alpine skiing, it can be taken up at a later age and novices can get a good deal of pleasure from it from the very beginning. Before setting out, however, it is wise to have learnt some navigation and have some understanding of weather conditions.

Many older people who have learnt Alpine skiing when young can still go on enjoying the sport, but the twisting and turning can become difficult.

There are also quite a number of dry ski slopes around the country which, as well as providing useful practice, can provide interesting sport in themselves.

English Ski Council
Area Library Building, Queensway Mall, The Cornbow, Halesowen, West Midlands B63 4AJ (Tel: 021-501 2314).

The Ski Council will be glad to send you a booklet, *Nordic Skiing*, which provides information on Nordic Clubs affiliated to the ESC, as well as details of where to buy or hire equipment. Information is also given on commercial facilities, schools and tour operators offering nordic skiing.

Ski Council of Wales
240 Whitchurch Road, Cardiff CF4 3ND (Tel: 0222-619637).

Mostly Alpine skiing, but there is some Nordic skiing in the Brecon area. All the ski slopes in Wales cater for older people. The Council will be glad to send you a leaflet, *Skiing in Wales*, which, as well as giving general information, also provides information on affiliated ski centres.

Membership fee for individuals is £7.50 per year. All members receive the *Ski Council of Wales Newsletter*.

=▶ *Scottish National Ski Council*
Caledonia House, South Gyle, Edinburgh EH12 9DQ (Tel: 031-317 7280).

Individuals can become Association Members of the SNSC or they can join a club. Benefits of membership can include: advice on equipment, ski schools, safety, organised club weekends, use of clubhouses and mountain huts.

=▶ *Northern Ireland Ski Council*
Secretary: Sarah Eames, 61 Warrenpoint Road, Nistrevan, Co. Down (Tel: 06937-38835).

Peter White, Chair, writes 'Skiing can be enjoyed by all ages from 5 to 85 and we therefore welcome any enquiry from older people regarding local facilities. We are mostly concerned with Alpine skiing at present but could advise on Nordic in appropriate cases.'

=▶ *The British Ski Club for the Disabled*
Springmount, Berwick St John, Shaftesbury, Dorset SB7 OHQ (Tel: 0747-828515).

The Club was formed to provide skiing facilities for disabled people. It is affiliated to the English Ski Council, the Ski Club of Great Britain and the British Sports Association for the Disabled.

Special training is often necessary and facilities and equipment have to be suitable if the maximum benefit and proficiency are to be achieved. The Club has sessions at ski centres in Britain and acts as an information and advisory centre to all interested in cross country (Nordic) and downhill (Alpine) skiing, sledging and skating. Skiing holidays are arranged annually.

Instructors and guides are always required, so the Club welcomes and needs able-bodied members willing to qualify. Membership per annum: individuals £10; family £15; affiliation £20.

Square dancing

=▶ *British Association of American Square Dance Clubs*
c/o Carole Last, 21 Baronsmead Road, High Wycombe, Buckinghamshire HP12 3PQ (Tel: 0494-439961).

Throughout the United Kingdom there are 206 clubs which meet weekly and hold special Saturday evening/weekend dances. Modern Californian-style square dancing is taught throughout, together with round dancing (a cross between ballroom and modern sequence). There are no standard charges and attendance fees are very inexpensive (about £1 to £1.50 per weekday night, up to £2 to £3 per Saturday night). The age range can be from under 16 to 80 plus.

Swimming

Amateur Swimming Association
Harold Fern House, Derby Square, Loughborough LE11 0AL (Tel: 0509-230431).

ASA is the National Governing Body for Swimming in England and has some 1,700 affiliated swimming clubs. A special awards scheme has been developed, the Swim Fit Award, with the adult in mind. Details of this award are available from the ASA. It is recommended that you should progress gradually with a gentle approach. There should be no feeling of acute discomfort either during or following a session. First sessions should last only for short durations; 20 minutes will be sufficient, gradually building up to approximately one hour if you feel you are able. To gain an award you would need to fill in a log card which you can obtain from the ASA Awards Centre, 1 Kingfisher Enterprise Park, 50 Arthur Street, Redditch, Worcestershire B98 8LG (Tel: 0800-220292 or 0527-514288).

Handicapped Divers Association
64 Stroud Crescent, London SW15 3EJ (Tel: 081-789 5158).

People with a wide range of disabilities are enjoying diving and swimming. For further details and for a copy of the newsletter *Sink and Swim* write to the above address.

Scottish Amateur Swimming Association
Holmhills Farm, Greenlees Road, Cambuslang, Glasgow G72 8DT (Tel: 041-641 8818).

The SASA is the parent body for amateur swimming in Scotland. It also comprises 165 Amateur Swimming Clubs in Scotland and covers competitive swimmers, synchro swimmers, water polo, diving, long distance swimming, and Masters swimming.

Welsh Amateur Swimming Association
Wales Empire Pool, Wood Street, Cardiff CF1 1PP (Tel: 0222-342201).

Tennis

The Veterans' Lawn Tennis Association of Great Britain
3 Gainsborough Road, London W4 1NJ (Secretary Valerie Walley).

One of the aims of the Association is to promote National, County and other championships and competitions for veterans. Events are held for singles and doubles in different age groups from 40 upwards. The affiliation fee for a club having over 12 bona-fide members over the minimum ages of 40 (women) and 45 (men) and having a name of which the Council approves is £10. A booklet listing the clubs, laying out the constitution and describing the events both at home and abroad is available to members.

Short tennis

This is using the skills of lawn tennis on a smaller scale. Special rackets and balls are used. Apart from a simplified points-only form of scoring and larger service areas, the rules are the same as for tennis. It is played indoors or out on a badminton-size court and with specially produced rackets, balls and nets. An information bulletin entitled *All You Need to Know about Short Tennis* is available from the respective associations listed below. It includes a list of local Short Tennis organisers. However, because Short Tennis was first developed for children as a practical way of introducing them to tennis, the information only refers to children. Nevertheless, we are informed that older people certainly do use the facilities and your local Leisure Centre or your local Short Tennis organiser will be able to tell you about facilities.

The Scottish Lawn Tennis Association
12 Melville Crescent, Edinburgh EH3 7LU (Tel: 031-225 1284).

The Lawn Tennis Association Trust
Short Tennis Department, Queen's Club, West Kensington, London W14 9EG (Tel: 071-385 4233).

Welsh Lawn Tennis Association
National Sports Centre for Wales, Sophia Gardens, Cardiff CF1 9SW (Tel: 0222-371838).

Irish Tennis Association
54 Wellington Road, Ballsbridge, Dublin 4 (Tel: 01-681841).

London theatres and concerts

Theatre and Concert Travel Club
PO Box 1, St Albans, Hertfordshire AL1 4ED (Tel: 0727-41115).

As a member, one telephone call allows you to discuss the shows or concert halls and book seats for any number of theatres or concert halls at the box office price or less. We are informed that there are hundreds of performances on which discounts are available. Also that staff are chosen for their interest in theatre and music and are happy to talk about the shows, as well as answer the hundred-and-one questions about theatre seat locations, how far the theatre or concert hall is from the underground station, what time the show ends, and places to eat. At the same time you can book your discounted rail tickets and sleeper tickets, and reserve seats if you wish. The Club can also book a hotel at discounted prices.

The Club provides a bi-monthly newsletter and Theatre Guide. For a monthly supplement you can receive the monthly Barbican Centre, South Bank Concert Halls and Wigmore Hall Diaries. Annual subscription £12/£15 including Diaries. You can also obtain discounts on overseas holidays and flights.

Windsurfing

▶ *Senior and Veteran Windsurfers Association – SEAVETS*
Secretary: Dennis Heywood, 34 Nash Grove Lane, Wokingham, Berkshire RG11 4HD (Tel: 0734-734634).

SEAVETS is affiliated to the Royal Yachting Association. It aims to encourage the not-so-young of all levels from beginners to advanced sailors to enjoy the challenge of windsurfing. In 1991 SEAVETS organised 31 sailing days of events, and took part in many national events. SEAVETS supports 'Research Into Ageing', which funds research into the disabilities of old age. Membership for Seniors (over 34), Veterans (over 49) and Supervets (over 59) is £8 a year or £11 for couples. The emphasis of their activities is enjoyment. It is usual for those who feel tired to drop out, and everyone still has a good day. The oldest member is 80 and he still enjoys racing. There are 350 members, 100 of whom are women and nearly 70 of whom are Supervets. A few non-windsurfing members like to go along and help.

Writing

Most areas have 'Writing Circles' where both new and experienced writers join together to encourage each other and to enjoy the pleasure of writing. Your local library will be able to give you details. There may also be evening or day classes in writing – again your local library would be able to give you information. In addition, some open learning colleges provide courses. For more information about open learning see Section 10. One such college is the National Extension College: *see* below.

▶ *National Extension College*
18 Brooklands Avenue, Cambridge CB2 2HN (Tel: 0223-316644).

The NEC Creative Writing course is aimed at anyone who wants to develop – or discover – his or her skills as a creative writer. It covers all the essential writing skills and helps the student to apply these to a wide range of different types of writing. At each stage, imaginatively chosen activities encourage students to develop their powers of self-expression and self-criticism, analyse and express their own experiences, communicate their ideas effectively in writing, and develop their own writing style. An accompanying audio tape features discussions with experienced writers and with a group of creative writing students – samples of whose work are included in the course. The course emphasises the unique pleasure and self-development to be gained from writing creatively. Price: £195 with tutor support.

Helpful organisations

=▶ *Age Concern England*
Astral House, 1268 London Road, London SW16 4ER (Tel: 081-679 8000).

=▶ *Age Concern Scotland*
54A Fountainbridge, Edinburgh EH3 9PT (Tel: 031-228 5656).

=▶ *Age Concern Wales*
4th Floor, 1 Cathedral Road, Cardiff, South Glamorgan CF1 9SD (Tel: 0222-371 566).

=▶ *Age Concern Northern Ireland*
6 Lower Crescent, Belfast BT7 1NR (Tel: 0232-245729).

Age Concern groups are established throughout the United Kingdom. As well as other services they provide welcome club facilities for older local people. In many parts of the country, Age Concern groups have also set up Pop-ins. These are open to local older people who may not want to join a club or formal group but who welcome the chance to meet others of their own age in an informal setting. Some Pop-ins have an emphasis on health and keeping fit – some run regular keep fit exercises, others provide facilities for the game of indoor bowls. Some local groups regularly have tea dances. Other activities in some groups include: archery, art classes, carpet bowls, cookery (some classes for men on their own), drama/play readings, keep fit classes, music, photography, poetry, table tennis, Tai Chi, self defence, yoga, snooker, cards, dominoes and darts.

The above national addresses will be able to give you details of your nearest group but will be unlikely to know what activities there are as every group is completely autonomous.

Age Concern England has a fact sheet, *Leisure Education*, giving information on local and national resources as well as special interest and study holidays, and a further reading list. To obtain a copy send a 6" × 9" s.a.e. to the address above.

=▶ *Age Resource*
1268 London Road, London SW16 4ER (Tel: 081-679 2201).

Age Resource aims to encourage projects and activities which involve the creative potential and participation of older people at all levels of community need and in all endeavours. The new annual Age Resource Awards identify such activities which have benefited the community. The best of the entries in each of the main categories in 1991/92 received £1,000 to devote to its activity or project as well as recognition and publicity for its achievements.

A newsletter is available which gives information on a wide range of activities, and the Awards brochure provides details of the award-winning activities and projects. Both make a wonderful read and provide an insight into the imaginative range of activities in which older people are involved.

Beth Johnson Leisure Association
Parkfield House, 64 Princes Road, Hartshill, Stoke-on-Trent ST4 7JL (Tel: 0782-44036).

Although this organisation is locally active only in North Staffordshire, and we normally only include information for national organisations, we felt our readers would be interested in the activities, especially because they are led by retired people, and because they may act as a model to copy elsewhere – Beth Johnson would be glad to give information.

The Beth Johnson Leisure Association is an organisation run by retired people. Its aim is 'to promote and maintain a spirit of comradeship among the members and to promote and encourage activities for recreation in order to improve the quality of life of people aged 50 years and over'.

There is a nominal membership fee. Swimming instruction is given at five pools. Some, never having tried to swim before, have gained certificates for their first completed width and then for a length. There is a rambling section, offering weekly walks of 10, 6 and 4 miles in the beautiful countryside surrounding Newcastle and the Potteries area. In the summer the ramblers go further afield at regular periods to walk around other beauty spots. Members join together for badminton, outdoor bowls and Keep-Fit. There are also social events – barn dances, coach trips, theatre outings, slide shows and other get-togethers. In the spring and autumn holidays are taken together, mainly in England. Also, specifically for the ramblers, there is a walking holiday in Wales in early summer. Anyone can ask for other activities to be provided and all requests are considered.

The British Sports Association for the Disabled
34 Osnaburgh Street, London NW1 3ND (Tel: 071-383 7277).

The BSAD exists to bring the joys of sport and physical recreation to people, young and old, with many different kinds of disability, who may not have thought they could experience them. The BSAD helps to inform statutory and voluntary agencies of what is already done in many sports and activities for disabled people and what still needs to be done. The BSAD is recognised by the Government and the Sports Council as the co-ordinating body for all types of sport for all types of disablement.

The BSAD has representatives throughout the country organising regional sport, and these agents are always glad to advise and instruct, and will arrange talks and lectures to clubs.

Support is given to local authorities and other bodies to form new sports clubs for disabled people to encourage integration into existing able-bodied sports clubs. For further details and advice on aids and equipment for sporting activities write direct to the above address.

The Countrywide Holidays Association
Birch Heys, Cromwell Range, Manchester M14 6HU (Tel: 061-225 1000).

Special interest holidays include: bird watching, bridge, crafts, dancing, food, homes, gardens and flowers, health and fitness, heritage and the countryside, history, music, painting, photography, railways and walking. For further details of Countrywide Holidays *see* page 311.

► *Dark Horse Venture*
Kelton, Woodlands Road, Liverpool L17 OAN (Tel: 051-729 0092).

The Dark Horse Venture for retired people over 60 is an exciting and totally novel idea. It has been created by Mary Thomas to help older people realise their hidden abilities and talents. It aims to provide new opportunities for individuals to try completely new activities, all of which are totally non-competitive, and to support them in their endeavours.

All you have to do is select an activity you have never tried before and become involved in it on a regular basis for just twelve months. During this time you will be able to benefit from the guidance and advice of a person of your choice – someone who has professional training or experience in the activity you have chosen. To enter you simply purchase a Personal Journal that contains details of what to do and space to record your achievements.

Dark Horse Venture Certificates are awarded on the basis of progress and performance for each activity. There is no limit to the number of single subject certificates that you can enter and win. Those who have been awarded one certificate from each of the three activity categories can apply for the Gold Seal Certificate. The three activity categories are as follows:

- Giving and sharing – practical help – dog-walking, flower arranging, shopping, staffing hospital canteens, fund raising, sharing skills with young people, qualifying in First Aid, Life-saving, etc.
- Learning and doing – acting, collecting, cooking, drawing, decorating, fishing, gardening, investing, playing a musical instrument, singing, talking, writing, etc.
- Exploring and exercising – bowling, dancing, playing, rambling, swimming, travelling, etc.

► *Disabled Living Foundation*
380–4 Harrow Road, London W9 2HU (Tel: 071-289 6111).

► *Disability Scotland*
Information Department, 5 Shandwick Place, Edinburgh EH2 4RG (Tel: 031-229 8632).

► *Disability Action*
2 Annadale Avenue, Belfast BT7 3JR (Tel: 0232-491011).

These three organisations have information on aids and equipment which can help older people with disabilities to continue to enjoy the leisure opportunities of their choice.

They will be glad to advise. They can also provide information on organisations concerned with particular sports, arts and leisure activities which provide special facilities for people with disabilities. Further details of these and of Disabled Living Centres are given in Section 4.

▸ *LinkAge*
237 Pentonville Road, London N1 9NJ (Tel: 071-278 6601).

LinkAge aims to develop and foster links between the alternating generations: between young and old. Older people and children are brought together in a range of activities for them to mutually enjoy each other's company and to form special friendships. In one of the projects, older volunteers have taken their skills into the classroom. Individual children or small groups are taught to knit, sew, cook or to plant small gardens. These are skills that many people learn from their grandparents, but for some children contact with natural grandparents is impossible or rare.

At present LinkAge projects exist in: Oxfordshire and Tower Hamlets (London). In addition, a Foster Grandparent Scheme is being considered in the United Kingdom, similar to the American model which brings older people to the aid of children with special needs.

A LinkAge Training and Information Pack is being produced as a method of disseminating the organisation's experience to those who are interested. The Information Section will equip the subscriber with the kind of information that will enable him or her to start a project with confidence. Contents include: Video Film; Story Tape; Activity Work Sheets; A Book List; National Curriculum Guidelines; Elderly People as Volunteers in Schools; How to Use Local Agencies and Resources.

To find out if there may be a project coming to your area, or if you would like to start a project, or if you would just like more information – contact LinkAge.

▸ *REMAP GB – Technical Equipment for Disabled People*
Hazeldene, Ightham, Sevenoaks, Kent TN15 9AD (Tel: 0732-883818).

Local REMAP panels of voluntary engineers, occupational therapists, etc. are much concerned with aids to assist in leisure activities. Local panels have helped people with disabilities to enjoy playing musical instruments, to take part in sporting activities and to engage in a wide range of leisure opportunities with the aids that have been custom-made for individuals. Aids have been devised to (for example) help an ice-axe user with a weak hand via an ice-axe specially strengthened to take the holding straps and vital cross-piece; to help individuals to play snooker; to make it possible for a man in his wheelchair to go on smoking his pipe when he could no longer hold it safely. Extra-large chess pieces have been made, and a life-long player of the French horn has been enabled to continue playing despite muscular deterioration which was preventing her from supporting the weight of the instrument.

▸ *Royal National Institute for the Blind*
224 Great Portland Street, London W1N 6AA (Tel: 071-388 1266).

The RNIB would be glad to advise blind and partially sighted people how they can take up or continue to enjoy a broad range of sporting and leisure activities. The RNIB links up with other organisations for activity holidays and other events.

The RNIB, together with Age Concern England, has produced a booklet, *The Age of Adventure*, providing health advice and leisure opportunities for older people with a visual impairment. It gives information on a wide range of leisure activities, from reading to rambling, wood carving to gardening. The guide points out that sight loss combined with being older does not mean the end of a fulfilled and busy life. With the right support and, for some, special equipment, retirement can, in fact, be the age of adventure. Price: £1.50. For further information contact the RNIB Sports and Recreation Officer.

Saga
Freepost, Folkestone, Kent CT20 1BR.

Saga, well known for its extensive range of holidays – described in the next section – also produces a range of books. One of these is the *Saga Leisure Guide* by Ray Johnstone. Published by Unwin Hyman Limited. Price: £3.50. A wide range of ideas is explored in this book, including caravanning, weekend breaks, university courses, charity work and new sports and pastimes. The author discusses staying fit and healthy so that you can enjoy all these activities, as well as the possibilities of working after retirement. Also included are a great many useful addresses.

Scottish Retirement Council
204 Bath Street, Glasgow G2 4HL (Tel: 041-332 9427).

The Council is concerned with promoting occupational activities for retired people. It encourages young retired people to assume responsibility in organising and administering the activities of clubs and other services for older people. They become involved in the activities of the Crafts and Hobbies Centres, the Retired Employees' Association – run in connection with a number of industrial firms.

Sports Councils

The Sports Council
16 Upper Woburn Place, London WC1H OQP (Tel: 071-388 1277).

The Council has a campaign *50+ All to Play For*, aimed at encouraging older people to become more involved in sport and physical recreation. A booklet, *50+ All to Play For*, a manual of ideas and suggestions available from the Sports Council, describes how successful schemes can be organised and maintained and where help and advice can be sought. The Council says:

An involvement in physical activity, not only as a player but as a coach, official, secretary, helper in a club or manager of a youth football team, can be enjoyable and satisfying as well as contribute to health and physial well being.

Sport is interpreted in the widest sense, encompassing athletics and angling, darts and dance and much else. People over 50 have much to offer in terms of experience, expertise and enthusiasm. A habit formed in middle age can also lead to a more active and healthier old age.

Through the Campaign a wide range of activities has been enjoyed by those who are over 50, disproving the view that only certain activities are suitable. Land yachting, water skiing, boardsailing, roller skating, gliding, sub-aqua, basketball, snooker and skiing have all been sampled, proving that if the facilities are there older people will try them.

The Sports Council also arranges coaching courses and activity holidays. They will be glad to send you details.

A publications list is available.

The Sports Council for Northern Ireland
House of Sport, Upper Malone Road, Belfast BT9 5LA (Tel: 0232-381222).

The Council will be glad to advise you on activities, if you have been unable to find out information locally.

Scottish Sports Council
1 Caledonia House, South Gyle, Edinburgh EH12 9DQ (Tel: 031-317 7200).

The Council organises outdoor training courses at Aviemore for those who are over 50. Activities include: hill walking, natural history, rock climbing, Canadian canoeing and kayaking.

The Scottish Sports Council also has a range of literature which it will be glad to send to anyone interested in continuing or taking up any sporting activities. It will be glad to advise you where you can take up your particular interest.

Sports Council for Wales
The National Sports Centre for Wales, Sophia Gardens, Cardiff CF1 9SW (Tel: 0222-397571).

The Sports Centre itself has a very lively programme for over 50s which is enthusiastically attended and which includes badminton, swimming, table tennis, squash, modern sequence dancing and Keep Fit classes.

The Council also has a team of Development Officers throughout Wales who develop sporting activities for all age groups.

Townswomen's Guilds

Townswomen's Guilds
Chamber of Commerce House, 75 Harborne Road, Edgbaston, Birmingham B15 3DA (Tel: 021-456 3435).

Townswomen's Guilds offer a common meeting ground to all women who wish to broaden their knowledge and experience of life. They provide an opportunity to share mutual interests and increase the influence of women through a progressive, national organisation concerned with the fundamental issues of the community.

TG is for all women regardless of politics, race, age, religion or circumstances. Each of the 1990 Guilds is autonomous. Activities range from patchwork to parachuting; music, arts and crafts to drama and sport. Mandated by its National Conference, TG mounts a strong political lobby on national and regional issues. Resolutions on HIV/AIDS education in secondary schools, humane transportation of live animals and registration of donor drivers were debated and passed in 1991. Current concerns include the culmination of a campaign to plant five native broadleaved woodlands in Great Britain in association with the Woodland Trust, as well as the effects of the single European Market, and breast cancer. A playground safety campaign is under way, and various environmental projects are planned.

A lively magazine, *Townswoman*, is available, price 40p. Annual subscription: £7.

SECTION THIRTEEN

Holidays

It seems that there is no end to the variety of holidays available to all of us – that is if we can afford them. There is no reason that as older people we should necessarily take specially designed holidays for the older age group, but some may prefer to do so, and in this Section we mostly describe holidays designed with the older person in mind. Those who prefer to take their holidays in the mainstream of holiday provision as they always have will be able to get information from travel agents and advertisements. Some older people continue to take very adventurous holidays which they plan themselves without relying on any package tour operator.

Whatever our inclination, it is a great refreshment to our imaginations and to our bodies to have a break – to see new faces and places and to do different things – if we can possibly manage to get away.

We hope you will enjoy planning your next holiday. Why not send for a whole range of brochures before you decide exactly which holiday you are going to choose?

Railcards

Details of these are given in Section 11.

Insurance

Most holiday firms now include details of insurance as part of their package deals. Some may have exclusion clauses relating to age or to 'pre-existing medical conditions'. It is worth browsing through the brochures, not only for the best holiday, but also for the best insurance deal. We would recommend you read the small print carefully. If you have to arrange your own insurance you could try the company you already deal with for household insurance. We give details of a few firms who you could approach so that you can compare terms most suitable to meet your needs.

Age Concern Insurance Services
Garrod House, Chaldon Road, Caterham, Surrey CR3 5YZ (Tel: 0883-346964).

Age Concern has added a holiday travel insurance policy to its list of policies for people aged 60 or over.

Europ Assistance Ltd
Sussex House, Perrymount Road, Haywards Heath, West Sussex RH16 1DN (Tel: 0444-440 202).

Europ Assistance has added a new policy, called Senior Traveller, to its existing range of travel insurance services.

Senior Traveller has been specifically designed for those who are over 65. The policy offers special extra features beyond comprehensive Personal and Medical protection. As well as providing cover against medical expenses, repatriation, cancellation, lost or stolen baggage and money, public liability and personal accident, Senior Traveller will also help you if you lose your spectacles or passport, or have trouble with your booked accommodation. This product has been aimed at making worldwide and long-term European travel protection more affordable for those who are over 65, and there is no doubling or trebling of premiums without an improvement in benefits.

Europ Assistance continues to offer both Motoring Breakdown protection (called Personal Motoring Service in the United Kingdom and Premier Service on the Continent) and a variety of Travel Insurance services. The motoring products offer a rapid response to breakdowns via a network of 15,000 contracted garages spread throughout Europe, as well as car hire, accommodation and, if necessary, repatriation benefits.

Europ Assistance now waives medical certificate requirements for short-term motorists and travellers (within Europe) who are over 70 years of age. Anyone with a disability should contact Europ Assistance directly.

Extrasure Holdings Ltd
Lloyd's Avenue House, 6 Lloyd's Avenue, London EC3N 3AX (Tel: 071-480 6871/488 9341).

This firm specialises in insurance for business and holiday trips worldwide. For persons up to age 69 years, the Extrasure Complete Travel Insurance has no pre-existing medical condition exclusions, provided you are not travelling against a doctor's advice, nor for the purpose of obtaining medical treatment, and are not terminally ill at the time of booking your trip or the insurance is issued.

Persons over the age of 70 years are not covered for Cancellation or Medical in respect of any medical condition for which they have sought advice or received medical treatment in the six months immediately prior to the date the Insurance Certificate is issued. Persons over the age of 76 years are required to complete a Health Questionnaire before insurance can be arranged.

A 24-hour emergency telephone service is operated for the benefit of insured persons, so that, in the event of an emergency, particularly medical, help and advice can be given. If necessary, emergency repatriation will be arranged.

Holiday Care Service
2 Old Bank Chambers, Station Road, Horley, Surrey RH6 9HW (Tel: 0293-774535).

Holiday Care Service aims to provide competitive travel insurance, particularly for elderly and disabled people, their friends and family. The policy is specifically designed to cover most pre-existing medical conditions.

Benefits include: medical expenses (amount unlimited); additional hospital benefits up to £500; cancellation charges up to £2,000; travel delay up to £60; missed departure up to £500; personal property up to £1,000 in all; personal accident up to £15,000; personal liability up to £1,000,000 including costs.

Exclusions include the following: each insured person must pay the first £25 of any claim in respect of cancellation, curtailment, medical expenses, personal baggage and personal money; property stolen from an unattended vehicle; permanent total disablement for insured persons aged over 70; travel contrary to medical advice.

For further details of the Holiday Care Service *see* page 319.

Saga's Insurance Service

Saga arranges good insurance cover through the Norwich Union for its very wide range of holidays. There is no upper age limit. You can insure yourself against personal accident, medical expenses up to £1 million, luggage loss and personal liability. Also included: cover against extended cancellation; missed departure; legal expenses; and the reimbursement of reasonable additional accommodation and travel expenses incurred owing to interruption of scheduled public transport or accident/mechanical failure to the car in which you are travelling, causing you to miss your booked UK departure.

C.R. Toogood & Co. Ltd
Duncombe House, Ockham Road North, East Horsley, Leatherhead, Surrey KT24 6NX (Tel: 048-65 4181).

This company informs us that it has facilities for placing travel insurance on a worldwide basis in the company market, without exclusion of pre-existing medical conditions. However, premiums double for holidaymakers over 70. Leaflets and details of cover and rates together with proposal forms are available on request. Cover includes sections for baggage and personal effects, personal liability, cancellation or curtailment, personal accident, and medical and other expenses.

Medical treatment overseas

Sickness Benefit during a temporary visit to a member country of the European Community

Most UK citizens, covered by the UK National Insurance scheme, and their dependants, are entitled to immediately necessary medical treatment if they become ill while visiting another EC country. Persons covered by the regulations who are on holiday or otherwise staying temporarily in a Community country will be entitled to medical treatment for sickness or accidents which require urgent attention on the same basis as insured nationals of that country.

It must be borne in mind, however, that treatment available in the Community countries is that provided under their own domestic legislation, and in some but not all of them persons receiving medical treatment have to pay part of the cost. Medical benefits available under these schemes are dependent upon certain insurance conditions.

To get emergency medical treatment while you are in an EC country, you will need to complete an application form and a certificate of entitlement form (E111) which is attached to leaflet T2 (obtainable from post offices). When completed, you hand the forms into the post office where the counter officer will stamp and sign the E111 and give it back to you. You must take this with you when you travel.

Leaflet T2, *Health Advice for Travellers Inside the European Community*, contains information about preparations you should make before travelling to an EC country as well as how to get emergency medical treatment in each of the EC countries if you fall ill while you are there.

Travelling to countries outside the European Community

The United Kingdom has made arrangements with some countries for urgently needed medical treatment to be provided at reduced cost, or, in some cases, free. The range of medical care available outside European Community countries is, however, often less than that provided by the NHS in Britain and, in some countries, some charges are made. Only urgently needed medical treatment will be provided, and you will only receive care on the same terms as residents of the country visited. The Department of Health cannot refund any medical costs incurred abroad. The type of treatment available and the documents required to obtain treatment in particular, as well as details of charges, are listed in Leaflet T3 for the following countries: Anguilla, Australia, Austria, British Virgin Islands, Bulgaria, Channel Islands, Czechoslovakia, the Falkland Islands, Finland, Hong Kong, Hungary, Iceland, Isle of Man, Malta, Monserrat, New Zealand, Norway, Poland, Romania, St Helena, Sweden, Turks and Caicos Islands, some countries in the former USSR, and former Yugoslavia.

Leaflet T3 (formerly T1), *Health Advice for Travellers Outside the European Community*, provides information and advice on considerations before you go abroad, and while you are away. It gives information on precautions you can take against a number of diseases including available vaccinations, and gives details of specific disease risk areas. It also provides information on how certain diseases are caught. The listed diseases are: HIV/AIDS, cholera, viral hepatitis A, viral hepatitis B, malaria, poliomyelitis, rabies, tetanus, tuberculosis, typhoid and yellow fever. Leaflet T3 can be obtained by phoning (free of charge) 0800 555 777.

Vaccination Certificate Requirements for International Travel and Health Advice to Travellers is published annually by the World Health Organisation and available from HMSO Books, 51 Nine Elms Lane, London SW8 5DR (Tel: 071-873 0011). Price: £5.75 including postage and packing.

This is an official handbook intended for those who have to advise travellers regarding the risks they might encounter when visiting other countries. The information is detailed and therefore not for the casual traveller who does not venture far afield. However, for the adventurous among us, it makes interesting armchair reading as well as providing practical information covering, in addition to vaccination requirements, some health risks to which travellers may be subject including environmental effects, risks from food and drink, sexually transmitted diseases, and hazards from insects and animals; geographical distribution of health hazards to travellers in Africa, the Americas, Asia, Europe and Oceania; precautions against certain diseases and injuries.

Your pension and going abroad

See Section 1.

Holidays with specialist organisations

Carefree Holidays Ltd
64 Florence Road, Northampton NN1 4NA (Tel: 0604-34301/30382).

These are holidays designed primarily for people who are over 55 and their friends both in the United Kingdom and abroad. Holidaymakers range from the fit and active who want a holiday without the hassle of having to organise everything themselves to those who are less able, perhaps no longer able to climb stairs or carry luggage, those on their own or holidaying for the first time after a bereavement. People with a disability are welcome, either alone or with family and friends. (The term disabled is used in its widest sense to cover not only those who use a wheelchair but also those who use walking aids, have problems with sight or hearing or need certain facilities – that is, the provision of oxygen during the holiday, insulin injections, etc.

A Door to Door service, at no extra charge, is offered for those living in the county of Northamptonshire, Leicester, Market Harborough and on selected holidays in the Oxford and Newbury areas.

Experienced Tour Escorts accompany each holiday and are on hand to deal with luggage, organise excursions and provide practical assistance or advice to anyone in the party while at the same time encouraging people to enjoy their holiday to the full in whatever way they choose.

Accommodation is varied, from homely family-run guest houses and small hotels to prestigious sea-front hotels and top class holiday villages. Holidays are also arranged over Christmas. A range of 'Short Breaks' has been added to the programme, with prices from £108 for five days' full board in popular holiday villages.

On all continental coach tours and on many holidays in the United Kingdom luxury coaches with side lifts are used for easy access. On air tours, taxis and conventional coaches are usually used, but assistance is available on boarding.

A fully comprehensive insurance scheme with no age limits or pre-existing condition exclusion clauses is available.

Prices vary from £108 for five days' full board at a holiday village to £554 for a twelve day tour to Paris and the French Riviera.

Saga Holidays Ltd

The Saga Building, Middelburg Square, Folkestone, Kent CT20 1AZ (Tel: SAGA Holiday Advisers (all calls are free) – United Kingdom, Europe and Mediterranean: 0800-300 500; Cruises: 0800-300 400; Travellers World, America and Canada: 0800-414 383; Saga Flights Service: 0800-414 444).

This firm specialises in providing holidays for people who are over 60. Holidays are arranged direct with the holidaymaker, cutting out the travel agent. This means that Saga is able to provide a personal service. Saga will also arrange insurance.

Saga has its own Saga Magazine Club which you can join for an annual subscription of £10.90 for ten issues. The aim is to help people make the most of maturity. The advantages of belonging to the club include savings on selected holidays, a penfriends and partnership service, and free information sheets explaining tax changes and pension rights. The magazine itself is also a very interesting read, having a wide variety of articles as well as holiday information.

There is a range of brochures available covering a wide choice of holidays, These include:

– University and College Centres.
– Short Breaks.
– Europe and the Mediterranean.
– Travellers World, including holidays to: Borneo, Australia, New Zealand, China and the Far East, Kenya, India, Nepal, South America, Egypt, South Africa, Namibia, the Seychelles, Mauritius, Jamaica, Barbados, Iceland, Greenland, Thailand, Bali, Indonesia, Sri Lanka, Malaysia.
– USA.
– Canada.
– The Saga Cruise Collection.
– European Highlights.

- Coach Holidays in Britain and Ireland.
- Great British Touring Centres.
- The Great British Collection, including hotel holidays, holidays at universities and college centres, coach tours in Britain and Ireland, Great British Touring Centres.
- Great Britain, including holidays afloat, Channel Islands, Voyage of the Vikings, Christmas holidays.
- Singles holidays.
- Saga Arts and Special Interest Holidays. Typical holidays have included: Boston Cultural Tour, Harrogate Spring Festival, Bath Festival, Exeter Festival, Bournemouth Festival, Three Spires Festival, Three Choirs Festival, Music and Country Houses, Music and Gardens, Welsh National Opera, Cities of Music Vienna and Salzburg. Also special interest holidays for the following: anniversaries, antique appreciation, ballet, bowls, bridge, creative writing, cycling in Holland, dancing, film, gardens and gardening, healthy living, music, opera, painting, photography, scrabble, walking, whist.
- Saga holiday villages.
- Saga study holidays – for details of these see Section 10.

Saga also has a number of books, including Saga Retirement Guides (£3.50 each and available in bookshops): *Saga Health Guide*, *Saga Rights Guide*, *Saga Money Guide*, *Saga Property Guide*, *Saga Healthy Eating Guide*, *Saga Leisure Guide*.

Winged Fellowship
Angel House, 20–32 Pentonville Road, London N1 9XD (Tel: 071-833 2594).

This organisation provides holidays and respite care for severely physically disabled people at five UK centres and overseas. Full care is provided if the carer does not wish to accompany the guest, and daily outings and evening entertainment are arranged. A team of trained staff and 4,000 volunteers a year from 16 to 75 years of age care for the guests.

Centres are in Southport, Nottingham, Chigwell, Redhill and Southampton. In addition, small groups of nine or so go on overseas holidays accompanied by a courier and tour operator. In 1992, the new 'Discovery' holidays were launched. These provide a low budget UK alternative for the more adventurous.

Winged Fellowship also run a series of special weeks for people who have Alzheimer's Disease and their carers.

Young at Heart holidays
Department of Tourism and Attractions, 1 Clifton Street, Blackpool FY1 1LY (Tel: 0253-25212).

During May and June, for certain periods, there are discounts available to holidaymakers who are over 55 years and staying for three nights or more in holiday accommodation in Blackpool. The discounts are off Blackpool Borough Council facilities (the Tower, the piers, waxworks, etc.); accommodation; and other facilities. For details, contact the above address.

Special interest holidays and courses

A wide range of special interest and educational courses is available (we describe a few below), including some with facilities for anyone with a disability. Details of these are published every January and August in *Time to Learn* by the National Institute of Adult Continuing Education, 19B De Montfort Street, Leicester LE1 7GE (Tel: 0533-551451). Price: £3.95 inclusive of postage and packing.

Subjects covered include: painting, music, crafts, yoga, cookery, wine tasting, china restoration, sociology, realising self-esteem, caring for antiques, modern languages, folk interests, pottery, arts, history, social science, flower arranging, archaeology, literature, education, gardening, architecture, photography, nature studies, writing, lace making and film making.

See also details of the English Tourist Board's guide *Let's Go!* on page 320. This has details of special interest short breaks from flying and gliding to golf and bridge, from birdwatching to classical music and vintage car excursions, and many more.

Arts

NADFAS Tours Ltd
Hermes House, 80/89 Beckenham Road, Beckenham, Kent BR3 4RH
(Tel: 081-658 2308).

NADFAS (The National Association of Decorative and Fine Arts Societies) arranges tours in the United Kingdom and abroad exclusively for NADFAS members and their families and friends. All tours have a high artistic, cultural or educational ingredient and, with high standards, are good value for money. They are led by an organiser and accompanied by a lecturer. NADFAS Tours covenants its profits to the parent organisation to help fund sponsorship or projects in keeping with the aims of the Association.

Tours in 1992 included: Study of Porcelain, The Brontë Country, The Isle of Wight, King's Lynn and North Norfolk, Anglesey and the tip of Wales, Splendours of the Lake District, Garden Festival and Welsh Valleys, Castles of Mar and Balmoral, Buildings of Delight/Chichester, Isle of Man, Land of the Prince Bishops, Great Houses of Derbyshire, Perth – Heart of Scotland, Island of Jersey. Tours abroad have included artistic centres throughout Europe, as well as Egypt, Thailand, Canada, Oman.

For further details of NADFAS and how to become a member *see* page 263.

Countryside and environment

BTCV (British Trust for Conservation Volunteers)
Room RS, 36 St Mary's Street, Wallingford, Oxfordshire OX10 0EU
(Tel: 0491-39766).

BTCV's Natural Break programme of conservation working holidays enables nearly 6,000 volunteers of all ages to spend a week in a spectacular setting, learning new and challenging conservation skills from the repair of drystone walls to the construction of steps and stiles. Around 600 holidays take place throughout the country, offering a great opportunity for individuals to make a practical contribution to the protection of the environment. Prices start at around £29 a week including food, simple accommodation and all training. A free brochure is available from the address above – a 48p stamp would be appreciated.

Ordinary membership costs £10, with concessions for retired people at £5.50.

The Countrywide Holidays Association
Birch Heys, Cromwell Range, Manchester M14 6HU (Tel: 061-225 1000).

This is a non-profit-distributing organisation aiming to provide good country holidays, not in hotels, but in a country house which was built to take advantage of a lovely location. For 100 years the Association has sought to provide value for money holidays to country lovers. You may stay in a castle, an Elizabethan manor or in one of a number of Victorian mansions. You may not have the frills of a luxury hotel but this may be more than made up for by the country house atmosphere where there will be lots of activities.

Special interest holidays include: bird watching; bridge; crafts; dancing; food; homes, gardens and flowers; health and fitness; heritage and the countryside; history; music; painting; photography; railways; walking. Price: around £200 for full board for a week.

Countrywide Holidays are also arranged abroad. Some of these are walking holidays where the walking is graded: hard, strenuous, moderate, easier mountain walking, and easy. There are also adventure and discovery holidays, and others for special interests.

In addition to the holiday programmes there are Countrywide Holidays Association Clubs in over a hundred principal cities and towns throughout the country. Weekly social programmes include rambles, weekends at centres and dances.

Kindrogan Field Centre
Enochdhu, Blairgowrie, Perthshire PH10 7PG (Tel: 0250-21 286).

The Centre is a Victorian estate house converted to provide comfortable accommodation with laboratory, library, lounge and bar facilities. Within a reasonable distance is an impressive range of habitats from rich pasture and woodland in the valley to heather moor and mountain tops over 3,000 ft. Slightly further afield is a great variety of highland and lowland countryside including loch, river, Caledonian forest of pine and birch, intensive modern agriculture and undisturbed plateau. The wildlife and plants of these include golden eagles and ptarmigan, wildcat and red deer, twinflower and spring gentian. The Centre will be glad to answer queries about other Field Study activities in Scotland. Prices about £200 for a week.

▸ *Peak National Park Centre*
Losehill Hall, Castleton, Derbyshire S30 2WB (Tel: 0433-620373).

Exploring the Peak District for the over 50s is a summer holiday which provides a chance to explore the beautiful Peak National Park in a leisurely way. These holidays combine visits, tours by coach and short strolls with an opportunity to take part in a variety of activities.

All Losehill Hall holidays offer an optional evening programme of talks and slide shows by guest speakers which are chosen to complement the daily programme.
Price: £259 for a week's programme.

In addition to the above programme, a wide range of subjects can be covered on holidays including: landscape painting and photography; great houses and gardens; walking; canals; learning more about mushrooms and toadstools; ferns; lichens; wildflowers, and so on.

▸ *YMCA National Centre*
Lakeside, Ulverston, Cumbria LA12 8BD (Tel: 05395-31758).

50 + Activity Holidays are arranged at YMCA Lakeside. Each participant can choose the activities that suit both interest and capability. Great care is taken to make sure that the various pursuits are conducted at your pace. Activity choices can include: fell walking; natural history; navigation and orienteering; archery; pony trekking; rock climbing; Canadian canoeing; and visits to places of interest such as Grizedale Forest, Stott Park Bobbin Mill and National Park Centre, Brockhole.

Plenty of options remain open during poor weather conditions. The evening programme includes crafts such as macrame, spinning and weaving, illustrated talks and films.

Vegetarians are catered for, as well as those needing special diets.
Price: £145 per person from Monday to Friday.

See also Saga on page 307, who arrange 'Gardens and Gardening' holidays; the Countrywide Holidays Association on page 311 for heritage and the countryside holidays.

Cycling

▸ *Cycling for Softies*
Susi Madron's Cycling Holidays Ltd, 2 and 4 Birch Polygon, Rusholme, Manchester M14 5HX (Tel: 061-224 0865).

These holidays are all in France. A great deal of concern and effort is put into matching the person with the holiday and the bicycle to ensure that the combination is just right. As they say, 'Some Susis [Softies] just love doing forty miles over hilly country, others just love doing ten miles on the flattest terrain we can find for them.' With your brochure you will receive a Holiday Planner to help you set down all your personal details and preferences for accommodation, choice of bicycle, etc. The price from approximately £390–£450 for 1 week includes: ferry or air fares; dinner, bed and breakfast; use of the bicycles and equipment; information packs, including maps, Susi Bags, Susi Guide and local information; and Representative's support.

Just Pedalling
9 Church Street, Coltishall, Norfolk NR12 7DW (Tel: 0603-737201).

The East Anglian countryside is relatively flat and ideal for cycling, with a wealth of quiet lanes, pretty villages and ancient churches. Age is no barrier in such conditions, providing you can ride a bicycle and are reasonably healthy. On all tours Just Pedalling provides: 7 nights' bed and breakfast accommodation, 3-speed touring cycle with lights, large luggage panniers, wet weather gear, cycle lock, basic repair kit, tools, brochures, booklets and maps. You will also be given descriptions and directions to your accommodation, which will be in a variety of guest houses located along the routes it offers. Usually in quiet villages and hamlets, they range from Elizabethan manor houses, flint cottages and working farms to real ale inns. There are various itineraries from which to choose, including a de luxe tour with accommodation in small halls originating from sixteenth-century houses of special interest. Prices range from £135 (low season) to £145 (high season) per person based on two people sharing a room.

See also Saga Holidays – Saga arranges cycling holidays in Holland.

See also the book *UK Activity Holidays* on page 316, which provides information on a number of holiday companies' cycling holidays.

Languages

British Institute of Florence
Palazzo Lanfredini, 9 Lungarno Guicciardini, 50125 Florence, Italy
(Tel: 010-39 055 284031).

The Institute, an officially sponsored joint Anglo-Italian institute of over 75 years' standing, runs 4–12 week graded Italian language courses throughout the year for learners of all ages and levels. There are also courses in English on the history of art and other subjects. Various events such as lectures and concerts are arranged by the Institute for students and local people. Accommodation can be arranged in local homes, pensioni and hotels: cost is from £11 per day. Teaching takes place in a thirteenth-century palazzo. Tuition fees vary according to the length and intensity of the course you choose: for example – £250 for 10 lessons a week for four weeks. The Florentine Renaissance courses (in English) last four weeks and cost £150. Discounts are offered for groups and for members of the University of the Third Age.

En Famille Overseas
The Old Stables, 60b Maltravers Street, Arundel, West Sussex BN18 9BG
(Tel: 0903-883266).

En Famille specialises in arranging individual visits to host families for people of all ages wishing to improve their knowledge of a foreign language. Such holidays can be arranged at any time of the year in many European countries including France, Germany, Italy and Spain. We are assured that many host families are pleased to accept senior citizens on an individual visit, who are also welcome at the house party centres. Every attention is paid to matching the intending visitor with the characteristics, background and interests of the host family. If you choose an individual visit you will be sent details of several suitable host families for you to indicate your preference.

En Famille also offers a range of language holidays in coaching or house party centres for adults at all levels, and intensive French home tuition where the host or hostess is a teacher. Special bargain prices apply at the North East France Centre and on the Tours Language Course. Prices at the Centre are approximately £127 per person per week, demi-pension, for families or couples with car; £148 per week for full board for guests without car, plus £31 per week for excursions and for being met.

Goethe-Institut
Postfach 800727, D-8000 München 90, Germany (Tel: 089-41868-200).

The Goethe-Institut has a range of language courses. There is also a special programme *Language, Culture and Leisure*, and it is this that was recommended to us as being particularly appropriate for older people. It is a four week course held at Staufen in the Black Forest. The language participants learn in small groups of 8 to 12 in these historic surroundings. There are plenty of leisure activities in the area, including: a wide range of sporting activities; taking part in the film programme at the institute; enjoying the varied cultural programme on offer in the nearby university town of Freiburg or in other cities such as Basle, Strasbourg or Stuttgart. Price: Just over £1,000 for the four week course including language course, accommodation, buffet breakfast and an extra-curricular cultural programme.

Music

Benslow Music Trust
Little Benslow Hills, Hitchin, Hertfordshire SG4 9RB (Tel: 0462-459446).

Benslow provides opportunities for the study and practice of music. There are weekend and other courses all the year for amateur players and singers. The programme covers chamber music, choral and solo singing, theory of music, Alexander Technique, jazz, piano, solo wind, and early music.

The standard fee for a weekend or two-day course is £67.50 with full board or £52.50 non-resident. Benslow now forms part of the EuroMusica network promoting an international programme of courses in France, Germany, Holland and Belgium.

See also Saga on page 307 and the Countrywide Holidays Association on page 311, who arrange music holidays.

Retreats

▶ *National Retreat Association (NRA)*
Liddon House, 24 South Audley Street, London W1Y 5DL (Tel: 071-493 3534).

The NRA is a federation of five denominational retreat groups – Anglican, Roman Catholic, Methodist, Baptist, and the United Reformed Church. An annual journal, *The Vision*, gives details of 160 Christian Retreat Houses in Britain and Ireland, and their programmes. Price: £2.50 including postage and packing. Free leaflets about different kinds of retreats are available on request.

Walking

▶ *HF Holidays Limited*
Imperial House, Edgware Road, London NW9 5AL (Tel: 081-905 9556).

This organisation specialises in walking and special interest holidays which can be enjoyed by all age groups. Especially suitable for the older holidaymaker are the HF Fellowship Weeks. These include gentle walks and rambles with coach excursions organised to places of local interest and beauty. HF houses aim to provide a special party atmosphere with a relaxing mix of fun, entertainment and good company. A Fellowship Week is designed to be equally enjoyable whether you go on your own or with a partner or friend.
Prices start from: £145 full board.

See also the publication *UK Activity Holidays* (page 316), Saga Holidays (page 307) and the Countrywide Holidays Association (page 311), who both provide walking holidays.

Publications

▶ *Central Bureau for Educational Visits and Exchanges*
Seymour Mews House, Seymour Mews, London W1H 9PE (Tel: 071-486 5101).

CBEVE have information on a wide range of educational and working holidays. We recommend you send for their publications list. We give details of two of their publications below:

1. *Working Holidays* – an international guide to seasonal job opportunities. This annual guidebook offers countless examples of ways to help protect the environment and restore our threatened heritage. From archaeology to yacht crewing, from Argentina to Zimbabwe, hundreds of employers in some 70 countries are listed, offering all kinds of paid and voluntary work. There are opportunities for all ages, lasting from a few days to a few months, available all year round. Price: £7.95 from bookshops or £8.95 from CBEVE.

2. *Home From Home* – an international guide to homestays, exchanges and term stays. If you're fed up with being herded around on package tours and want to find out what really makes another country tick, then why not try immersing yourself in another life-style, language and culture by staying with a family abroad? Or try swapping your home with a partner family to see what it's like to live just like them. A homestay or a home exchange treats you as a guest, a friend of the family, part of the local community. You can always reciprocate the hospitality by inviting the family back to your own home. This guide lists reputable agencies arranging stays in some fifty countries, and offers tips on making the most of your visit. Price: £6.99 from bookshops or £7.99 from CBEVE.

For details of *Study Holidays* from CBEVE, *see* page 244.

⇒ *RAC Activity Holiday Guide Great Britain and Ireland*
RAC Publishing, 39 Milton Park, Abingdon, Oxfordshire OX14 4TD (Tel: 0235-834885).

Whether it's excitement, fun and adventure you want, or a chance to develop your interests and talents, activity holidays offer you an opportunity to get the most value out of your breaks away. This new RAC guide helps you to find exactly the right holiday by providing detailed information on numerous activities and leisure pursuits in an attractive easy-to-use format. An informative introductory article describes the trends, opening up many new opportunities.
Price: £5.99 including postage and packing.

We recommend you also send for the RAC publications list with details of other holiday guides as well as map books.

⇒ *Royal Association for Disability and Rehabilitation*
25 Mortimer Street, London W1N 8AB (Tel: 071-637 5400).

The Association publishes two very good annual guides for people who have any form of disability: *Holidays for Disabled People* covering the United Kingdom (price: £4.50 including postage and packing) and *Holidays and Travel Abroad* (price: £3 including postage and packing). The UK guide includes a wealth of information on all kinds of holiday accommodation such as hotels, apartments, nursing homes and holiday centres, and grades the extent of their suitability to match an individual's needs. It contains a section on accommodation with nursing care. There are large sections on transportation, and activity holidays, as well as details of voluntary and commercial organisations involved in holiday provision for people with disabilities.

Holidays and Travel Abroad provides suggestions on planning and booking a holiday abroad. There is information on insurance, helpful voluntary organisations, sport and outdoor activity holidays/courses, transportation and international accommodation guides, as well as country-by-country information.

UK Activity Holidays
Published by Rosters Ltd, 23 Welbeck Street, London W1M 7PG
(Tel: 071-935 4550).

This guide brings together a wide range of activity holidays from all over England, Wales and Scotland. It covers holidays as diverse as mountaineering and watercolour painting, learning to drive and white water rafting. General headings include: cooking, crafts, cycling, flying, gardening, learning to drive, multi-activity holidays, riding, walking and watersports.

Each activity lists the various holiday companies which provide facilities in a wonderfully easy format. Each entry includes information on whether previous knowledge or experience is necessary, the cost per person, equipment guests would be expected to provide themselves, whether vegetarian meals are provided, and whether there is access for disabled people.
Price: £6.95.

Home exchange

Maybe you are tired of impersonal hotels and of having to conform to their way of doing things and would prefer to try staying in somebody else's home, in fact a home from home in another area in the UK or abroad. There are a number of agencies who may be able to help you and details of these are given in the book *Home From Home – see* 'Publications' above. We give details of one agency below to give a flavour of what you can expect.

Intervac
International Home Exchange Service, 6 Siddals Lane, Allestree, Derby DE3 2DY
(Tel: 0332-558931).

As the brochure says, Intervac unlocks the door to rent-free holidays worldwide. 'Swap homes, swap lifestyles' is their slogan. In 1991 they had 8,500 families joining from 45 countries. The application form seeks the sort of information which will help members to choose the kind of exchange best suited to their preferences. Included is a question about the suitability of a member's home for disabled visitors. It would then be up to an intending visitor to check that any facilities were in fact suitable for individual needs. Intervac was very positive that it wanted to encourage home exchanges which included those using wheelchairs or having mobility difficulties. All kinds of homes are offered, from modest bed-sitters to mansions.

Each year, Intervac publishes three Holiday Directories. Your details would be listed in one of these. You receive each of the three books as they are published. After publication of Book 3, a 'late exchange service' provides computer print-outs to anyone still looking for a holiday. Those offering accommodation which may be suitable for disabled people are indicated by the use of the wheelchair symbol. Holidays are arranged by contacting other members by telephone or letter. The international code used helps to reduce language problems, and, in any case, most members speak English. The annual membership fee is £43.

Holiday cottages and homes

▪▶ *Care Home Holidays Ltd*
Wern Manor, Porthmadog, Gwynedd LL49 9SH, Wales (Tel: 0766-513322).

Care Home Holidays have established a holiday network of specialist care homes capable of dealing with the special needs of older people. These are private homes and we understand that each home depicted in the brochure has been individually inspected. Prices range from about £150 to £295 a week.

▪▶ *Forestry Commission*
For information phone or write to: Forest Holidays (VI), 231 Corstophine Road, Edinburgh EH 12 7AT (Tel: 031-334 0303 during office hours; or 031-334 0066 – 24-hour answerphone).

You can spend a few days in a forest cabin or cottage or you can take your own caravan or tent to one of the Forestry Commission campsites. The various sites in England, Scotland and Wales blend in well with the surroundings and there are plenty of opportunities to enjoy outdoor activities, to suit everyone's tastes.

▪▶ *The National Trust*
36 Queen Anne's Gate, London SW1H 9AS (Tel: 071-222 9251).

The National Trust now has a wide variety of holiday cottages and houses in many areas of England, Wales and Northern Ireland with varying accommodation for 2 to 10 people. The Trust will be glad to send you a leaflet *Holiday Cottages*, which will give you the addresses of whom to contact in the area in which you are interested. The leaflet briefly describes the sort of accommodation available in each area, and also shows those which may be suitable for disabled people.

▪▶ *The National Trust for Scotland*
5 Charlotte Square, Edinburgh EH2 4DU (Tel: 031-226 5922).

Holiday accommodation is available in a variety of cottages and flats throughout Scotland. Information is given on sporting and leisure facilities in the area.

All properties are priced according to their style, size and situation, with prices varying according to the season. Details can be obtained from the Holiday Department at the above address.

The NTS also runs a variety of Thistle Camps, which help to conserve and maintain properties.

Helpful organisations

▶ *Association of British Travel Agents*
55–7 Newman Street, London W1P 4AH (Tel: 071-637 2444).

You would be well advised to seek out those travel agents who are members of ABTA, which means they will conform to a common code of practice. In the event of difficulties with your holiday arrangement made through a travel agent, and if the agent has proved uncooperative over a complaint, you may then approach the Consumer Affairs Department of ABTA, which will advise you on the options open for resolution of your dispute, including low cost, binding arbitration.

▶ *Age Concern England*
Astral House, 1268 London Road, London SW16 4ER (Tel: 081-679 8000).

▶ *Age Concern Wales*
4th Floor, 1 Cathedral Road, Cardiff CF1 9SD (Tel: 0222-371566/371821).

▶ *Age Concern Scotland*
54A Fountainbridge, Edinburgh EH3 9PT (Tel: 031-228 5656).

▶ *Age Concern Northern Ireland*
6 Lower Crescent, Belfast BT7 1NR (Tel: 0232-245729).

Some Age Concern local groups arrange annual holidays for their members. Contact your local group for details. The national offices above will be able to give you the address of your nearest group, but as each group is autonomous, the national offices are unlikely to know whether a particular group is involved in arranging holidays or not.

▶ *ARP Over 50 (The Association of Retired People Over 50)*
Greencoat House, Francis Street, London SW1P 1DZ (Tel: 071-895 8880; Travel Club Hotline 0800-585 871).

The ARP Over 50 Travel Club brings a range of services to members. By ringing the Hotline you can get expert travel advice, details about the latest holiday offers, and a comprehensive booking service. You can also get discounts on package arrangements provided by tour operators. For example, holidays with a value up to £700 would have a discount of 3.5 per cent; a holiday with a value between £1,501 and £2,500 would have a discount of 4.5 per cent. There are also discounts available on travel insurance, international air and charter flights and car hire, as well as domestic air and all ferries. For details of membership of ARP and other services *see* page 327.

▶ *Cruse – Bereavement Care*
Cruse House, 126 Sheen Road, Richmond, Surrey TW9 1UR
(Tel: 081-940 4818).

Holiday Ideas from Cruse – a selection of holidays specially compiled to help bereaved people find a holiday to suit their needs. Published annually (January) it is not specifically for older people, but nevertheless it is used a great deal by older members of Cruse to help them find holidays when they are on their own. Price: £2.35.

▸ *50 Forward*
The Manor House, 46 London Road, Blackwater, Camberley, Surrey GU17 0AA (Tel: 0276-34462).

This organisation provides discounts on a range of items including travel. For further information on *50 Forward* see page 338.

▸ *Holiday Care Service*
2 Old Bank Chambers, Station Road, Horley, Surrey RH6 9HW (Tel: 0293-774535).

This service has established itself as a most valuable resource, providing a wide range of free information and advice on holidays for people who are elderly or disabled, with low income, or who are lone parents or who are carers. The holiday information given may relate to: an independent hotel holiday in the Highlands; a self-catering cottage in Wales with boating and fishing; a package tour to Europe or the United States; or a holiday camp with activities and entertainments.

Holiday Care Service can help with travel insurance (for further information see the beginning of this section), transport information, where you may be able to get help with paying for a holiday, and names of organisations which can provide a short-term carer to go into the home. An extensive range of leaflets is available to enquirers. Holiday Care Service cannot, however, make reservations or bookings.

▸ *National Trust for the Welfare of the Elderly*
Kauri House, 33 Hook Road, Goole, North Humberside DN14 5JB (Tel: 0405-763149).

The Trust provides rent-assisted holidays for elderly people in self-catering chalets and mobile homes at Reighton and Withernsea.

▸ *Travel Companions (UK) Ltd*
110 High Mount, Station Road, London NW4 3ST (Tel: 081-202 8478).

This is a small group of people who have experienced the difficulties of travelling alone and have decided to do something about it. They run a service for people aged 30 to 75 who enjoy travel and who are looking for an agreeable companion. They say, 'Some people enjoy extended far-away holidays, others choose short breaks nearer home. Some like adventure and activity while others prefer leisure in the sun. What is important is to share the experience with another person of similar interests.'

The charge is £40 a year, and for this the group will put you in touch with members who have similar interests. In addition, it can assist you in planning your holidays.

▪▶ *Travelmate*
6 Hayes Avenue, Bournemouth BH7 7AD (Tel: 0202-393398).

Travelmate is an introduction agency for travellers. On joining you will receive a list of potential travel companions who match up to your requirements as given on your application form. Travelmate caters for all who wish to find a travel or holiday companion, be it for a Round the World trip, trekking in the Himalayas, a fortnight in the sun, or just a weekend break. You can even form your own group or party from the listings.

Membership is valid for one year with a registration fee of £25. On joining, new members receive a list of members in their classification which is based on area of travel and/or special interest as well as the sex and age group specified. A new member's name and details will be sent out to other members on the same basis. Updated lists are available throughout the period of membership, on request.

Addresses are not divulged, and contact is made either by telephone or through a box number.

Tourist Boards

The Boards for each country within the United Kingdom will be glad to give information about accommodation, from farmhouses and bed and breakfasts to guest houses and hotels, as well as other facilities and interests to tourists within their areas. They all have a range of publications, some of which are free.

England

▪▶ *English Tourist Board*
Dept D, 24 Grosvenor Gardens, London SW1W OET.

ETB has a wide range of publications, including the following titles (to order by telephone, using a credit card, tel: 071-824 8266):

1. *Let's Go!* – a selected listing of hotels in England offering special short breaks. Also included, 'Special Interest Breaks', featuring such interests as: French regional gourmet weekends; golfing breaks; medieval banquets; Mexican, Polynesian, Dixieland, Swiss and party weekends; painting; photography; birdwatching; 'murder'; wine appreciation; hot air ballooning; clay pigeon shooting; vintage car excursions. Available free.
2. Where to Stay Guides–England: *Hotels and Guesthouses* (ref: CO58OM), price £8.50; *Bed and Breakfast, Farmhouses, Inns and Hotels* (ref: CO581M), price £6.99; *Self Catering Holiday Homes* (ref: CO582M), price £5.99. Also in the Where to Stay series: *Camping and Caravan Parks in Britain*, with descriptions of towns, comprehensive indexes, maps and features on the English regions (ref: CO583M), price £5.75.

3. *Let's Do It!* – information on holidays afloat, action and sports, outdoor pursuits, arts and crafts, special interests, and holidays for children (ref: CO362M). Price: £3.75.
4. *Stay on a Farm.* Published in association with the Farm Holiday Bureau UK and the National Tourist Boards, this guide has details of farm holiday accommodation on nearly 1,000 working farms. Accommodation includes B and B, half-board, self-catering (ref: CO531M0). Price: £5.99.
5. *Visit Britain at Work* – a guide to hundreds of interesting workplaces, from visits to breweries and broadcasting studios to piano workshops and power stations (ref: CO843M). Price: £3.95.
6. *Family Leisure Guides* – a series of directories with an emphasis on outdoor pursuits and short-break visits to other places of interest based around the chosen activity. The first two titles in the series are *Golf* and *Horse Racing*. Future titles to include *Bird Watching* and *Horse Riding* (CO381M). Price: £10.99.

England's regional Tourist Boards

▶ *The London Tourist Board and Convention Bureau*
26 Grosvenor Gardens, Victoria, London SW1W ODU (Tel: 071-730 3488).

Telephone Accommodation Booking Service 071-824 8844. Whatever your budget, LTB can find you somewhere to stay throughout the London area. All the accommodation offered has been inspected by LTB.

A number of free publications, including *Markets in London, London Restaurant Guide, London Holiday: The official guide to London, Take Time to Discover the River Thames* and *London Accommodation for Budget Travellers*, are obtainable from LTB by post or at their main information centre, situated on Victoria Station forecourt.

The LTB booklet *Where to Stay in London: The official guide to hotels, guest houses, apartments, and bed and breakfast* is available from: The Publications Division, Automobile Association, Fanum House, Basingstoke, Hampshire RG21 2EA. Price: £2.95.

▶ *Cumbria Tourist Board*
Ashleigh, Holly Road, Windermere, Cumbria LA23 2AQ (Tel: 05394-44444).

▶ *East Anglia Tourist Board*
(Essex, Suffolk, Norfolk, and Cambridge).
Toppesfield Hall, Hadleigh, Suffolk IP7 5DN (Tel: 0473-822922).

▶ *East Midlands Tourist Board*
(Derbyshire, Leicestershire, Lincolnshire, Nottinghamshire, Northamptonshire).
Exchequergate, Lincoln LN2 1PZ (Tel: 0522-531521).

▸ *The Heart of England Tourist Board*
(Warwickshire, Gloucestershire, Staffordshire, Shropshire, Herefordshire, Worcestershire, the West Midlands).
Woodside, Larkhall Road, Worcester WR5 2EF (Tel: 0905-763436).

▸ *Northumbria Tourist Board*
(Cleveland, Durham, Northumberland, Tyne and Wear).
Aykley Heads, Durham DH1 5UX (Tel: 091-384 6905).

▸ *North West Tourist Board*
(Cheshire, Greater Manchester, Lancashire, Merseyside, High Peak of Derbyshire).
Swan House, Swan Meadow Road, Wigan Pier, Wigan WN3 5BB
(Tel: 0942-821222).

▸ *South East England Tourist Board*
(East Sussex, Kent, Surrey, and West Sussex).
The Old Brew House, Warwick Place, Tunbridge Wells, Kent TN2 5TU
(Tel: 0892-540766).

▸ *Southern Tourist Board*
(Hampshire, Dorset, Isle of Wight, Dorset, and South Wiltshire).
40 Chamberlayne Road, Eastleigh, Hampshire SO5 5JH (Tel: 0703-620555).

▸ *Thames and Chilterns Tourist Board*
(Bedfordshire, Berkshire, Buckinghamshire, Hertfordshire, and Oxfordshire).
The Mount House, Church Green, Witney, Oxfordshire OX8 6DZ
(Tel: 0993-778800).

▸ *West Country Tourist Board*
(Avon, Cornwall, Devon, Somerset, Western Dorset, Wiltshire, and Isles of Scilly).
60 St Davids Hill, Exeter, Devon EX4 4SY (Tel: 0392-76351).

▸ *Yorkshire and Humberside Tourist Board*
(North Yorkshire coast and Humberside, Yorkshire Dales, Yorkshire Moors, West and South Yorkshire).
312 Tadcaster Road, York YO2 2HF (Tel: 0904-707961).

Northern Ireland

▸ *Northern Ireland Tourist Board*
St Anne's Court, 59 North Street, Belfast BT1 1NB (Tel: 0232-231221).

The Board has a number of very interesting publications. The one entitled simply

Northern Ireland is a fascinating magazine to read in its own right. It gives details of all the places of interest. It also gives details of painting, craft and steam train holidays. In addition, many other activities are mentioned including rambling and walking, golfing, painting, and pony trekking and riding. Another publication, *Where to Stay in Northern Ireland*, describes accommodation available.

Scotland

Scottish Tourist Board
23 Ravelston Terrace, Edinburgh EH4 3EU (Tel: 031-332 2433).

STB has a range of publications, including a very informative free guide describing over 300 holidays. It also has some useful general information and advertisements providing helpful information.

The following publications are available from: Scottish Holidays, 118 Elderslie Street, Glasgow, G3 7AW. Or tel. 0800-636 660 (24-hours, free) quoting the items you require and your credit card details. *Scotland: Where to stay hotels and guest houses*, £6.30; *Scotland: Where to stay bed and breakfast*, £4.60; *Scotland: Self-catering accommodation*, £4.95; *Enjoy Scotland Pack*, £7.70; *Scotland's Touring Map*, £3.20; *More Than 1,001 Things To See in Scotland*, £4.40.

Wales

Wales Tourist Board
Brunel House, 2 Fitzalan Road, Cardiff, South Glamorgan CF2 1UY
(Tel: 0222-499909).

The free holiday brochure is packed with a huge selection of holiday accommodation – hotels, guest houses, farmhouses, self-catering, caravan holiday home parks and touring caravan and camping sites. There is also a section on activity and special interest holidays. Accommodation featured in this brochure has been checked by the Wales Tourist Board. The Wales Holidays brochure also contains information on a range of attractions of interest to holidaymakers, a gazetteer of towns, villages and resorts, and a full colour map of Wales. There is also a publications list, featuring a wide range of guides available on the Principality. Other guides include:

1. *Wales Hotels, Guest Houses and Farmhouses* – an annual guide to over 250 hotels, guest houses and farmhouses in Wales. Price: £2.50.
2. *Wales Bed and Breakfast* – an annual guide to budget accommodation in Wales, featuring over 500 hotels, guest houses and farmhouses, all with one thing in common – they offer bed and breakfast at an all inclusive price of £18 or under per person per night. Price: £2.50.

SECTION FOURTEEN

Helpful organisations

The following organisations offer help to older people in various ways. In the main, we have excluded those concerned with specific disabilities (for which see our companion volume *Directory for Disabled People* – see page 356). However, we have included a few concerned with disabilities which particularly affect elderly people.

Age Concern England (National Council on Ageing)
Astral House, 1268 London Road, London SW16 4ER (Tel: 081-679 8000).

Age Concern is a national organisation established in 1940 to promote the welfare of older people. The governing body includes representatives of over 87 national organisations and several government departments. There are around 1,100 independent local groups in England which provide a wide range of services. Age Concern England also works closely with its national counterparts in Scotland, Wales and Northern Ireland (*see* below).

Age Concern provides services to elderly people with the help of over 180,000 volunteers; campaigns with and on behalf of elderly people; stimulates innovation and research; and works in partnership with other relevant statutory and voluntary bodies.

The wide range of services provided by Age Concern groups includes day care, visiting housebound people, lunch clubs, over-60s clubs, and specialist services for physically and mentally frail elderly people. The Fieldwork Department of Age Concern England provides direct assistance to local groups and volunteers working with elderly people throughout the country. Grants are made to new projects undertaken by local Age Concern groups.

Each year, nearly 100,000 people contact Age Concern England direct for advice. In addition, a series of fact sheets is published, single copies of which are available free of charge in response to a 9" × 6" s.a.e. (*see* page 351 for details). A wide range of advisory publications are also made available. These are referred to throughout this Directory, under relevant subject headings. Local groups also offer advice and information on a whole range of topics and problems.

Age Concern England offers advice in a number of fields: housing, residential care, community care, transport and mobility. Local groups offer a wide range of community services and many leisure and social activities. A free booklet, *Age Concern At Work*, provides more detailed information concerning the numerous support services provided by this organisation.

⇒▶ *Age Concern Greater London*
54 Knatchbull Road, London SE5 9QY (Tel: 071-737 3456).

There are approximately 1.2 million people of pensionable age living in Greater London, nearly 17 per cent of the population. This regional organisation is thus an important part of the Age Concern movement. Its dual function is to offer development and support services to the 65 autonomous local Age Concern groups throughout the capital, and to campaign for the rights and needs of elderly people in London by promoting issues and co-ordinating policy discussions.

Particularly valuable is Age Concern Greater London's research report, *Older People in London* (November, 1990), price £5 including postage and packing. Other reports have looked at bathing services, homelessness and chiropody services. Also available are guides to setting up and improving services to support carers and to leisure activities in and around London, with special reference to those that are free or where concessions are available.

⇒▶ *Age Concern Northern Ireland*
6 Lower Crescent, Belfast BT7 1NR (Tel: 0203-245729).

In Northern Ireland, more than a quarter of elderly people depend on Income Support. Many live in unsatisfactory housing conditions, and hundreds of elderly people die prematurely because of hypothermia and cold-related ill health.

Age Concern (NI) is the centre for a network of independent local groups providing direct services to elderly people. It functions as 'watchdog', social advocate and campaigning body, and provides a resource centre, an information centre, and support for local community initiatives. A team of development officers support and help to set up new Age Concern branches.

Age Concern (NI) also organises campaigns and projects, conferences and seminars, holidays and outings, advice centres, home-visiting schemes, carers' relief schemes, research work and public education. A wide range of publications and training materials is available.

⇒▶ *Age Concern Scotland*
54A Fountainbridge, Edinburgh EH3 9PT (Tel: 031-228 5656).

Age Concern Scotland aims to improve services for older people and campaign on their behalf. A network of over 250 local groups provide practical services and friendships for older people in Scotland. Age Concern Scotland co-ordinates these groups and brings together in membership many national organisations as well as individuals. Age Concern Scotland also campaigns for better services for elderly people, lobbying government, local authorities, health boards and private companies.

An information service answers enquiries from individuals and organisations concerned with older people, and publishes a two-monthly newsletter, *Network Notes* for members, and a newssheet, *Adage*, available on subscription to a wider readership. In addition, a team of trained volunteers run a personal advice and counselling service for older people and their carers from the Edinburgh office, Monday to Friday, 10 a.m. to 4 p.m. (Tel: 031-228 5467).

Age Concern Scotland stocks relevant books and pamphlets, including the annually updated *Your Rights* and *Your Taxes and Savings*. Policy reports and practical guides to help local groups develop new services are also produced. A publications list is available in response to a s.a.e.

A particular area of concern is housing. A Housing Officer answers enquiries on housing issues, and campaigns to improve housing policies, organising conferences, lobbying on legislation, and producing publications to keep policy-makers and older people well informed.

Age Concern Scotland is also involved at local level. Central to this work is its team of Development Officers. They encourage and support local groups working with old people. These groups, run by volunteers, have established services for older people in their areas. These may include good neighbour schemes, sitting services for the relief of carers, and information services. Many groups run lunch clubs and day centres, and some provide a visiting service for those who are lonely.

Age Concern Scotland is committed to improving standards of service and the quality of life for older people in Scotland. Its Training Officers run courses, seminars and conferences, and produce training materials for professionals and volunteers. There is also an Enterprise Fund which gives financial support to local organisations setting up or developing services for older people. The aim is to fund projects where relatively small amounts of money can make a significant contribution.

Age Concern Wales (Cyngor Henoed Cymru)
4th Floor, 1 Cathedral Road, Cardiff CF1 9SD (Tel: 0222-371566).

Age Concern Wales was formed in 1947 as the national voluntary organisation specialising in the welfare of the elderly in Wales. Through its central office in Cardiff and around 250 local Age Concern groups or Old People's Welfare Committees, it provides a wide range of voluntary services and promotes relevant local schemes.

The organisation campaigns on behalf of elderly people and works to educate public opinion through reports, conferences, publicity and exhibitions. It stimulates innovation and research for the benefit of elderly people and provides opportunities for them to contribute their skills and experience to society; many of Age Concern's voluntary workers are themselves elderly.

Age Concern Wales provides a wide-ranging advice and information service with a Welsh orientation, and is able to respond bilingually to requests. In addition to being directly contactable by letter or telephone, it makes available many relevant publications. These include fact sheets on specific issues, up-to-date bulletins, a directory of services for elderly people, and leaflets. There is also an extensive library in Cardiff. Publications are those of Age Concern England.

Ageing
See Research into Ageing.

Alzheimer's Disease Society
158–60 Balham High Road, London SW12 9BN (Tel: 081-675 6557).

Alzheimer's disease is a condition which causes intellectual disturbance by damaging some of the cells in the brain. The cause is unknown, and the treatment is, at present, limited to amelioration of its effects.

The Society, founded in 1979, aims to give support to families by linking them through membership; to provide information about the disease and available aids; to ensure that adequate nursing care is available when it becomes necessary; and to promote research and the education of the general public. A newsletter, information sheets, advice sheets and booklets are published; meetings and symposia are arranged.

ADS has a network of relatives' self-help groups and contact people throughout the United Kingdom. Recommended subscription £7 per annum.

ARP Over 50 (The Association of Retired Persons Over 50)
Greencoat House, Francis Street, London SW1P 1DZ (Tel: 071-895 8880; Fax: 071-233 7132).

This is a self-financing membership association which aims to change basic attitudes to age and to enhance the quality and purpose of life, both for those planning retirement and the retired, harnessing their growth and social strength.

There are 60 local Friendship Centres and event organisers throughout Great Britain and more are planned. Members receive a quarterly magazine, *050*, and have access to a series of Helplines, which offer impartial legal and consumer rights advice. There is also a number to call, round the clock, in the event of unforeseen domestic emergencies such as blocked drains or burst pipes: ARP will locate the nearest reputable tradesperson, and agree a guaranteed pre-set price with you before arranging an immediate call-out.

ARP provides free insurance for all members, irrespective of age, which provides £30 per day payment for up to 100 days during any period of hospitalisation exceeding 24 hours following an accident, and a lump sum of £1,000 should you be the victim of a reported assault or mugging which leaves you needing medical treatment. ARP has also negotiated discounted terms for other insurance cover, car hire, vehicle breakdown, private health care and international travel with leading companies.

The membership fee is £10 a year (£8 when paid by direct debit), with partner/spouse paying half price.

Arthritis Care
18 Stephenson Way, London NW1 2HD (Tel: 071-916 1500).

This is the only national charity devoted solely to helping people cope with the problems caused by rheumatism and arthritis. There are over 500 branches throughout the United Kingdom which hold regular social meetings and organise group holidays. In addition, a team of volunteers visit housebound people, mainly in areas where there is no branch. There are five specially adapted holiday centres and 14 self-catering holiday units. A residential home provides 24-hour nursing care. Information and advice is available from the address above, and financial grants are sometimes available in cases of special need. There is a quarterly newspaper, *Arthritis News*, which is sent free to members.

Membership subscription £3 per annum.

The Arthritis and Rheumatism Council

Copeman House, St Mary's Court, St Mary's Gate, Chesterfield, Derbyshire S41 7TD (Tel: 0246-558033; Fax: 0246-558007).

The Council aims to inspire and encourage medical research into the causes and cure of arthritis and rheumatism, ensure that the beneficial results of the research are made available to sufferers as quickly as possible and raise the funds necessary for the research to continue. It publishes a quarterly magazine called *ARC Magazine*, which can be obtained for a nominal annual subscription and which contains many short articles on interesting aspects of medical research and arthritis.

Association of Carers

See Carers' National Association.

Association of Crossroads Care Attendant Schemes Ltd

10 Regent Place, Rugby, Warwickshire CV21 2PN (Tel: 0788-573653).

This scheme became a national organisation in April 1977. It represents a bold, imaginative (though totally practical) and much-needed strategy to improve the care of disabled people within the community. The scheme's primary objective is to relieve stress in the families or carers of disabled people and to avoid their admission to hospital or residential care should a breakdown or other failure occur in the household. To achieve this objective the Association promotes the establishment of domiciliary support services in local areas, managed by local committees and staffed by 'care attendants' who are paid for their time and provided with appropriate training. Attendants are not professional people, but act rather as substitute relatives, providing care in a homely and friendly way, in a manner to which the disabled person is accustomed. An important aspect of an attendant's work is that attendance is provided on a flexible basis, if necessary outside what are considered normal working hours. The Association emphasises that such teams supplement and complement, and do not replace, existing statutory services and work closely with them, striving for the highest possible standards of care.

Many physically handicapped people are able to live at home only because of the support they get from other people – friends, housekeepers or relatives. Those who care for disabled people in this way are often under great strain themselves and the support provided by care attendants can make all the difference. Equally, if for any reason a breakdown occurs in normal support, the help of a care attendant, for a few hours a week, can fill the gap and save the situation.

In addition to the main office, there are eight regional offices. Details of these and of places where the scheme operates are available from the above address. A useful publications list is also available free on request.

Back pain
See National Back Pain Association.

The Beth Johnson Foundation
Parkfield House, 64 Princes Road, Hartshill, Stoke-on-Trent, Staffordshire ST4 7JL (Tel: 0782-44036).

The Foundation, which was established in 1972, is a charitable trust concerned with the promotion of the quality of life of older people. It is particularly involved in the field of self-health care and maintenance and in leisure activities, together with the promotion of educational activities for older people and those involved with their welfare. Its aim is to sponsor and encourage innovative work, locally and nationally, for the benefit of the over-60s, although the vast majority of the Foundation's income is now used in the development of its activities in the North Staffordshire area.

From its earliest days, the Foundation has sought to support projects which enable opportunities and services to be established on a sure footing, so that they remain viable when the Foundation withdraws its financial involvement. Projects have included the development of day centres, transport services for frail older people, rural community facilities and neighbourhood-based support schemes for elderly mentally infirm people.

In more recent years, the Foundation has directly developed a number of schemes for which older people themselves have taken on the management responsibility. The emphasis has shifted to the encouragement of projects based on self-help and self-health care. The Foundation is also convinced of the importance of monitoring and recording innovative work and of sponsoring research related to ageing.

The Foundation plays an active role in extending knowledge about old age and expanding educational opportunities for older people both by encouraging the provision of education for older people and by sponsoring courses and seminars on old age for those who work with the over-60s.

Since 1989, the Foundation's work has expanded into advocacy for old people in a variety of care settings and into locally-based reminiscence therapy work.

A publications list is available on request.

Blindness and Partial Sight
See: Optical Information Council; Partially Sighted Society; Royal National Institute for the Blind.

Breakthrough: Deaf–Hearing Integration
Birmingham Centre, Charles W. Gillett Centre, 998 Bristol Road, Selly Oak, Birmingham B29 6LE (Tel: 021-472 6447; Text: 021-471 1001; Fax: 021-471 4368).

Breakthrough is a voluntary organisation which encourages integration between deaf and hearing people of all ages through varied programmes of social activities and practical projects.

Programmes and services organised from the Birmingham Centre include Total Communication workshops and courses, a reference and loans library, an electronic mail service for deaf and deaf-blind subscribers, and a self-help integration programme.

British Association of the Hard of Hearing
7–11 Armstrong Road, London W3 7JL (Tel: 081-743 1110 (voice and minicom); Fax: 081-742 9043).

BAHOH is a national organisation for those who have lost all or part of their hearing after acquiring normal speech and language and who communicate via a hearing aid and/or lipreading (sign language is rarely used in BAHOH). It was founded in 1947 by hard-of-hearing people, who continue to guide its policies and know the problems associated with hearing loss from personal experience.

BAHOH has over 200 social clubs throughout the United Kingdom, run by hard-of-hearing people for hard-of-hearing people, where lip-reading and clear speech are encouraged. The various regions have annual rallies. There are also pen circles you can join.

The Association co-operates with statutory and voluntary bodies to advance measures to prevent and cure deafness and to secure the provision of better services for hard-of-hearing people.

BAHOH's Information Service covers relevant equipment, local clubs, lip-reading classes, and voluntary visiting schemes (which train volunteers to visit elderly hearing aid users). There is a range of relevant publications, including a quarterly magazine, *Hark*. Membership subscription £4 per annum.

British Association for Service to the Elderly
119 Hassell Street, Newcastle under Lyme, Staffordshire ST5 1AX
Tel: 0782-661033).

BASE is a registered charity which provides opportunities for those who care for elderly people, either professionally or privately, to meet together in an informal atmosphere. It is hoped that the exchange of ideas and experience will assist in furthering better care for the elderly.

Anyone may join who is concerned in some way to improve the quality of life for elderly people, and members come from many areas of work. Thus, for example, health and social services staff, remedial therapists, and residential care staff are eligible for membership. People without professional training or the backing of a statutory organisation are also welcome.

Members receive the Association's quarterly journal, *Baseline*, and have an opportunity to attend meetings, study days, workshops and conferences organised by BASE. The annual membership subscription costs £15 (unwaged £5).

The British Deaf Association
38 Victoria Place, Carlisle CA1 1HU (Tel: 0228-48844 (voice and minicom); 0228-28719 (Vistel)).

The Association has local branches throughout the country. It organises a variety of group activities for deaf people, and is able to advise individuals and parents on development and education. Special holidays for deaf and elderly people are arranged, with financial assistance in suitable cases. The Association also organises courses for school leavers, outdoor and adventure courses for young deaf people, and an annual summer school and short special interest courses for all age groups. Educational material (including sign language video tapes) and a monthly news magazine are available. A publications list will be provided on request.

British Diabetic Association
10 Queen Anne Street, London W1M 0BD (Tel: 071-323 1531).

BDA seeks to safeguard the interests of diabetics, provides information and advice, and raises money for research. A bi-monthly magazine, *Balance*, is sent free to all members; cassette versions are provided for people with sight problems. A wide range of literature and books is produced; catalogue available on request.

British Nursing Association (a Nestor-BNA company)
North Place, 82 Great North Road, Hatfield, Hertfordshire AL9 5BL (Tel: 0707-263544).

With 115 branches in England, Scotland and Wales, BNA provides fully qualified nurses and also carers or auxiliaries to private patients for care in their own homes. As well as specialised care, the company offers twilight visits and 'sleeper' duties for those who need only limited assistance, and escort services for patients who cannot travel alone.

A nurse or carer (male or female) can be provided for any period from one to 24 hours a day. BNA has a national branch network and is able to respond at short notice, seven days a week, round the clock to cover routine and emergency needs. Contact the above address or see Yellow Pages for your nearest local branch.

British Pensioner and Trade Union Action Association (BPTAA)
Norman Dodds House, 315 Bexley Road, Erith, Kent DA8 3EZ (Tel: 0322-335464).

BPTAA has many thousands of pensioners organised in over 400 branches, sometimes known as Pensioner Action Groups. It has 32 trade unions in affiliation and works to encourage them to support action to bring about improvements in the provision made for older people. A quarterly journal, *British Pensioner*, is published.

The British Red Cross Society
9 Grosvenor Crescent, London SW1X 7EJ (Tel: 071-235 5454).

The British Red Cross Society gives skilled and impartial care to people in need and crisis, in their own homes and in the community, at home and abroad. In the United Kingdom, it operates through over 90 county branches and 1,200 neighbourhood centres. Its extensive range of services includes escort help for people with mobility difficulties, 425 ambulances, over 1,000 medical loan depots (*see* page 114), and over 700 clubs for elderly and/or disabled people (including 41 stroke clubs).

The British Red Cross also runs 10 residential care homes, and provides over 5,000 holidays for people with disabilities.

British Tinnitus Association
Room 6, 14–18 West Bar Green, Sheffield S1 2DA (Tel: 0742-662806).

The British Tinnitus Association helps to form self-help groups throughout the country, of which there are currently over 60. They provide mutual support and offer varying degrees of counselling. Many encourage development of relaxation through classes and tape lending services.

The Association publishes a quarterly journal, *Quiet*, which includes information on new research, a postbag feature, and news about tinnitus organisations in other countries. It also campaigns for more clinics and better services for people with tinnitus. An information pack is available on request, price £2. The annual membership subscription is £3.

Campaign for Equal State Pension Ages (CESPA)
'Constables', Windsor Road, Ascot, Berkshire SL5 7LF (Tel: 0344-21167), or 19C Kingsweston Road, Henbury, Bristol BS10 7QT (Tel: 0272-509810).

CESPA was formed in August 1986 as a result of increasing concern at the government's failure to take steps to equalise the different state pension ages for men and women in the United Kingdom and to remove resulting anomalies in pension age benefits and concessions. CESPA is an association of concerned people who campaign through local or regional groups and nationally on behalf of older people who face discrimination in pension and other entitlements. Annual subscription: £4.

Canine Concern Scotland Trust
East Lodge, Caldarvan, Gartocharn, Strathclyde (Tel: 038-983 325).

CCST is establishing a pet visiting service (Therapet) in Scotland to provide a voluntary service of dog owners who, with their dogs, are willing to spend an hour or two regularly visiting homes, hospitals or single, lonely, housebound elderly people who can no longer care for a dog themselves.

Carers
See Association of Crossroads Care Attendant Schemes, British Nursing Association, Carers' National Association, United Kingdom Home Care Council.

Carers' National Association
29 Chilworth Mews, London W2 3RG (Tel: 071-724 7776; Fax: 071-723 8130). Scotland: 11 Queens Crescent, Glasgow G4 9AS (Tel: 041-333 9495).

Formerly Association of Carers and the National Council for Carers and their Elderly Dependants.

The Association provides information and support for people caring for sick, disabled or frail elderly relatives or friends. A range of free leaflets is available and local contacts can give local information and put carers in touch with one another.

Centre for Policy on Ageing
25–31 Ironmonger Row, London EC1V 3QP
(Tel: 071-253 1787; Fax: 071-490 4206).

CPA is an independent think-tank examining public policy and how it affects older people; its work is aimed mainly towards professionals and academics.

CPA aims to promote informed debate about issues concerning older age groups, stimulate awareness of their needs, formulate and promote effective policies and encourage the spread of good practice. Recent published work has looked at risk-taking, media attitudes to older people, advocacy and information networks for community care. Particularly relevant publications are *Home Life* (1984, price £5), a code of practice for residential care, and Eric Midwinter's *The Wage of Retirement* (1985, price £6), which calls for a radical overhaul of the social security system. A full catalogue is available. A European directory of old age is planned for 1992.

CPA's Information Service houses the United Kingdom's foremost reference library on social gerontology, and offers a current awareness and other library services.

Chartered Society of Physiotherapy
14 Bedford Row, London WC1R 4ED (Tel: 071-242 1941; Fax: 071-831 4509).

In the United Kingdom today there are approximately 23,000 chartered physiotherapists. They treat injury and disease by improving and assisting the body's own natural healing mechanism. Although the majority of practitioners work in the NHS, a growing number now work in private practice. Physiotherapy is very important in the areas of pain relief, healing and rehabilitation, and can be very important in overcoming mobility problems as we get older. It is beneficial for the treatment of a wide range of specific impairments, including sciatica, lumbago, arthritis, and swollen or stiff joints.

All chartered physiotherapists have spent a minimum of three years full-time studying for their degree or diploma in physiotherapy. But 'physiotherapist' is not a protected title and some people who practise physiotherapy do not have the same training, knowledge and experience as a chartered physiotherapist.

Many GPs can now refer you directly to a chartered physiotherapist at your local NHS hospital. In some areas, if you cannot get to a hospital, a community physiotherapist may be able to treat you in your own home. Alternatively, if you want and are able to afford private treatment, the names of chartered physiotherapists in private practice can be obtained from your doctor, Yellow Pages, your local library or the Organisation of Chartered Physiotherapists in Private Practice, 50 Mannering Gardens, Westcliff-on-Sea, Essex SS0 0BQ (Tel: 0702-352113).

A publications list is available from The Chartered Society of Physiotherapy at the Bedford Row address. This is mainly of professional interest, but includes some advisory leaflets, such as *Look After Your Back*, *Take the Strain Out of Gardening* and *Mobility is a Must*.

Chest, Heart and Stroke Association
See under new name, The Stroke Association.

The Cinnamon Trust
Poldarves Farm, Trescowe Common, Germoe, Penzance, Cornwall TR20 9RX (Tel: 0736-850291).

The Trust has established a network of volunteers to provide help for elderly pet owners at home – for example walking the dog or fostering pets when elderly owners are temporarily hospitalised. The aim is to make it possible for the owner and pet to remain together for as long as possible in spite of any difficulties that may arise. The Trust also provides a sanctuary for companion animals whose owners have died or been admitted to residential homes. Elderly owners can thus be relieved of anxiety about their pets and be given the confidence to have a new pet when an 'old faithful' dies.

No charge is made for the Trust's services, but it naturally hopes that pet owners who benefit from its work will, if possible, make a contribution towards the cost. Those who wish to support the Trust can become members; the subscription rates are £7.50 per annum (OAPs and under 16s, £3), life membership £75. Members receive free twice-yearly newsletters.

Citizens Advice Bureau Service
Administration: National Association of Citizens Advice Bureaux (NACAB), 115–23 Pentonville Road, London N1 9LZ (Tel: 071-833 2181; Fax: 071-833 4371).

Local Citizens' Advice Bureaux (CABs) provide information and advice, free of charge, on every subject. There are over 1,000 CAB outlets in the United Kingdom, and in 1990–1 they dealt with over seven million enquiries. Eighty per cent of these enquiries related to social security and welfare benefit problems, money matters including debt and credit, housing and consumer complaints, and employment and legal tangles. Over half the bureaux offer sessions with local solicitors in attendance, and one-third have qualified accountants on hand. Fifteen per cent have specialist debt counsellors, but all CAB workers are trained to deal with money problems. All bureaux also have a community information system which includes everything from the address of the nearest library or tax office to details of local self-help groups and the names of local solicitors. As well as giving you information and advice, the CAB will write or telephone on your behalf, if you wish.

CAB is an independent organisation – not part of local or central government – and does not support any political party. Ninety per cent of its workers are volunteers who go through an extensive training programme lasting up to one year. CABs have extensive information on local support groups, social service contacts, etc.

Consult your telephone directory or local library for the address and telephone number of your nearest CAB. If necessary, please check that the CAB office is accessible before you go; many are not.

Compassionate Friends
See Section 8, 'Planning for Death and Coping With Bereavement'.

Counsel and Care for the Elderly
Twyman House, 16 Bonny Street, London NW1 9LR (Tel: 071-485 1550 (administration); 071-485 4513 (appeals); 071 485 1566 (casework – Mondays to Thursdays, 10.30 a.m. to 3.00 p.m.)).

This charity (formerly known as the Elderly Invalids Fund) was founded in 1954. From very modest beginnings it has become a nationwide service for elderly people which provides all its services free of charge and regardless of race, religion, colour or background. It has had its present name since 1977, reflecting its widening role. CCE offers help in a variety of ways:

- It provides, through a team of professional caseworkers, an information and advice service to elderly people and those concerned with their welfare. The service answers some 10,000 enquiries every year and provides help and information on a variety of subjects including homes, statutory benefits and services, help with bills, respite care, and lump sum grants for special needs. It publishes a number of free fact sheets concerning residential care, statutory benefits and charitable help which will be sent in response to a large s.a.e.
- As far as possible, it makes available lump sum grants for items to improve the quality of life of elderly people, for example one-off expenses such as telephone installation, household items, aids and respite care. (Note: These grants are made from trusts administered by CCE. Where clients are not eligible for such help, CCE can advise on alternative sources of help.)
- It operates, through caseworkers, a scheme of annual visits to all private and voluntary homes in Greater London, gathering information on the facilities they provide. Caseworkers are then able to suggest suitable homes to meet the individual needs and

preferences of each enquirer. (Note: If people are seeking care outside the London area, CCE can put them in touch with other organisations that can help.)

▸ *Crossroads Care Attendant Schemes*
See Association of Crossroads Care Attendant Schemes.

▸ *Cruse – Bereavement Care*
See Section 8, 'Planning for Death and Coping With Bereavement'.

▸ *Deafness*
See Hearing Impairment.

▸ *Debt*
See Section 2, page 56, National Debtline.

▸ *Dementia*
See Alzheimer's Disease Society, Scottish Action on Dementia.

▸ *Depressives Associated*
PO Box 5, Castle Town, Portland, Dorset DT5 1BQ
(Tel (answerphone): 081-760 0544).

The Association does not claim to have an instant cure for depression, nor does it offer itself as an alternative to medical help, but it does provide a fund of practical advice, sympathy and understanding from people who have themselves experienced this illness. Depressives Associated aims to:

— help those who are depressed by putting sufferers in touch with one another to form self-help groups for mutual support;
— provide information about the nature of depression and how it may be overcome;
— educate public opinion towards a better understanding of depression;
— co-operate with the caring professions and provide a back-up to medical treatment;
— help relatives to understand and cope with the problems that arise when a family member is depressed;
— promote and encourage research into the causes and cure of depression.

The Association offers understanding and personal replies to your enquiries, and believes that it can offer hope, contact and friendship. It publishes a quarterly newsletter containing up-to-date information, helpful suggestions and other material designed to help you to gain a measure of relief and understanding. The Association also has a selection of booklets and fact sheets on subjects which are frequently of concern.

Joan Gibson, the Correspondence Secretary, is the author of *Look for Rainbows* (Gateway Books, Bath, 1987, price £3.95), which covers loneliness, bereavement, depression and fear of old age or death. Written in a friendly and personal way, it should be of particular help to older people.

Diabetes
See below and British Diabetic Association.

Diabetes Foundation
177a Tennison Road, London SE25 5NF (Tel: 081-656 5467).

This organisation was formed in 1982. Its main aims are:
- to fund research into the causes and complications of diabetes, including blindness, heart and kidney disease, and gangrene, with the primary objective of finding a cure for diabetes;
- to provide a programme of public awareness and education;
- to raise funds to supplement hospitals with equipment and other help required for diabetic care;
- to represent the interests of all diabetics in the United Kingdom.

The Foundation issues an interesting quarterly magazine, *Diabetic Life*, for the understanding of diabetes, with regular mailings to members of the most recent progress in diabetic research work. In addition, the Foundation has a panel of doctors and allied members of the medical profession who are able to give general help and advice to diabetics.

A 24-hour telephone helpline is operated on the above number to give non-medical advice, with co-ordinators appointed throughout the country as local contacts. The annual membership subscription is £3.50 (£2 for pensioners).

Distressed Gentlefolk's Aid Association
Vicarage Gate House, Vicarage Gate, London W8 4AQ (Tel: 071-229 9341).

DGAA's provision falls broadly into two parts: firstly, direct financial help to assist people to stay in their own homes or to help them to cover the cost of fees in private nursing homes; and, secondly, 376 places in thirteen homes, some offering residential care and some offering full nursing facilities.

The Association's terms of reference stipulate that its resources must be used 'to alleviate need and distress among *gentlefolk* of both sexes of British or Irish nationality...'. In practice, it offers help to people of professional or similar background or their dependants, as well as to those whose once-sheltered life has left them ill-equipped to deal with subsequent hardship and poverty. Applications for a place in DGAA's homes cannot be considered from people who are blind or likely to become blind, or who are mentally confused or who have a history of psychiatric illness or alcoholism. Fees are related to ability to pay.

Euthanasia
See Voluntary Euthanasia Society.

Feminists
See Older Feminists Network.

50 Forward
The Manor House, 46 London Road, Blackwater, Camberley, Surrey GU17 0AA (Tel: 0276-34462; Fax: 0276-32990).

This 'club' for people over 50 offers, through a quarterly magazine (*see* page 357), a variety of special offers on a range of goods and services, including travel. Subscription £7.50 a year.

Friends of the Elderly and Gentlefolk's Help
42 Ebury Street, London SW1W 0LZ (Tel: 071-730 8263).

From small beginnings in 1905, this voluntary organisation now runs twelve homes for elderly people, five with nursing wings. It strives to combine the provision of care with the preservation of independence. There is no fixed rule about applicants' ages, but 75 would nowadays be a recommended minimum age.

The Society also provides, on a limited scale, grants to help with personal needs.

Hearing Impairment
See British Association of the Hard or Hearing, British Deaf Association, Royal National Institute for Deaf People.

Help the Aged
St James's Walk, London EC1R 0BE (Tel: 071-253 0253).

Help the Aged works to improve the quality of life of elderly people in the United Kingdom and internationally, particularly those who are frail, isolated or poor. By identifying needs, raising public awareness, and through effective fund raising, Help the Aged promotes and develops aid programmes of a high standard which are practical and innovative.

In the United Kingdom, Help the Aged funds projects such as minibuses, day centres, day hospitals, hospices and community alarms.

The charity also publishes a wide range of advice leaflets and information sheets which are referred to in the relevant sections of this Directory.

SeniorLine is Help the Aged's free national information service for senior citizens, their relatives, carers and friends. Trained advice workers can give general information on welfare and disability benefits, housing, health, support for carers, mobility, community alarms, sources of local practical help and other voluntary organisations. Freephone 0800-289 404, 10 a.m. to 4 p.m. Monday to Friday.

Immigrants
See Joint Council for the Welfare of Immigrants.

Jewish Care
Stuart Young House, 221 Golders Green Road, London NW11 9DQ (Tel: 081-458 3282; Fax: 081-455 7185).

Jewish Care is the largest Anglo-Jewish social work agency in the United Kingdom. It provides services for elderly, visually impaired, physically handicapped and mentally ill people and their families.

The extensive services include sixteen residential homes, eight day centres, two special day care units, two hostels, six group homes, a mental health centre, social work teams, and flatlet schemes.

Joint Council for the Welfare of Immigrants
115 Old Street, London EC1V 9JR (Tel: 071-251 8706).

JCWI is a national organisation dealing solely with immigration and nationality law. It provides a service of advice and representation to those who are adversely affected by UK law and practice in this area, and campaigns for change, producing information for individuals and organisations and training other advice workers in immigration and nationality law. Its many publications include a reform briefing paper on the position of elderly parents and other relatives.

The National Association of Widows
54–7 Allison Street, Digbeth, Birmingham B5 5TH (Tel: 021-643 8348).

The Association was set up in 1971 to help widows to cope with the loneliness, isolation and financial difficulties which are almost always the result of bereavement. It aims to offer information, advice and friendly support to all widows and to all those who are concerned to help widows overcome the problems they face in society today. The Association's head office offers a free advice and information service, and a network of branches throughout the country provides the basis of a supportive social life for widows. The Advice and Information Service is free and completely confidential and includes help with housing problems, social security, pensions and taxation. Enquiries are usually dealt with by telephone and letters, but callers are welcome at head office or at any of the local Advisory Service offices.

National Association of Widows' advisors also represent widows at appeals tribunals and have won cases for many widows.

Another key task is to provide information about issues affecting widows and their families. The Association constantly works to monitor the actions of central and local government, and regularly comments on government policies. On several occasions, the Association has been consulted by government departments and has successfully campaigned around the issues of widows' and taxation and widows' entitlement to benefits.

Throughout the country there are branches of the National Association of Widows, each of which is run by widows for widows. Each local branch is different, responding to the needs of its members, but they are all based on the same principles and have the same aims: to provide a friendly social life for widows, and a place where widows can share their experiences with others, and to offer relevant information and advice.

The Association publishes information leaflets for widows and professionals and a regular newsletter.

National Back Pain Association
31–3 Park Road, Teddington, Middlesex TW11 0AB (Tel: 081-977 5474; Fax: 081-943 5318).

The NBPA is the only national charity devoted to back pain. Its aims are:
- to fund scientific research into the causes and treatment of back pain;
- to educate people to use their bodies sensibly and thus reduce the incidence of back pain;
- to help form and support branches through which back pain sufferers and those who care for them may receive information, advice and mutual help.

The National Osteoporosis Society
PO Box 10, Radstock, Bath BA3 3YB (Tel: 0761-432472).

Osteoporosis is the name given to a condition in which the bones have become porous and brittle as a result of calcium deficiency. It affects one in forty men and one in four women, particularly after the menopause, when calcium is lost more rapidly. Typically, bones may break easily. Those in the spine may become compressed, causing loss of height. Eventually, they may fracture and collapse, causing the curve of the spine sometimes described as 'dowager's hump'.

The NOS offers (free to members): information about osteoporosis, regular newsletters, and in some areas the opportunity to join local groups. The Society also seeks to increase public awareness of the prevalence and the serious effects of this bone disease, to encourage the medical profession, the government and relevant organisations to work towards improved methods of prevention and treatment, and to assist appropriate research.

Ordinary membership £10 a year (please send s.a.e.); medical/health care professionals £20.

Northern Ireland Widows Association
The Ozinam Centre, William Street, Lurgan, Northern Ireland (Tel: 0762-323224).

The Association is concerned with the care, counselling, welfare and education of widows in Northern Ireland. It is able to make grants and loans for the relief of poverty, suffering and distress among widows and their families, and through an extensive branch structure provides information, advice and opportunities for social contact.

Nursing
See Carers.

Older Feminists Network
c/o Wesley House, 4 Wild Court, Kingsway, London WC2 or 54 Gordon Road, London N3 1EP (Tel: 081-346 1900).

The OFN was formed in 1982 and has met regularly ever since. Its newsletter (£5 for six issues; £3 for those on a low income) reaches women throughout the country.

Meetings, which include discussion groups on chosen subjects, are held on the second Saturday of each month at Millman Street Community Rooms, Millman Street, 34–6 Alleyway, London WC1 (nearest tube: Russell Square) from 11 a.m. to 5 p.m. (bring cold food to share).

▶ *Optical Information Council*
57A Old Woking Road, West Byfleet, Weybridge, Surrey KT14 6LF
(Tel: 0932-353283).

The Council publishes a number of free leaflets giving information on the help available for the visual problems of the partially sighted, the use of low-visual aids, and methods of protecting the eyes against glare.

▶ *Osteoporosis*
See The National Osteoporosis Society.

▶ *Parkinson's Disease Society of the UK*
22 Upper Woburn Place, London WC1H 0RA
(Tel: 071-383 3513; Fax 071-383 5754).

The Society has three aims:
— To help those with Parkinson's Disease, and their relatives, with the problems which arise from the disease.
— To collect and disseminate information on Parkinson's Disease.
— To encourage and provide funds for research into Parkinson's Disease.

Information, help and advice are available at headquarters and through over 200 branches.

▶ *Partially Sighted Society*
Registered Office (and Editor of *Oculus*): Queens Road, Doncaster DN1 2NX
(Tel: 0302-368998).
National Low Vision Advice Centre: Dean Clarke House, Southernhay East, Exeter EX1 1PE (Tel: 0392-210656).
Greater London office: 62 Salusbury Road, London NW6 6NS (Tel: 071-372 1551).

The Society offers assistance to all people with impaired vision. Its services include information and advice, publications (including a bi-monthly magazine, *Oculus*, in large print), a special printing and enlargement service, and aids to vision.
The society has 32 local branches in the United Kingdom offering direct support and contact. Nationally, the Society represents the interests of partially sighted people to government bodies and other organisations. Membership is open to all: full £17.50 (£15 if by banker's order); supporters £7.50; organisations £15.

Pensioner organisations

See below, and Association of Retired People Over 50 (ARP), British Pensioner and Trade Union Action Association, 50 Forward, and Saga. There are also many organisations linked to pensioners' previous employment.

Pensioners for Peace International
16 Sandy Lane, Petersham, Richmond upon Thames TW10 7EL
Tel: 081-940 2611).

This organisation is affiliated to the Campaign for Nuclear Disarmament and works with it while developing its own contribution to peace and international goodwill. It seeks to provide pensioners with opportunities not readily available to them through CND, while nevertheless helping pensioners to co-operate in CND's aims.

PPI is managed on a national basis, but with regional organisations wherever possible, corresponding to the CND regions. A network of local groups, again normally co-terminous with CND's local groups, is being developed.

The national subscription is 'a minimum of £3 a year (£4 for a couple) wherever possible'. The intention of this is that members shall pay what they can afford, be it as little as 50p a year.

Pensioners' Voice (National Federation of Retirement Pensions Associations)
Melling House, 14 St Peter Street, Blackburn, Lancashire BB2 2HD
Tel: 0254-52606).

The Federation was founded in 1939, and immediately began campaigning for an increase in the 'old age pension'. A newsletter, *The Pensioner* (now *Pensioners' Voice*), first appeared in February 1940. The Federation now has over 600 branches throughout the United Kingdom and a large and growing number of individual members. The Federation's objects are:

– to organise pensioners and supporters throughout the United Kingdom;
– to organise public support for the aims and objects of the Federation;
– to bring pressure to bear on government, local authorities, and Members of Parliament on behalf of pensioners.

The Federation is a pressure group, not a charity. Its finance is drawn from pensioners, non-pensioner supporters, trades unions, industry and commerce. It stands to ensure that pensioners shall have not just enough to make life tolerable, but a sufficiency. It campaigns for a better quality of life for older people, especially through improvements in state retirement pensions, health care, and facilities for education and leisure, and for heating allowances for all pensioners.

People's Dispensary for Sick Animals
Whitechapel Way, Priorslee, Telford, Shropshire TF2 9PQ
(Tel: 0952-290999; Fax: 0952-291035).

The PDSA was founded in 1917 to provide free veterinary treatment for sick and injured animals whose owners could not afford private veterinary fees. The Society provides this same service to eligible pet owners today, many of whom are elderly or lonely people who rely upon their pets for companionship.

There are now 50 PDSA Veterinary Centres in this country, and in addition to this the PDSA Pet Aid Scheme is available through private practices in a further 64 communities.

In 1990 the PDSA performed 1.4 million treatments on sick and injured pets.

Pet Concern
Animal Welfare Trust, Tyler's Way, Watford By-pass, Watford, Hertfordshire WD2 8HQ (Tel: 081-950 8215 or 081-950 0177).

Pet Concern was established in 1979 to care for the pets of elderly people during hospital treatment or convalescence. If within easy reach of the Trust's rescue centres (in Birmingham, Bristol, Ipswich, Somerset and London), dogs may be boarded at £2.50 a day and cats at £1.50 a day. In other areas, small grants may be considered; applications must be in writing.

Pets

See Canine Concern Scotland, The Cinnamon Trust, People's Dispensary for Sick Animals, Pet Concern.

The Pre-Retirement Association of Great Britain and Northern Ireland
Nodus Centre, University Campus, Guildford, Surrey GU2 5RX (Tel: 0483-39323).

The PRA is the major organisation within Great Britain and Northern Ireland promoting awareness of the needs of those preparing for retirement and requiring assistance in retirement. The Association provides educational back-up, planning and support services that relate to the successful transition from an increasing diversity of employment patterns.

In addition, the PRA assists people facing redundancy or early retirement.

Relate: Marriage Guidance
Herbert Gray College, Little Church Street, Rugby CV21 3AP (Tel: 0788-73241).

Relate services are available to all, of any age, of either sex, in any circumstances, who are worried about personal relationships, regardless of whether they are married or not. It can be a couple or a woman or man alone.

Counselling normally takes place in Relate premises. Sessions are usually arranged weekly to last for an hour, free from interruptions, spread over a few weeks or several months – whatever is necessary for clients to talk through their problems. If there is a sexual problem as distinct from purely a relationship problem, it may be appropriate, with the client's agreement, to seek the help of one of Relate's sexual therapists. The theory behind Relate's methods of sexual therapy is that through carefully developed learning methods, most sexual difficulties can be completely overcome.

Counselling is described by Relate as a 'learning process which allows people to reach their own solutions while giving them the emotional strength and confidence to carry on'.

There is no obligatory charge for counselling help, but naturally Relate, as a voluntary organisation, hopes that clients will contribute to the cost of the work and this is something the counsellor will discuss with you.

Relate operates in England, Wales, and Northern Ireland. It is independent and is not attached to any sectarian, denominational or cultural institution. Some counsellors have specialist knowledge of disability where this is needed.

To make an appointment, telephone, write or call in to your local Relate office. Telephone numbers and addresses for Relate are listed in telephone directories under 'Marriage Guidance'.

Research into Ageing

49 Queen Victoria Street, London EC4N 4SA
(Tel: 071-236 4365; Fax: 071-489 0384).

Founded in 1976 (as Action Trust), Research into Ageing is a charity dedicated to improving the health and quality of life of elderly people through the initiation, funding and support of medical research. Activities include:

– Funding medical and scientific research into the diseases and disabilities that affect elderly people, and into the ageing process itself.
– Encouraging and enabling promising students of ability to enter and work in the fields of gerontology and geriatric medicine.
– Co-ordinating information and research and promoting education in these areas, and stimulating planning and action.

Since 1978, Research into Ageing has committed over £2 million to more than 120 research projects to improve knowledge of the ageing process and disabilities associated with age. Research covers a range of subjects including dementia and Alzheimer's disease, cataracts, incontinence, osteoporosis, the improvement of nutrition, and the maintenance of mobility.

Retirement

See The Pre-Retirement Association, The Retirement Association of Northern Ireland, Scottish Retirement Council.

The Retirement Association of Northern Ireland

Room 11, Bryson House, 28 Bedford Street, Belfast BT2 7FE (Tel: 0232-321324).

This Association offers pre-retirement courses, lectures and voluntary services. It is concerned with all social aspects of life for active retired people.

Rheumatism
See Arthritis Care, Arthritis and Rheumatism Council.

The Royal National Institute for the Blind (RNIB)
224 Great Portland Street, London W1N 6AA (Tel: 071-388 1266).

RNIB works for the better education, training, rehabilitation, employment and general welfare of Britain's blind people. It runs schools, training colleges, two rehabilitation centres, homes for elderly blind people and hotels for holidays. It sells specially adapted goods, publishes braille and Moon books and magazines, and provides services for producing individual items in braille, Moon and on tape. RNIB runs braille and tape libraries and a Talking Book library. It helps blind people find commercial and professional jobs and funds research into the prevention of blindness. It publishes a monthly magazine, *New Beacon*, in print and braille, and also publishes leaflets and information sheets on blindness and services for blind people.

The Royal National Institute for Deaf People (RNID)
105 Gower Street, London WC1E 6AH
(Tel: 071-387 8033, Fax: 071-388 2346, Minicom: 071-383 3154, Querty: 071-388 6038).

The RNID is a voluntary organisation representing the interests of deaf, deaf-blind and hard of hearing people. It ensures that their needs are properly recognised by both government and the general public, and that facilities and services for deaf people are continually improved.

RNID provides a wide range of direct services including residential and rehabilitation centres, training, interpreting services, information and advice, and environmental aids. It also runs a national telephone relay service for deaf people, and a helpline on tinnitus, 0345-090210, 10 a.m. to 3 p.m. Monday to Friday.

Saga Club
The Saga Building, Middelburg Square, Folkestone, Kent CT20 1AZ
(Tel: 0303-857526).

Subscribers to *Saga Magazine* (*see* page 358) automatically become members of the Saga Club, whose members enjoy a number of benefits, including special Saga holiday offers at discounted prices, access to a members-only Penfriends and Partnerships contact service, a range of special offers, a series of free advisory leaflets (referred to in the relevant sections of this Directory) and a telephone advisory service (currently charged at 48 pence a minute, or 36 pence a minute cheap rate).

The Samaritans
10 The Grove, Slough SL1 1QP (Tel: 0753-532713 – for administrative purposes only).

The Samaritans have branches in many parts of the United Kingdom, all of which are dedicated to helping despairing or suicidal people. They are particularly keen to ensure that their services are made as available as possible to older people, and they have a team of volunteers currently reaching out to these groups.

Samaritans are ordinary people from all walks of life who devote part of their spare time to help people in distress. They are carefully chosen and prepared, and work under the guidance of a volunteer director. The branches can be contacted at any hour of the day or night by telephone, or by personal visit any day or evening. Some people also make contact by letter, and a few are visited, when it seems particularly necessary, in their own homes. The service is absolutely confidential and free. The telephone numbers of local branches are in telephone directories.

Scottish Action on Dementia
33 Castle Street, Edinburgh EH2 3DN (Tel: 031-220 4886).

Dementia is a term used to describe various forms of disease which gradually destroy the brain cells. It is more common in older age groups and is nearly always incurable.

SAD is a voluntary organisation which seeks to unite everyone concerned about the plight of people with dementia and their carers. It works in partnership with other major charities including Alzheimer's Scotland, Age Concern Scotland and the Scottish Association for Mental Health. SAD works to:

— stand up for the rights of sufferers and carers to the highest possible quality of life, and for services to meet the needs of individuals;
— provide principles against which plans, services and standards can be measured;
— promote the development of local services;
— keep well informed and to pass on that information;
— monitor financial allocations and services;
— promote education and training for both professional and lay carers;
— raise public awareness through publicity and discussion papers;
— organise conferences and workshops;
— lobby the government and statutory authorities.

SAD has a number of relevant publications and produces a periodical bulletin, *Dementia – Update* (free to members). Membership costs £10 a year (£5 if unwaged; £70 for life).

The Scottish Retirement Council
204 Bath Street, Glasgow G2 4HL (Tel: 041-332 9427).

The SRC promotes education for retirement in co-operation with employers and appropriate statutory and voluntary bodies. It publishes relevant literature, provides information and advice services, and runs a number of crafts and hobbies centres.

Sex and Personal Relationships

See Relate, SPOD.

SPOD: Association to Aid the Sexual and Personal Relationships of Disabled People
286 Camden Road, London N7 OBJ (Tel: 071-607 8851).

SPOD provides information on disability and sexuality, including a range of publications. It has a countrywide network of counsellors and can usually put anyone with a disability in touch with a counsellor near to their home. SPOD also organises a range of study days and workshops on various aspects of sexuality.

The Stroke Association
CHSA House, Whitecross Street, London EC1Y 8JJ
(Tel: 071-490 7999; Fax: 071-490 2686).

The Stroke Association was launched in November 1991 when the Chest, Heart and Stroke Association (CHSA) handed on its work in chest and heart disease to other charities, enabling it to concentrate the whole of its resources on strokes. The Association works to prevent strokes happening (both by encouraging research into their causes and by the application of existing knowledge about the risk factors), funds research in new methods of treatment, and provides practical help for those affected by strokes and their families. It publishes many helpful booklets, leaflets and videos (list available), and can refer enquirers to local stroke centres.

The Volunteer Stroke Service (VSS), set up with the co-operation of speech and language therapists, uses trained volunteers to visit stroke families at home to give help with speech and communication. The Stroke Association is also committed to providing, through its Stroke Family Support Service, a visiting service for all stroke families.

A network of 500 affiliated stroke clubs, run on a voluntary basis, provide social activities. Welfare grants are made through Social Services Departments for hospital visiting fares, respite or convalescent holidays, and special clothing or equipment (e.g. food processors for those with swallowing problems).

Sue Ryder Foundation
Cavendish, Sudbury, Suffolk CO10 8AY (Tel: 0787-280252).

The Foundation has 24 homes in the United Kingdom, open or in the course of being established. Domiciliary visiting and bereavement counselling are undertaken from several of these homes. The Foundation is also active in a number of overseas countries.

Tinnitus
See below and British Tinnitus Association.

Tinnitus Helpline
0345-090210.

This helpline is run by the Royal National Institute for Deaf People.

United Kingdom Home Care Council
206 Worple Road, London SW20 8PN (Tel: 081-946 8202).

This Association represents private and voluntary organisations providing domiciliary care to elderly or disabled people. It is primarily concerned with promoting high standards. Its members work to a Code of Practice.

The Association publishes documents dealing with all aspects of running domiciliary services and is working on such issues as training and insurance.

The Association also provides a forum for discussion and negotiation with relevant authorities in central and local government and forms links with other professional voluntary or charitable organisations with similar interests. It is in the process of building up a database on the services and resources of the independent domiciliary care sector.

Voluntary Euthanasia Society
13 Prince of Wales Terrace, London W8 5PG (Tel: 071-937 7770).

The Society was founded in 1935. Its principal object is to promote legislation which would allow an adult person, suffering from a severe illness to which no relief is known, to receive an immediate painless death if, and only if, that is their expressed wish. A free booklet, *The Last Right*, discusses the surrounding issues. Among other things, this explains that individuals can make an advance declaration on a form available from the Society and to be lodged with their doctor, which makes the following declaration:

If there is no reasonable prospect of my recovery from physical illness or impairment expected to cause me severe distress or render me incapable of rational existence, I request that I be allowed to die and not be kept alive by artificial means and that I receive whatever quantity of drugs may be required to keep me free from pain or distress even if the moment of death is hastened.

Membership costs £10 a year (£15 for couples), and a newsletter, *VES*, is published approximately quarterly.

Wales Pensioners
Transport House, 1 Cathedral Road, Cardiff CF1 9SD (Tel: 0222-225141).

Wales Pensioners seeks to provide an information and support service for all pensioners throughout the Principality, circulating leaflets and other information received from appropriate services. The organisation is seeking to establish a county structure throughout Wales.

The War Widows' Association of Great Britain
P.R.O., 17, The Earl's Croft, Coventry CV3 5ES (Tel: 0203-503298).

The Association has about 4,500 members and represents war widows throughout Great Britain. There are 50 areas, each with a regional organiser. Its main aims are to work with various organisations on behalf of members, keeping them and the government informed of problems of which it has become aware, to provide members with information about any current legislation affecting them, and to help members in matters concerning their welfare, putting them in touch with those who can assist financially.

The Association seeks, through the presentation of well-founded and well-argued cases, to improve conditions for war widows and their families and to end present anomalies in pension provision, and tries to ensure that members receive the full range of benefits to which they are entitled. It has helped many war widows in their efforts to get war widows' pensions when their husbands have died through war injury. A news sheet, *Courage*, is published. The Association takes part in all national commemorative events. There is an enrolment fee of 50 pence, and a life membership subscription of £5. Associate members – relatives and interested friends – are welcome.

Widows

See Cruse, National Association of Widows, War Widows Association.

Wireless for the Bedridden Society (Inc.)

159A High Street, Hornchurch, Essex RM11 3YB (Tel: 0708-621101).

Provides, on free loan, radio and television sets to needy invalids and the aged poor. Maintenance is covered, and in some cases the licence fee.

Women's Royal Voluntary Service

234–44 Stockwell Road, London SW9 9SP (Tel: 071-416 0146).
Scotland: 19 Grosvenor Crescent, Edinburgh EH12 5EL (Tel: 031-337 2261).
Wales: 26 Cathedral Road, Cardiff CF1 9YJ (Tel: 0222-228386).

The WRVS, first formed in 1938 in anticipation of wartime needs, now provides a wide variety of help to people in need – particularly those who need support to remain in their own homes. This includes a range of help for elderly people. Welfare services are also provided for people in hospital, residential homes and sheltered housing.

WRVS works independently, initiating its own services, as well as in partnership with local authorities and voluntary organisations. It has over 160,000 members regularly serving in various capacities, and in an emergency several thousand more could be deployed. The range of activities varies in every locality and includes welfare services for elderly people (such as luncheon clubs for those who are active and meals on wheels for those who are not), arranging holidays for elderly people to relieve their relatives, shopping for housebound people, supplying clothing and bedding, a books on wheels service (approximately 2,000 schemes), and providing escorts for journeys. To give an idea of the scale of the work, in 1987 WRVS delivered 15,221,887 meals and served 2,657,861 meals in luncheon clubs; over $2\frac{1}{2}$ million garments were issued from WRVS clothing stores; emergency teams were called out to 245 incidents; WRVS runs

2,080 day and evening clubs, 52 stroke clubs, 18 registered care homes and one nursing/convalescent home, while WRVS members work in 1,100 hospitals, giving the NHS gifts to a value of nearly £1½ million each year.

Anyone in need of help or advice can contact their local WRVS office (listed in your telephone directory) or the above address.

SECTION FIFTEEN

Selected further reading

Books and other literature relating to specific sections of this Directory are referred to in those sections. The following titles are generally of wider interest. We hope that when you read this, the books listed in this section will still be in print and readily available. Should you, however, need to locate an out-of-print book, you may find it helpful to use the Out of Print Book Service, 13 Pantbach Road, Birchgrove, Cardiff CF4 1TU (Tel: 0222-627703). This covers both fiction and non-fiction and while they cannot guarantee to find a book, they have wide contacts with the second-hand book trade. If successful, you will receive full details of price (there is a minimum of £6) and condition; a book is not dispatched unless and until a firm order follows. No charge is made for the service itself, but a stamped addressed envelope should be included with requests. An explanatory leaflet giving further details of the service will be sent in response to a s.a.e.

Some of the more specialist books listed in this section are not generally available at booksellers. Though any good retailer will order particular titles for you, we have included publishers' addresses in case you have difficulty or need to order direct. The listing is very much a selection – largely of those books we have actually seen. We think, anyway, that it can be more helpful to limit the number of books put before you: long lists can easily be counter-productive in their effect. Quite certainly, however, many fine books will have been omitted. If you want a wider resource reference, you will find the publications lists of Age Concern England, Astral House, 1268 London Road, London SW16 4ER (Tel: 081-679 8000) and the Disabled Living Foundation (Library Resource List, *Elderly*), 380–4 Harrow Road, London W9 2HU (Tel: 071-289 6111), particularly helpful.

Age Concern England fact sheets

▶ *Age Concern England*
Astral House, 1268 London Road, London SW16 4ER.

351

Age Concern England produces the following fact sheets:

1. *Help with Heating*
2. *Sheltered Housing for Sale*
3. *Television Licence Concessions*
4. *Holidays for Older People*
5. *Dental Care in Retirement*
6. *Finding Help at Home*
7. *Making Your Will*
8. *Rented Accommodation for Older People*
9. *Rented Accommodation for Older People in Greater London*
10. *Local Authorities and Residential Care*
11. *Income Support for Residential and Nursing Homes*
12. *Raising Income or Capital from Your Home*
13. *Older Home Owners: Financial help with repairs*
14. *Probate: Dealing with someone's estate*
15. *Income Tax and Older People*
16. *Income Related Benefits: Income and capital*
17. *Housing Benefit and Community Charge Benefit*
18. New title forthcoming
19. *Your State Pension and Carrying on Working*
20. *National Insurance Contributions and Qualifying for a Pension*
21. *The Community Charge (Poll Tax) and Older People*
22. *Legal Arrangements for Managing Financial Affairs*
23. *Help with Incontinence*
24. *Housing Schemes for Older People*
25. *Income Support and the Social Fund*
26. *Travel Information for Older People*
27. *Arranging a Funeral*
28. *Help with Telephones*
29. *Finding Residential and Nursing Home Accommodation*
30. *Leisure Education*

Single copies are available free in response to a 9" × 6" s.a.e.

Multiple copies or a selection of fact sheets cost 26 pence per copy (13 pence to Age Concern groups or other voluntary agencies).

Fact sheets are revised and updated throughout the year. A complete set of factsheets in a ring binder, including a year's updating, is available for £30. The current price for updating after the first year is £12 a year. (If you are outside the United Kingdom, the subscription rates are higher.)

Caring

Call for Care
By Yasmin Gunaratnam (King's Fund Centre Carers Unit with the Health

Education Authority, 1991), price £1.95 plus 80 pence postage and packing. Available from Distribution Department, HEA, Hamilton House, Mabledon Place, London WC1H 9TX,

Information for Asian carers of elderly people. It covers such topics as housing and welfare benefits, coping with death, and racial discrimination and violence. It also includes useful contacts and addresses.

Call for Care is published in English, Bengali, Gujarati, Punjabi and Urdu.

▶ *Caring for Elderly People*
By Susan Hooker (Routledge, 11 New Fetter Lane, London EC4P 4EE, 3rd edition 1990), price £10.99.

A guide for anyone dealing on a day-to-day basis with elderly people. This updated and revised edition contains information on financial help and services and on new technology available.

The book is primarily concerned with elderly people who live either alone or with relatives.

▶ *Caring at Home*
By Nancy Kohner (King's Fund Carers' Unit, 126 Albert Street, London NW1 7NF (Tel: 071-267 6111), mail orders for single copies to Bailey Distribution Ltd, Dept D/KFP, Warner House, Folkestone, Kent CT19 6PH, 3rd edition, 1989), price £3 plus 50 pence postage and packing.

An easy-to-read guide to available services, help in the home, money and legal matters, time off, day-to-day caring skills and the problem of coping with feelings.

The King's Fund Carers' Unit also has details of a number of books for carers in black and ethnic minority communities.

▶ *Caring for Parents in Later Life*
By Avril Rodway (Consumers' Association with Hodder & Stoughton, 1992), price £9.95. Available from Consumers' Association, Castlemead, Gascoyne Way, Hertford X, SG14 1LH.

Offers advice on the emotional, practical, financial and legal aspects of care.

▶ *Caring for the Person with Dementia*
(Alzheimer's Disease Society, 158–60 Balham High Road, London SW12 9BN, 1989), price £2.50 including postage and packing.

The Alzheimer's Disease Society has a wide range of relevant literature.

▶ *Common Problems with the Elderly Confused*
A series of books published by Winslow Press, Telford Road, Bicester, Oxfordshire OX6 0TS.

Selected further reading

▶ *Coping with Ageing Parents*
By Chris Gilleard and Glenda Watt (W & R Chambers, 43-5 Annandale Street, Edinburgh EH7 4AZ, 1983), price £3.95 plus 60 pence postage and packing.

▶ *In Touch Care Guides*
(Broadcasting Support Services, PO Box 7, London W3 6XJ), price £1.75 each.

These booklets are available in large print or braille (or on audio cassette from RNIB, PO Box 173, Peterborough PE2 0WS). Current titles are:

— *Pleasures of Listening*
— *Partners or Helpers*
— *Coping with Sight Loss at 80+*
— *Home, School and Away*
— *Getting About Safely*
— *Learning to Live with It*

▶ *Taking a Break: A guide for people caring at home*
By Maggie Jee (mail orders to Taking a Break, Newcastle upon Tyne X, NE85 2AQ), free to carers, 60 pence to others.

This booklet provides information on all types of breaks, both at home and away from home. It will assist all carers, regardless of the age or disability of the person for whom they care.

▶ *Taking Good Care*
(Age Concern England, 1989, available from Central Books, 99 Wallis Road, London E9 5LN (Tel: 081-986 4854)), price 6.95.

Written for all those concerned with caring for older people in a residential setting, this book covers such vital issues as communication skills, the medical and social problems encountered by carers, the role of the care assistant, the older person's viewpoint, and activities and group work.

▶ *The 36-hour Day*
By Nancy L. Mace and Peter V. Rabins (Age Concern with Edward Arnold, 1985, available from Central Books, 99 Wallis Road, London E9 5LN (Tel: 081-986 4854)), price £7.50 [new edition due September 1992].

Specifically written for those who are involved in the care of confused elderly people at home. Originally written for the United Sates, the British edition has been extensively revised and updated by Beverly Castleton, Christopher Cloke and Evelyn McEwen, and takes account of legal and social differences in the United Kingdom.

Common disabilities

=▶ *After the Stroke*
By May Sarton (The Women's Press Ltd, 34 Great Sutton Street, London EC1V 0DX, 1988), price £4.95.

May Sarton, after a long career as a novelist, essayist and poet, was disabled by a stroke at the age of 75. This is a personal account, in the form of a journal, of its aftermath as she faced severe physical limitations, pain, loneliness and depression, and of her fight back to health and independence.

=▶ *Coping with Dementia: A Handbook for Carers*
(Health Education Board for Scotland, Woodburn House, Canaan Lane, Edinburgh EH10 4SG, 1987).

A clear, well-designed guide including basic information about dementia, coping with the task of caring generally, facing the particular problems associated with dementia, and support services and benefits.

=▶ *Coping with Disability*
By Millicent Isherwood (W & R Chambers Ltd, 43-5 Annandale Street, Edinburgh EH7 4AZ, 1986), price £3.95.

=▶ *Coping with Disability*
By Peggy Jay (Disabled Living Foundation, out of print but a new edition due in 1992).

This guide has always provided a great deal of practical information, backed up by extensive illustrations, designed to show disabled people how to get help from the health and social services, from voluntary organisations and others. Previous editions have contained advice on how to make life easier in the home: how to get in and out of a bath and manage independently in the lavatory, how to cope with problems of clothes and dressing, cooking, eating, housework and laundry; with sections on mobility, on keeping in touch, on getting out and about, and on pastimes and leisure activities.

=▶ *Dementia and the Family*
(Mental Health Foundation, 8 Hallam Street, London W1N 6DH, 1991).

An introductory free leaflet.

=▶ *In Touch Handbook*
By Thena Heshel and Margaret Ford (Broadcasting Support Services, PO Box 7, London W3 6XJ), price £12.50 (print, tape or braille versions).

A wide-ranging guide to aids and services for blind and partially sighted people.

Directories

▪▶ *Directory for Disabled People*
By Ann Darnbrough and Derek Kinrade (Harvester Wheatsheaf, Campus 400, Maylands Ave, Hemel Hempstead, Herts HP2 7EZ, 6th edition 1992), price £19.99.

This directory brings together all kinds of basic information relevant to people with disabilities, including the infirmities of age. It is intended primarily for use by disabled people themselves, and its philosophy is rooted in the belief that knowledge empowers and that information conveys independence and personal choice. It is both a handbook of opportunity and a guide to services in all aspects of daily living.

It covers motoring and mobility, statutory services, financial benefits and allowances, equipment, housing, education, employment, holidays in Britain and abroad, sports and leisure, sex and personal relationships, legislation, contact and tape clubs, and organisations offering a variety of mostly voluntary services.

▪▶ *Directory of Services for Elderly People in the UK*
Edited by Kate Lodge (Longman Industry and Public Service Management, Westgate House, The High, Harlow, Essex CM20 1YR, in collaboration with the Centre for Policy on Ageing, 1991), price £40.

This directory is one of a number of Longman Community Information Guides. It brings together information on where elderly people, their relatives or service providers can seek specialist advice and services, including accommodation, benefits information or assistance in respect of illness or handicap.

▪▶ *Good Retirement Guide*
By Rosemary Brown (Kogan Page Ltd, 120 Pentonville Road, London N1 9JN, 1992), price £12.99.

A really valuable guide which is extremely wide-ranging, managing to say a little about most services and quite a lot about those subjects which are vital to people who want to plan for a constructive, active and financially secure retirement. The organisation of information is commendably systematic and clear.

Hospices

▪▶ *Tears and Smiles*
By Martyn Lewis (Michael O'Mara Books Ltd, 9 Lion Yard, 11-13 Tremadoc Road, London SW4 7NF, 1989), price £9.95.

This handbook brings together and signposts a mass of information about the hospice movement. Particularly valuable are sections on the function of hospices (which is wider than generally supposed), how to obtain admission to a hospice, how hospice charities can help, and a directory of hospices in the United Kingdom and the Republic of Ireland.

Legal aid

⇒ *Legal Aid Guide and Getting Legal Help*
(Legal Aid, 5th and 6th floors, 29-37 Red Lion Street, London WC1R 4PP).

Free leaflets offering general guidance, intended for people seeking help on legal matters and for advice workers. The *Legal Aid Guide* contains financial eligibility information and a self-assessment section so that laypeople can work out whether they qualify. The leaflet *Getting Legal Help* is available in several foreign languages, including five Asian languages.

⇒ *Solicitors' Regional Directory*
(Law Society, annually).

This directory can be consulted in reference libraries. It lists firms which undertake legal aid work and the particular areas of legal work in which they specialise. It also contains information on duty solicitors and Mental Health Review Tribunal members.

Loneliness

⇒ *Loneliness: How to overcome it*
By Val Marriott and Terry Timblick (Age Concern England, 1988), available from Central Books, 99 Wallis Road, London E9 5LN (Tel: 081-986 4854), price £3.95.

A source of practical advice on ways to relieve isolation.

Magazines

⇒ *Choice*
(Choice Publications Ltd, Subscriptions, 3 and 4 Hardwick Street, London EC1R 4RY (Tel: 071-833 5793)), price £1.75 per copy.

This is a monthly magazine marketed as 'Britain's magazine for successful retirement'. It is closely connected to the Pre-Retirement Association (see Section 14). Wide-ranging and well presented.

⇒ *Fifty Forward*
(DCA Publications, 29 Daventry Street, London NW1 6TD).

The magazine for members of the 50 Forward Club (*see* page 338). It combines feature articles and commercial advertisements of goods and services with a variety of special discount offers.

=▶ *The Oldie*
(26 Charlotte Street, London W1P 1HJ (Tel: 071-636 3686)), price £1.40 per copy, available on subscription.

A fortnightly general interest magazine, where readers will find a wide range of subjects from current affairs and politics to the arts, food and history. While not excluding any interested reader, the magazine focuses on the interests, tastes and culture of those in middle and old age, rather than the 'youth culture' purveyed by so many newspapers and magazines. With Richard Ingrams as its editor, there is no threat of piety in *The Oldie's* approach.

=▶ *Saga Magazine*
(Saga Publishing Ltd, The Saga Building, Middelburg Square, Folkestone, Kent CT20 1AZ), price £1.25 per copy, available on subscription (which gives automatic membership of the Saga Club).

This seems to us a much better read than other magazines of its kind. It is full of relevant information, with holiday bargains and a section of advertisements for penfriends and partnerships (limited to members of Saga Club).

Retirement guides

=▶ *Approaching Retirement*
(Consumers' Association, Castlemead, Gascoyne Way, Hertford X, SG14 1LH), price £8.95.

A practical guide to forward planning. The emphasis is financial: pensions, investments, how to generate additional income; but there is also useful advice on such matters as where to live, fitness, health and leisure, and work after retirement, all presented in a very crisp and methodical format.

=▶ *Coping with Change: Focus on retirement*
By Allin Coleman and Anthony Chiva (Health Education Authority, Hamilton House, Mabledon Place, London WC1-9TX, 1991), price £7.95.

A complete programme for use in pre-retirement courses and guidance that can be used with people from all walks of life. It aims to help people: analyse their understanding of change and transition; explore their feelings and reactions; identify the key issues of their retirement; consider their choices and options; assess their skills and the resources available to them to put their plans into action.

=▶ *Good Retirement Guide*
See heading Directories.

=▶ *Living and Retiring Abroad*
By Michael Furnell (Kogan Page Ltd, 120 Pentonville Road, London N1 9JN, 5th edition, 1991), price £8.99.

This *Daily Telegraph* Guide is essential reading for anyone, young or old, planning to buy an overseas property for holidays or for retirement. The regions covered include southern Europe, the Caribbean, North America (especially Canada and Florida), Australia and New Zealand. The guidance provided is very wide-ranging and includes procedures for purchase in the various locations, financial and tax implications, letting your UK home, health benefits and insurance, education overseas, and the rules concerning taking pets into other countries.

=▶ *Making the Most of Your Retirement*
By Keith Hughes (Kogan Page Ltd with Legal & General, 120 Pentonville Road, London N1 9JN, second edition, 1989), price £4.99.

The author is retirement counselling manager for Legal & General. His guide presents a wealth of information in a concise and direct style for those who see their retirement as a time of opportunity and enjoyment.

=▶ *Management Retirement Guide*
(Newhall Publications Ltd, Newhall Lane, Hoylake, Wirral L47 4BQ), free.

Published twice a year, this guide has a wide variety of useful information interspersed (and not always unconnected) with relevant commercial advertisements.

Women

=▶ *As We Are Now*
By May Sarton (The Women's Press Ltd, 34 Great Sutton Street, London EC1V 0DX, 1983), price £3.95.

A novel which illuminates the plight of a woman of independent spirit and lively intellect who is abandoned in 'a concentration camp for the old...where people dump their parents or relatives exactly as though it were an ash can'. The author penetrates a hidden nightmare world in which personal dignity is constantly under assault. There can be no 'happy ending', but this is a story of courage in which there is a final personal triumph.

=▶ *Look Me in the Eye: Old women, aging and ageism*
By Barbara Macdonald with Cynthia Rich (The Women's Press Ltd, 34 Great Sutton Street, London EC1V 0DX, 1984), price £2.95.

First published in the United States, this book brings together a series of essays written by two women about the ageing of women and the factors which relegate them, despite their numbers, to the fringes of society: the conspiracy of silence (in which old women themselves collude) which draws a veil over reality and hides them from view. The authors, who have each experienced the exclusivity of prejudice, confront the subject with rare and revealing understanding.

Sixty Years On: Women talk about old age
By Janet Ford and Ruth Sinclair (The Women's Press Ltd, 34 Great Sutton Street, London EC1V 0DX, 1987), price £4.95.

This interesting book draws on interviews with a few of the millions of women in Britain over pensionable age. They tell of their difficulties in adjusting to old age, how they overcome such problems as loneliness and immobility, how they try to hold on to their independence while needing and accepting help, and how they strive to maintain a sense of purpose without the routine of a working day. As is so often the case, the words of others bring a clearer recognition that problems we internalise as intensely personal are, in reality, shared problems in a common experience.

What Every Woman Should Know About Retirement
Edited by Helen Franks (Age Concern England, 1985, available from Central Books, 99 Wallis Road, London E9 5LN (Tel: 081-986 4854)), price £4.50.

A handbook written from a woman's point of view with sections on money matters, coping with your partner's retirement, personal relationships, retiring alone, feeling good and looking good.

INDEX

Abbeyfield Society, 76-7
Able to Garden, 274-5
Action on Coronary Heart Disease in Asians, 192
Action Resource Centre, 217
Action on Smoking and Health (ASH), 163, 182-3
acupuncture, 174-5
administration of an estate, 204-6
Adult Bedwetting, 180
adult education, 233-44
   helpful organisations, 242-4
   home study courses, 235-9
   local classes, 234
   open learning, 234
   publications, 244
   retirement courses, 241
   study holidays and courses, 240
   television education, 245
   travelling fellowships, 241-2
   universities and colleges, 235
After the Death of Someone Very Close, 209
After the Stroke, 355
Age Concern, 73, 75, 101, 181-2, 217, 295, 324-7
   advice on
     alcohol, 162-3
     dental care, 168
     education, 242
     funerals, 199, 203
     health, 190
     housing, 101, 103-4
     incontinence, 179
     keeping warm, 137-8
     probate, 206
   Care with a Chair scheme, 256
   fact sheets, 351-2
   holidays, 318
   Insurance Services, 100-1, 138, 250
Age Exchange, 284
Age Resource, 217-95
Age Well, 190
AIDS and You, 192
air travel
   assistance, 248
   concessions, 247
AL-ANON, 163, 182
alarms
   burglar, 152-3
   community, 143-6
   personal, 147
alcohol, safe limits, 162
Alcohol Concern, 162-3
Alcoholics Anonymous, 162, 182
All England Netball Association, 283
Almshouses Association, 75, 102
Alzheimers Disease Society, 327
Amateur Rowing Association, 288-9
Amateur Swimming Association, 292
Anchor, 62-3, 77
annuities, 35-6
antiques, 259
Approaching Retirement, 358
archaeology, 260
archery, 260
Architectural Heritage Society of Scotland, 279
ARP Over 50, *see* Association of Retired People Over 50
Arranging a Funeral, 199, 203, 209

Arthritis Care, 327–8
Arthritis and Rheumatism Council, 328
Articles Specially Designed or Adapted for Blind People, 113
arts, 260–1
Arts Boards (regional), 261–2
Arts Councils, 261
As We Are Now, 359
ASH, *see* Action on Smoking and Health
Association to Aid the Sexual and Personal Relationships of Disabled People, 347
Association of British Insurers, 54, 101
Association of British Travel Agents, 318
Association of Charity Officers, 43, 96
Association of Crossroads Care Attendant Schemes, 328–9
Association of Retired People Over 50, 18, 327
Astra Housing Association, 77–8
At Home in a Home, 98
Attendance Allowance, 1–3, *see also* Disability Living Allowance

bank deposit accounts, 33
BASE, *see* British Association for Service to the Elderly
basket-making, 265
Basketmakers' Association, 265
Be Sure Who's At the Door, 149
Beat the Burglar, 153
Benslow Music Trust, 313
Bereavement, 200–1
  helpful organisations, 206–9
  publications, 209, 210, 211–12
Bereavement, 209
Bereavement Care, 210
Beth Johnson Foundation, 183, 217, 329
Beth Johnson Housing Association Limited, 63, 78
Beth Johnson Leisure Association, 296
Beyond Grief, 210
birdwatching, 270
blindness, *see* visual handicap
Blunt Fin Limited, 287
BODY, *see* British Organ Donor Society
Bogus Callers: The knock code, 151
bones, care of, 173–4
bowling, 266

brass rubbing, 266
Breakthrough Deaf-Hearing Integration, 117, 330
British Acupuncture Association & Register, 174–5
British Antique Dealers Association, 259–60
British Association of American Square Dance Clubs, 291
British Association of Friends of Museums, 277
British Association of the Hard of Hearing, 173, 330
British Association for Local History, 278
British Association of Numismatic Societies, 283
British Association for Service to the Elderly, 330–1
British Chess Federation, 266–7
British Chiropractic Association, 175
British Correspondence Chess Association, 267
British Correspondence Chess Society, 267
British Deaf Association, 331
British Diabetic Association, 331
British Executive Service Overseas, 218
British Federation of Care-home Proprietors, 96
British Federation of Film Societies, 272
British Federation of Sand and Land Yacht Clubs, 290
British Footwear Manufacturers' Federation, 172
British Gas
  budget accounts, 129
  Code of Practice, 130
  complaints, 128
  difficulty in paying bills, 128–9
  free safety checks, 128
  Home Service Advisers, 127
  installation and servicing, 135
  prepayment meters, 129
  publications, 132
  savings stamps, 129
British Heart Foundation, 157, 183–4
British Homeopathic Association, 175–6
British Humanist Association, 198
British Institute of Florence, 312
British Jigsaw Puzzle Library, 281

British Judo Association, 281
British Music Education Yearbook, 282
British Numismatic Society, 283–4
British Nursing Association, 331
British Nutrition Foundation, 157, 184
British Organ Donor Society, 199, 206
    fact sheets, 199, 200
British Orienteering Federation, 285
British Pensioner and Trade Union Action Association, 331–2
British Postal Chess Federation, 267
British Rail travel concessions, 245–7
British Red Cross Society, 114, 218, 255, 332
British Ski Club for the Disabled, 291
British Sports Association for the Disabled, 296
British Tinnitus Association, 173, 332
British Trust for Conservation Volunteers, 310–11
British Wireless for the Blind Fund, 286
BT Guide For People Who Are Disabled Or Elderly, 110
buggies, 248–9
building society savings, 33
BUPA
    health plan, 190
    Medicall, 184
burglar alarms, 152–3
burglary, safeguards against, 150–3
burial at sea, 203–4
bus fare concessions, 245
But Can I Bring My Cat?, 98
Buyer's Guide to Sheltered Housing, 73
Buying a Home, 104
Buying and Selling a Home, 38

Call for Care, 352–3
Campaign for Equal State Pension Ages, 332
Cancer: A guide to reducing your risks, 192
Canine Concern Scotland Trust, 332–3
capital gains tax, 31–2
Care with a Chair, 256
Care Home Holidays Limited, 317
Care and Repair Limited, 63, 139
Care and Repair schemes, 62–4
Carefree Holidays Limited, 306–7
Carelink, 247
Carers National Association, 333

Caresearch, 97
Caring for Elderly People, 353
Caring at Home, 353
Caring for Parents in Later Life, 363
Caring for the Person with Dementia, 353
Castle Rock Housing Association Limited, 78–9
cataracts, 169
Cavity Foam Bureau, 134
Centre for Accessible Environments, 102
Centre for Policy on Ageing, 333
Charity Made Clear, 43–4
Charity Search, 44
Chartered Society of Physiotherapy, 333–4
chess, 266–7
chiropodists, 171–2, 189
chiropody treatment, 171–2
Chivers Press Publishers Limited, 288
Choice magazine, 357
cholesterol, 161
Chosen Heritage Limited, 199
Christians Abroad, 218
Chronically Sick and Disabled Persons Act, 1970, 3
Church of Ireland Housing Association (NI) Ltd, 79
Church Missionary Society, 219
Cinnamon Trust, 334
Citizens Advice Bureaux Service, 138, 334–5
Civic Trust, 219, 277
clothing, to keep warm, 123–5
coach fare concessions, 245
Coldwatch, 138
College of Health, 181
Colleges, 235
Come Gardening, 109, 276
Coming Home: A guide to dying at home with dignity, 210
Common Problems with the Elderly Confused, 353
communication aids centres, 116
community alarm systems, 143–6
community nurses, 188–9
community psychiatric nurses, 189
Community Service Volunteers, 70–1, 219
community transport schemes, 253–6
Compassionate Friends, 206
concessionary fares, 245–7

continence management, 177–81
  Age Concern leaflets, 179
  cleanliness and smell, 178–9
  clinics, 178
  clothing, 178
  DLF advice, 178, 179–80, 191
  equipment, 178
Coping with Ageing Parents, 354
Coping with Change: Focus on retirement, 358
Coping with Dementia: A handbook for carers, 355
Coping with Depression, 191
Coping with Disability(Chambers), 355
Coping with Disability(DLF), 355
Coping with Ear Problems, 173
Coping with Rheumatoid Arthritis, 190–1
Coping with Sight Loss at 80+, 113
CORGI, see Council for Registered Gas Installers
Coronary Prevention Group, 184–5
  advice on diet, 158–61
  advice on looking after your heart, 167, 184–5
  advice on smoking, 163–4
Council for the Accreditation of Correspondence Colleges, 242
Council for British Archaeology, 260
Council for the Protection of Rural England, 269
Council for Registered Gas Installers, 135
Counsel and Care for the Elderly, 96, 97, 335–6
  housing publications, 104
country dancing, 267–8
Country Houses Association Limited, 79–80
Countrywide Holidays Association, 296–7, 311
Court of Protection, 53–4
Cremation Society of Great Britain, 206–7
Criminal Injuries Compensation Board, 155
croquet, 268
Croquet Association, 268
Cruse – Bereavement Care, 207, 318–19
Cutting the Cost of Keeping Warm, 137
Cycling for Softies, 309–10
Cyngor Cymru I'r Anabl
  information service, 115

Dangerous Cold, 123, 126, 138
Dark Horse Venture, 297
day centres, 70
deafness, *see* hearing impairment
death
  funerals, *see* separate heading
  planning for, 197–200
  practical arrangements, 201–6
  registering, 204
  wills, *see* separate heading
Deathing, An Intelligent Alternative for the Final Moments of Life, 210
debt, 55–6, 141
Debt: A survival guide, 56
Dementia and the Family, 355
dental care, 167–8
Dental Care in Retirement, 168
dental charges, concessions, 13–14
dentist, finding a, 168
Departments of
  Energy (Home Energy Efficiency scheme), 133
  Social Security (*Freephone* advice), 26
Depressives Associated, 336
Derwent Housing Society Limited, 80
Designed for Living, 117
Diabetes Foundation, 337
Dial-a-Ride schemes, 253–4
diet, 125–6, 157–62
Directory
  of Continence and Toiletting Aids, 180
  for Disabled People, 356
  of Hospice Services, 208
  of Independent Hospitals and Health Services, 97
  of National Voluntary Organisations for Scotland, 231
  of Services for Elderly People in the UK, 356
Disability Action, 297–8
Disability Handbook, 3, 6
Disability Living Allowance, 1, 4–7
Disability Rights Bulletin, 26
Disability Rights Handbook, 26
Disability Scotland
  information service, 115
  leisure activities, 297
Disabled Facilities Grants, 68
Disabled Housing Trust, 80–1

Disabled Living Centres, 116, 179, 249
Disabled Living Centres Council, 116
Disabled Living Foundation (DLF)
    clothing and footwear advisory service, 172, 191
    continence advisor, 178, 179–80, 191
    footcare leaflets, 172
    health care publications, 191
    information service, 115
    Information Service Handbook, 118
    leisure activities, 297
Disabled Person's Railcard, 246–7
Distressed Gentlefolk's Aid Association, 337
district nurses, 70, 188–9
DLF, *see* Disabled Living Foundation
Domestic Coal Consumers' Council, 139
donating body/organs for medical research, 199–200
Don't Leave Your Money to Chance, 53
draught proofing, 132–3, 135
Draught Proofing Advisory Association, 135
drinking for health, 162–3
driving, 249–53
driving licences, 250–1

East Regional Health Authority Linkline, 156–7
Eat Well...Live Well, 158, 184
Eat to Your Heart's Content, 157
eating for health, 157–62
Ecology Building Society, 31
Elderly Accommodation Counsel, 96, 102
    database, 73, 75, 97, 208
Electrical Contractors' Association, 135
electric blankets, 124–5
electricity
    approved contractors, 137
    budget accounts, 129
    Code of Practice, 130
    difficulty in paying bills, 128–9
    installation and servicing, 135, 137
    regulation, 141
    savings stamps, 130
Electricity Association publications, 131
Embroiderers' Guild, 268
embroidery, 268
En Famille Overseas, 312–13
Enduring Powers of Attorney, 53

Energy Action Grants Agency, 133–4
Energy Action Northern Ireland, 122, 133, 134, 139
Energy Action Scotland, 133, 139
energy projects, 133
English Bowling Association, 266
English Churches Housing Group, 81
English Courtyard Association, 81–2
English Ski Council, 290
English Vineyard Association, 269
Enjoy Healthy Eating, 158, 192
environment, 268–71
equipment for daily living, 107–20
    alarms, 143–6, 147
    bathroom, 108
    bedroom, 108–9
    books and publications, 117–20
    buggies, 248–9
    centres
        for communication aids, 116
        for deaf/hearing-impaired people, 117
        for disabled living, 116
        for visually handicapped people, 116
    chairs, 109
    continence management, 178
    gardening, 109
    hearing impairment, 109–10, 173
    home adaptations, 65
    household, 110
    information services, 115
    kitchen/eating, 110–11, 169
    lifts, 112
    on loan, 114
    from local authorities, 113
    low speed vehicles, 248–9
    on mail order, 114
    mobility, 111
    from the NHS, 114
    personal hygiene, 108
    pressure relief, 111
    purpose-made, 111–12
    rising seats, 109
    scooters, 248–9
    stairlifts, 112
    visual handicap, 112–13, 169
Equipment for Disabled People, 118–19
escort services, 255
estate, administering, 204–6

Ethical Investment Research Service, 31
Ethical Investor, 31
Eurisol UK Mineral Wool Association, 135
Europ Assistance Limited, 303
euthanasia, *see* Voluntary Euthanasia Society
Everyday Aids and Appliances, 119
exercise, 164–6, 258–9
  to keep warm, 126
Exercise. Why Bother?, 165, 192–3, 258
EXTEND – Exercise Training Ltd, 166
External Wall Insulation Association, 135
Extrasure Holdings, 303–4
Eye Care, 170
Eye Care Information Bureau, 170
eyes, care of, 168–70

Family Finance: How to make your money go further, 37
family histories, 271
fats, varieties of, 160–1
Federation of Family History Societies, 271
Federation of Private Residents' Associations Limited, 102–3
feet, care of, 171–3
feminists, *see* Older Feminists Network
ferry concessions, 246
50 Forward, 319, 338
  magazine, 357
films, 272
film making, 272
Financial Services Act 1986, 30, 36
Finding Residential and Nursing Home Accommodation, 95, 97
Fire, 150
fire prevention, 149–50
  Central Office of Information leaflets, 150
first aid courses, 154
Five Counties Housing Association Ltd, 82
flower arranging, 272
Fold Housing Association, 82
food, *see* diet
Food Should be Fun, 157
Foot Care Book – An A–Z of fitter feet, 173, 191
Forestry Commission, 270, 317
Friends of the Earth, 220, 269
Friends of the Elderly and Gentlefolk's Help, 82–3, 338

Friends of Historic Scotland, 279
Friends of the National Museums of Scotland, 279
Fuel Rights Handbook, 130–1
funerals, 197–9, 202–4
  Age Concern fact sheet on, 199
  do-it-yourself, 203
  prepayment, 198–9
  publications, 203, 209, 210–11, 212
  secular, 198
Funerals, 210
Funerals: And how to improve them, 203, 210–11
Funerals Without God, 211
further education, *see* adult education

Galpin Society, 282
gardening, 272–6
  equipment for, 109
Gardening, 272
Gardening for Disabled Trust, 273
Gardening is for Everyone, 274
Gardening in Retirement, 273
Gardening Without Sight, 275
Gardens of England and Wales, 273
gas, *see* British Gas
Gas Consumers Council, 128, 140
  publications, 131–2
Gay Bereavement Project, 208
genealogy, 271
General Consumer Council for Northern Ireland, 140
Georgian Group, 278
Getting About Safely, 111, 256
glasses, voucher scheme, 14–15
glaucoma, 169, *see also* International Glaucoma Association
Goethe Institut, 313
Going Into Hospital, 181
golf, 276
Golf Club Great Britain, 276
Good Book Guide, 287
Good Retirement Guide, 105, 356
Grand National Archery Society, 260
grants
  for facilities for disabled people, 68
  for home improvements, 66–8
  for insulating your home, 133–4

grants (*continued*)
  from charities, 42–4
Green Party, 269
Greenpeace, 220, 270
Growth Point, 109
Guardian Housing Association Limited, 83
Guide for Blind and Partially Sighted People, 27
Guide to Grants for Individuals in Need, 44
Guide to Housing Benefit, 9
Guide to Medicines and Drugs, 191–2
Guide to Non-contributory Benefits for Disabled People, 27
Guide to Reviews and Appeals, 27
Guinness Trust, 83

Handbook for Receivers, 54
Handicapped Divers Association, 292
Hanover Housing Association, 84
Hanover Housing Limited, 84
Hanover (Scotland) Housing Association Limited, 84
Hardy Plant Society, 273–4
Health and Beauty Exercise, 166
health care, 156–96
  alternative, 174–7
  diet, 157–62
  information, 156–7, 181, 185
  private health plans, 189–90
  professionals, 188–9
Health Directory, 192
Health Education Authority
  publications, 158, 163, 165, 167, 192–3
Health Education Board for Scotland, 140, 185
  publications, 157, 173, 174, 193
Health and Healthy Living, 193
Health Information Network, 185
Health Search Scotland, 185
health visitors, 189
Healthcall Directory, 181
Healthy Living Holidays, 166
Healthy Wise: An intelligent guide for the over 60s, 193
hearing impairment
  centres, 117
  equipment, 109–10
heart, looking after your, 167

heating
  financial help, 121–2
  in the home, 127–30
  installing and servicing, 135, 136
Heating and Ventilating Contractors' Association, 136
Help and Advice on Leg Problems, 173
Help the Aged, 338
  community alarms, 144, 145, 146
  Housing and Care Division, 84–5
  publications, 170, 171
  Winter Warmth Line, 140
Help with Daily Living, 119
Help with Heating, 138
Help with Incontinence, 179
Help for People Who Live in Residential Care Homes or Nursing Homes, 98
Help When Someone Dies, 211
heritage, 277–81
Heritage Housing Ltd, 85
Heritage in Wales, 280
HF Holidays Limited, 314
Hip Replacement Operation, 181
Historic Houses Association, 277
Historic Houses, Castles & Gardens, 278
Historical Association, 277–8
history, 277–81
History Today, 278
Holiday Care Service, 304, 319
holidays, 302–23
  activity, 259
  antique appreciation, 259
  arts, 309
  bowling, 266
  cottages and homes, 317
  countryside and environment, 310–12
  cycling, 309–10
  healthy living, 166
  helpful organisations, 318–20
  home exchange schemes, 316–17
  insurance, 302–4
  languages, 312–13
  medical treatment overseas, 305–6
  music, 313
  painting, 260
  publications, 314–16
  retreats, 314
  Saga, *see* separate heading

holidays (*continued*)
  special interest and courses, 309–14
  with specialist organisations, 306–8
  tourist boards, 320–3
  walking, 314
Holidays for Disabled People, 315
Holidays and Travel Abroad, 315
home adaptations, 65
home care service, 69
Home Energy Efficiency scheme, 133
home exchanges, 75–6
Home from Home, 315
Home from Home schemes, 94
home, help in, 69–71
home improvement grants, 66–8
Home Improvements, 65
home income plans, 38–9
home maintenance, 67–8, 70
home, providing income from your, 37–42
home reversion schemes, 39–40
home security, 150–3
home study courses, 235–9
Homesitters, 152
hormone replacement therapy, 174
Horticultural Therapy, 274
Hospice Information Service, 208
hospices, 208
hospital
  effect on state benefits, 7
  Eye Service, 15
  travelling expenses when visiting, 7–8
Housewatch Ltd, 152
housing,
  adaptations, 65
  care and repair schemes, 62
  contractors, 64–5
  Disabled Facilities Grants, 68
  exchange schemes, 75–6
  heating, 127–30, 135, 136
  improvement grants, 66–8
  improvements, 64–5
  independent living projects, 70–1
  insulating, 132, 134, 135, 136–7
  insulation grants, 133–4
  insurance, 100–1, 153
  living with a host family, 94
  local authority housing, 59
  mobility housing, 61
  paying for renovations and alterations, 66
  planning permission, 65–6
  private developments, 60
  renovation grants, 67–8
  repairs etc, 67–8, 70
  selling up, 38, 74
  sheltered housing, 60–1, 71–4
  staying put, 38, 62
  wheelchair housing, 61
housing associations, 59–60, 76, 93
Housing Benefit, 8–9
Housing Corporation, 72, 74
Housing Options for Older People, 73, 76, 104
Housing Organisations Mobility and Exchange Services, 75–6
Housing Rights Guide, 105
Housing Year Book, 105
How to Cope with Doorstep Salesmen, 149
How to Cut the Cost of Keeping Warm, 138
How to Direct Your Own Funeral, 211
How to Eat a Healthy Diet, 157
How to Lose Weight and Keep Fit, 194
How to Take Care of Your Heart, 193–4
hypothermia, 122–3

Improvement Grants, 66–8
In Control: Help with incontinence, 179
In Touch Bulletin, 113, 169, 194
In Touch Care Guides, 354
In Touch Handbook, 113, 169, 171, 194, 355
In Touch at Home, 194
In Touch kitchen, 169
income from your home, 37–42
Income Support, 9–11
Income Tax, 44–8
  allowances, 47–8
  further information, 48
  on interest, 45
  on investment income, 32, 44–5
  on lump sums, 46
  on motor mileage allowances, 216
  on pensions, 45
  on state benefits, 46–7
incontinence, see continence management
Incontinence (tape), 181
Incontinence and Stoma Care, 180

Incontinence: Your problems answered, 180
Incorporated Society of Registered Naturopaths, 176
Independent Living Projects, 70-1
Inheritance Tax, 48-50
  further information, 50
  gifts, 49-50
Inheritance Tax, 50
Inheritance Tax and Capital Gains Tax, 32, 50
Inland Revenue leaflets
  Capital Gains Tax, 32
  Income Tax, 45
Institute of Amateur Cinematographers Limited, 272
Institute for Complementary Medicine, 174, 176
Instructions for My Next of Kin and Executors Upon My Death, 52
insulating your home, 132, 134, 135, 136-7
insulation grants, 133-4
insurance, 54-5
  through Age Concern, 100-1, 138
  buildings, 100-1
  contents, 100-1, 153
  holidays, 302-4
  household emergencies, 138
  motoring, 249-50
  for pets, 55
  through Saga, 101
International Cooperation for Development, 220-1
International Glaucoma Association, 185-6
International Voluntary Service, 221
Intervac, 316-17
intestacy, 204-5
intruder alarms, 152
Invalid Care Allowance, 11-13
Invent-Heat, 124
investment bond income schemes, 40-1
investments, 30-7
  annuities, 35-6
  banks, 3
  building societies, 33
  compensation scheme, 36-7
  ethical, 30-1
  further information, 37
  gilts, 35
  for growth, 34-5
  National Savings, 33-4
  protection, 36-7
  for safety, 32-3
Irish Lawn Tennis Association, 293
ISIS large print, 287
It's Never Too Late, 166

James Butcher Housing Association, 85-5
Jephson Homes Housing Association Limited, 86
Jewish Care, 338-9
jigsaw puzzles, 281
Joint Council for the Welfare of Immigrants, 339
judo, 281
Just Peddling, 310

Keep Able Catalogue, 119
keep fit, 164-6, 258-9
Keep Moving, Keep Young, 165
Keep Warm, Keep Well, 140
Keep Warm this Winter, 125, 138, 140
Kindrogan Field Centre, 311
Kirk Care Housing Association Limited, 86-7

large print books, 287-8
laundry service, 69
Lawn Tennis Association Trust, 293
legal aid guides, 357
legs, care of, 173
leisure activities, 258-94
  helpful organisations, 295-301
letters of administration, 204-5
LinkAge, 222, 298
Living in Homes, 98-9
Living and Retiring Abroad, 105, 359
local authority services
  alarm systems, 145, 146
  equipment for daily living, 113
  housing, 59
  leisure activities, 259
  residential care homes, 95
London Anatomy Office, 200
London Appreciation Society, 278
Loneliness: How to overcome it, 357

Look Me In the Eye: Old Women Aging and Ageism, 359
Love and Sex After 60, 201

Magic of Movement, 165, 195
Making and Changing Your Will, 52
Making the Most of Your Retirement, 359
Making Your Will, 52
Management Retirement Guide, 359
marking possessions, 152
Marriage Counselling Scotland, 222
meals-on-wheels, 70
Medau Society, 166–7
Merseyside Improved Homes, 87
meteorology, 281
Methodist Homes for the Aged, 87
mobility, 245–57
Mobility, 257
Mobility Allowance, *see* Disability Living Allowance
mobility housing, 61
money management, 29
Money Management Council, 56–7
Monumental Brass Society, 266
motoring, 249–53
Motoring and Mobility for Disabled People, 249, 251, 256
music, 281–3

NACRO, *see* National Association for the Care and Resettlement of Offenders
National Adult School Organisation, 242–3
National Approval Council for Security Systems, 153
National Art Collections Fund, 262
National Assistance Act 1948, 171
National Association for the Care and Resettlement of Offenders, 222
National Association of Decorative and Fine Art Societies, 263, 309
National Association of Estate Agents, 103
National Association of Flower Arrangement Societies of Great Britain, 272
National Association of Funeral Directors, 202
National Association of Leagues of Hospital Friends, 223

National Association of Loft Insulation Contractors, 136
National Association of Prison Visitors, 223
National Association of Victims Support Schemes, 223–4
National Association of Volunteer Bureaux, 224
National Association of Widows, 339
National Association of Women's Clubs, 243
National Back Pain Association, 340
National Cavity Insulation Association, 136–7
National Deaf Children's Society
  hearing impairment equipment centre, 117
National Debtline, 56, 141
National Extension College, 235–6, 270, 294
National Federation of Housing Associations, 72, 74
National Federation of Music Societies, 282
National Health Service charges concessions
  dental services, 13–14
  glasses, 14–15
  prescription charges, 15–16
  sight tests, 14–15
National House Building Council Sheltered Housing Code of Practice, 73
National Inspection Council for Electrical Installation Contracting, 137
National Institute of Medical Herbalists, 177
National Library for the Blind, 288
National Music and Disability Information Service, 282
National Osteoporosis Society, 165, 174, 340
National Philatelic Society, 285
National Retreat Association, 314
National Savings, 33–4
National Secular Society, 198
National Society of Allotment and Leisure Gardeners, 275
National Trust, 279, 317
National Trust for Scotland, 280, 317
National Trust for the Welfare of the Elderly, 319
National Welfare Benefits Handbook, 27
Nationwide Housing Trust Limited, 88
Natural Death Centre, 208–9
Natural Death Handbook, 209

Neighbourhood Energy Action, 141
netball, 283
New Design for Old, 120
New Horizons Trust, 224
North British Housing Association Group, 63–4, 88
North Housing, 88
Northern Counties Homes, 89
Northern Counties Housing Association Limited, 89
Northern Ireland Co-ownership Housing Association Limited, 89–90
Northern Ireland Federation of Housing Associations, 73, 75
Northern Ireland Housing Executive, 64
Northern Ireland Information Service for Disabled People, 115
Northern Ireland Ski Council, 291
Northern Ireland Widows Association, 340
Norwich Union Fire Insurance Society Limited, 250
Notes on Bowel Problems, 180
numismatics, 283–4
nursing homes, 94–100

Occupational Pensions Advisory Service, 57
Office of Electricity Regulation, 141
Office of Fair Trading publications, 38, 56, 65, 101, 149
Office of Gas Supply, 141–2
Older Feminists Network, 340–1
Oldie, 358
Open College, 239
Open College of the Arts, 236
Open Learning Map of Scotland, 244
Open University, 237–8
Operations, 181
Optical Information Council, 113, 170, 341
oral history, 284
Oral History Society, 284
Orange Badge Scheme, 251–3
Orbit Housing Association, 64, 90
Orbit Spa Housing Association Limited, 91
organ donation, 199–200
orienteering, 285
osteoporosis, 173, *see also* National Osteoporosis Society
Overseas Hospice Services, 208

Owner's Guide: Your home in retirement, 104
Owning Your Flat, 105
Oxfam, 224–5

parking, 251–3
Parkinson's Disease Society of the United Kingdom, 341
Partially Sighted Society, 113, 169, 186, 287, 341
  National Low Vision Centre, 116, 186, 341
PDSA, *see* People's Dispensary for Sick Animals
Peak National Park Centre, 311–12
Pensioners for Peace International, 342
Pensioners' Voice, 342
pensions
  income tax liability, 45
  retirement pension, state, 21–5
People's Dispensary for Sick Animals, 342–3
Pet Concern, 343
Pet Protect Limited, 55
philately, 285
photography, 285–6
Planning: A householder's guide, 66
planning permission, 65–6
Police advisory publications, 155
power of Attorney, 53–4
  enduring, 53
Practical Ways to Crack Crime, 143, 155
Pre-Retirement Association of Great Britain and Northern Ireland, 343
Presbyterian Housing Association (NI) Limited, 91
prescription charges, concessions, 15–16
Preventing Heart Disease, 195
Principal Registry of the Family Division, 204
Private Health Partnership, 189–90
private health plans, 189–90
Private Patients Plan, 190
probate, 204–6
Probate: Dealing with someone's estate, 206
Problems Afoot: Need and efficiency in footcare, 172

Quaker Social Responsibility and Education, 91–2

372 Index

QUIT! National Society of Non-smokers, 163, 186–7

RAC Activity Holiday Guide, 259, 315
radio, 286
Rail Europ Senior Card, 246
Rail fare concessions, 245–7
rail travel, assistance, 247
Railway Correspondence and Travel Society, 286
railways, 286
Ramblers Association, 286–7
rambling, 286–7
RC Heated Products, 125
REACH, *see* Retired Executive Action Clearing House
reading, 287–8
Registered Nursing Homes Association, 98
Rehabilitation Engineering Movement Advisory Panels, 111–2, 298
 Yearbook, 120
Relate: National Marriage Guidance, 225, 343–4
Relaxation for Living, 187
Religious Society of Friends, 225
REMAP, *see* Rehabilitation Engineering Movement Advisory Panels
reminiscing, 284
renovation Grants, 67–8
Rented Accommodation for Older People, 76
repairs Grants, 67–8
Research into Ageing, 344
Residential Care – Is it for me?, 99–100
residential care homes, 94–100
Resource Unit to Promote Black Volunteering, 226
Retired Executives Action Clearing-House, 226
Retired and Senior Volunteer Programme, 226
Retirement Association of Northern Ireland, 344
retirement courses, 241
Retirement Education Centre, 241
Retirement Homes and Finance, 73, 75, 105
Retirement Lease Housing Association, 92

retirement pension, *see* state retirement pension
Rights Guide for Homeowners, 106
Rights Guide to Non-means-tested Social Security Benefits, 27
Rights to Repair guides, 106
RNIB, *see* Royal National Institute for the Blind
RNID, *see* Royal National Institute for Deaf People
roll-up loans, 41–2
rowing, 288–9
Royal Air Forces Association, 92
Royal British Legion
 Housing Association Limited, 92–3
 property repair loan scheme, 66
Royal Horticultural Society, 275
Royal Meteorological Society, 281
Royal National Institute for the Blind, 345
 equipment for visual impairment, 113, 116
 leaflets, 170
 leisure activities, 298–9
Royal National Institute for Deaf People, 110, 173, 345
Royal Photographic Society, 285–6
Royal Scottish Country Dance Society, 267–8
Royal Society for the Protection of Birds (RSPB), 270
Royal Yachting Association, 289
running, 289
Running Sixties, 289
RUBV, *see* Resource Unit to Promote Black Volunteering

Safe Home Income Plan Campaign, 38
Safer Drinking for the Over 60s, 162–3
safety, 127, 143–55
Safety in Your Home, 148
Saga Food Guide, 195
Saga Health Guide, 195
Saga Services Ltd
 bowling, 266
 buildings/contents insurance, 101
 Club, 345
 holiday insurance, 304
 holidays, 166, 240, 259, 299, 307
 magazine, 358

Saga Services Ltd (*continued*)
  motor insurance, 250
  private health care plan, 190
  publications, 195
sailing, 289-90
St John Ambulance
  ambulance services, 255
  first aid courses, 154, 187
Saltire Society, 280
Save the Children Fund UK, 227
savings, see investments
scooters, 248-9
Scotland's Gardens, 275
Scottish Action on Dementia, 346
Scottish Amateur Swimming Association, 292
Scottish Civic Trust, 219
Scottish Conservation Projects, 227-8
Scottish Council on Alcohol publications, 163, 196
Scottish Federation of Housing Associations, 72, 75
Scottish Language Society, 280
Scottish Lawn Tennis Association, 293
Scottish National Ski Council, 291
Scottish Netball Association, 283
Scottish Retirement Council, 299, 346
Scottish Sports Council, 300
Secret Flowers: Mourning and the adaptation to loss, 211
Securities and Investment Board, 36-7
Security in Your Home, 153
Security Systems, 152-3
Senior Railcard, 245-6
Senior and Veteran Windsurfers Association, 294
Severe Disablement Allowance, 16-18
SHAC (London Housing Aid Centre), 103
Shape Network and affiliates, 263-5
Share Owner's Guide, 37
Shelter - National Campaign for Homeless People, 103
sheltered housing
  buying, 71-3
  further information, 73
  renting, 74-5
Sheltered Housing Services Limited, 73
Shires Housing Association Limited, 93
Sick or Disabled?, 27

Sight tests, concessions, 14-15
Simple Guide to Planning Applications, 66
Simple Solutions, 120
Simple Relaxation, 165, 196
Sixty Years On: Women talk about old age, 360
Ski Council of Wales, 390
skiing, 290-1
Skill: National Bureau for Students with Disabilities, 243
Skillshare Africa, 228
smoke detectors, 150
smoking, 163-4
Smoking and Your Heart, 163
So You Want to be a Volunteer, 232
Social Fund, 18-21
social workers, 69
Socially Responsible Investment, 31
Society of Chiropodists, 172
Society of Genealogists, 271
Society for Horticultural Therapy, 109
Society for One-Armed Golfers, 276
Society of Recorder Players, 282-3
Society of Voluntary Associates, 228
Solicitors Regional Directory, 357
Sound Advantage plc
  equipment for hearing impairment, 117
SOVA, *see* Society of Voluntary Associates
SPOD: *see* Association to Aid the Sexual and Personal Relationships of Disabled People
Sports Council, 299-300
Sports Council for Northern Ireland, 300
Sports Council for Wales, 300
square dancing, 291
state benefits and concessions, 1-28
  further information, 26-8 (*see also* under the individual benefits)
  effect of voluntary work on, 215-16
  and income tax, 46-7
  helpful organisations, 26
  when someone dies, 212
State Retirement Pension, 21-5
  income tax on, 45
Stress Incontinence, 180
Stroke Association, 347
Study Holidays, 244
study holidays and courses, 240

Sue Ryder Foundation, 347
Sutton Housing Trust, 93
swimming, 292

Taking a Break: A guide for people caring at home, 354
Taking Good Care, 354
Talking About Bereavement, 211
Talking Newspaper Association, 288
Talman Limited, 147
taped books, etc, 288
Tax and Pensioners, 48
Tears and Smiles, 356
teeth, looking after your, 167-8
television educational programmes, 235
television licence concessions, 100
tennis, 292-3
Theatre and Concert Travel Club, 293-4
theatres and concerts in London, 293-4
therapeutic earnings, 17
36-hour Day, 354
Through Grief: The bereavement journey, 211-12
Time to Learn, 309
tinnitus, see British Tinnitus Association
Tinnitus Helpline, 347
Toogood, CR & Co, 304
tourist boards, 320-3
Townswomen's Guild, 301
trade associations, 134-7
travel, assistance with, 247-8, see also Tripscope
Travel Companions, 319
travelling fellowships, 241-2
Travelmate, 320
Tripscope, 248

UK Activity Holidays, 316
Ulster Cancer Foundation - Stop Smoking Group and Advice Centre, 163, 187-8
Ulverscroft Large Print Books, 288
Understanding Incontinence, 180
Undertaken with Love, 203, 212
Unit Trusts: A guide for investors, 37
United Kingdom Home Care Council, 348
universities, 235

University of the Third Age, 239-40
unknown callers, 148-9
Using Your Home as Capital, 42

Vegan Society, 162, 188
vegan and vegetarian diets, 161-2
Vegetarian Society (UK) Limited, 162, 188
Veterans' Lawn Tennis Association of Great Britain, 292
Victim Support, 154
Victim Support Scotland, 154
visual handicap (*see also* In Touch)
    centres for visually impaired people, 116
    equipment, 112-13
    gardening, 275-6
    registration, 170-1
VMM, 188
Voluntary Agencies Directory, 231
Voluntary and Community Transport Schemes Directory, 255
Voluntary Euthanasia Society, 348
Voluntary Service Overseas, 228-9
Voluntary work, 214-32
    drivers, 254-5
    effect on state benefits, 215-16
    motor mileage allowance, liability to tax, 216
    organisations welcoming volunteers, 216-31
Volunteer Bureaux Directory, 231-2
Volunteer Centre UK, 229
Volunteer Reading Help, 229
Volunteer Stroke Service, 230
Volunteer Work, 232
VSO, *see* Voluntary Service Overseas

Waiting List Helpline, 181
Wales Council for the Disabled, *see* Cyngor Cymru I'r Anabl
Wales Pensioners, 348
walking in wintry conditions, 147-8
Warm Toes Burnt Fingers?, 106
war pensioners
    concessions on sight tests and glasses, 14-15
War Widows' Association of Great Britain, 348-9
waste disposal, 69-70

Way Around Disability Living Allowance and Disability Working Allowance, 7
Welsh Amateur Swimming Association, 292
Welsh Federation of Housing Associations, 72, 75
Welsh Lawn Tennis Association, 293
Welsh Netball Association, 283
What to Do After a Death, 212
What to Do After a Death in Scotland, 212
What to Do When Someone Dies, 212
What Every Woman Should Know About Retirement, 360
wheelchair housing, 61
wheelclamping, exemption, 253
Which Benefit?, 27
Which Way to Save and Invest, 37
Who Dies? An investigation of conscious living and conscious dying, 212
Which Way to Save Tax, 32, 48, 50
Widows' Benefits and Tax, 48
Widow's Bereavement Tax Allowance, 48
Wildfowl and Wetlands Trust, 271
wills, 51–3, 197, 205–6
Wills and Probate, 52–3, 205–6, 213
windsurfing, 294
Winged Fellowship, 308
Winston Churchill Memorial Trust, 241–2
Winter Warmth Lines, 122

Wireless for the Bedridden Society, 349
women, advice on personal safety, 155
Women's League of Health and Beauty, 166
Women's Royal Voluntary Service, 230, 349–50
  escort services, 255
Workers' Educational Association, 243–4
Working Holidays, 314
writing, 294
WRVS, *see* Women's Royal Voluntary Service

YMCA National Centre, 312
yoga, 165–6, 177
Yoga for Health Foundation, 177
You and Your GP, 196
You and Your Heart, 167
You and Your Pension, 25
Young at Heart Holidays, 308
Your Benefit (1989), 27
Your Eyes, 170
Your Health in Retirement, 196
Your Heating in Retirement, 137
Your Prostate Operation, 180
Your Rights, 28
Your State Pension and carrying On Working, 25
Your Taxes and Savings, 37, 48
Youth Clubs UK, 231